Robotic Colorectal Surgery

Peter Coyne · Jim Khan
Editors

Robotic Colorectal Surgery

Complete Manual of Surgical Techniques

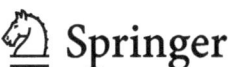 Springer

Editors
Peter Coyne
Newcastle Hospital NHS Foundation Trust
Newcastle upon Tyne, UK

Jim Khan
Queen Alexandra Hospital
Portsmouth, UK

ISBN 978-3-031-15197-2   ISBN 978-3-031-15198-9 (eBook)
https://doi.org/10.1007/978-3-031-15198-9

This Springer imprint is published by the registered company Springer Nature Switzerland AG
The registered company address is: Gewerbestrasse 11, 6330 Cham, Switzerland

Introduction

Surgery is a vast and ever-evolving field. New developments and technologies are frequently created to improve outcomes and the quality of surgery. Robotic surgery has seen exponential growth over the last decade and is rapidly becoming the standard for the care of complex colorectal pathology. Minimally invasive surgery truly began with the first laparoscopic cholecystectomy in 1977. Multiple studies across surgical disciplines have shown a vast array of improvements in outcomes—including length of stay, complications, return to function and oncological outcomes.

Within Colorectal surgery, laparoscopic colectomy saw a wider adoption for both oncology and benign resections for the above-mentioned reasons. However, technical, oncological and training challenges in laparoscopic surgery have resulted in the ceiling effect with stagnation for major resection in many countries. Within the UK, the 2020 National Bowel Cancer Audit (NBOCA) reported around 64% usage of laparoscopic surgery in colorectal cancer. Robotics has the potential ability to overcome some of the challenges of laparoscopic surgery. Technological advances, better training programs and improved access to robotic platforms have resulted in increased uptake of robotic surgery.

Robotic surgical platforms offer improved optics and vision (including 3D and HD), increased precision and dexterity, elimination of fulcrum and tremor, scaling of motion, endo-wristed instruments compared to straight standard laparoscopic, integrated use of advanced technologies such as ICG for perfusion/lymph node harvest, reduced need for surgical assistance and improved surgical ergonomics.

In 2019, there were approximately 30 hospitals using robotic surgery for colorectal and general surgery in the UK. This number has risen to over 160. The market has also opened up and there are now multiple systems from different manufacturer with improved costs (once seen as a major barrier to robotics) and are continuing to drive technological development.

This manual aims to look at the commonly performed robotic colorectal surgical procedures. It is not an exhaustive list but does cover the spectrum of procedures and diseases encountered and highlight where robotic surgery can assist and be of value. The book is designed to highlight the key steps and tips and tricks from a world-renowned faculty on robotic surgery. The aim is to not only provide a text that can be used to inform those starting off on their robotic journey but also stimulate debate and discussion with those experts in the field. For that reason, we have included a few different interpretations of some of the commonly performed procedures such as anterior resection to allow the reader to read and understand different ways of safely performing such operations.

The first segment of the manual details some basic steps—docking, port placement and ergonomics as well as some of the systems on the market—even this is changing with new competitors coming to market within the next 12–18months. We have included a chapter on the role of surgical care practitioner (SCP) and how vital they are to a program as well as how they are trained to give an insight into this developing role vital to the implementation of a successful program.

The second and third segments look at different colorectal resections and techniques for both rectal and colonic surgery. Looking at some of the standard and complex resections performed using the system, the expert tips and tricks we hope users will find useful and the stepwise manner of text allow readers to visualise each step or modular element of the procedure itself. It is designed to be a manual—taking the reader through the required elements and highlighting where problems can arise and using the expertise of the authors to show the range of help robotic platforms can give us.

The final segments look at the role of robotic surgery within other fields—emergency surgery, when a reader may be called to a robotic case within another specialty such as urology—with their procedures explained to give background knowledge to the colorectal surgeon and what they may encounter. We also include a segment of hernia surgery for the colorectal surgeon highlighting how para-stomal and perineal hernias can be tackled.

We hope to supplement this text with live interviews and case discussions over the next 12 months with the aim of producing a structured expert-led way of viewing robotic colorectal procedures safely.

We are very lucky to have had collaborators from around the world who worked with us on this project. We would like to thank all of our authors for taking the time during a very demanding period amidst a pandemic, for their hard work and efforts to bring this project to fruition.

We hope you enjoy reading this book and it provides good insight and technical tips for success with robotic colorectal surgery.

Peter Coyne
Jim Khan

Contents

Part I
Basics

Chapter 1
Robotic Port Positioning

Eleanor Rudge and Irshad Shaikh

Abstract Robotic colorectal surgery has become increasingly embraced because of the benefits that robotic surgery can reportedly provide, both to patients and surgeons. To make the most of these advantages, optimal robotic port placement, along with correct patient positioning, are both paramount to ensuring patient safety and facilitating smooth and efficient surgery. This chapter will discuss and detail our suggested port positions, along with patient positioning tips, for two colorectal procedures: robotic anterior resection and robotic right hemicolectomy.

Keywords Robotic · Port placement · Port positioning · Patient positioning · Robotic anterior resection · Robotic right hemicolectomy

Introduction

The introduction of robotic surgical systems has recently been gaining great momentum. Robotic colorectal surgery has become increasingly embraced because of the benefits that robotic surgery can reportedly provide, not only to patients, but also to the operating surgeons [1]. Robot-assisted surgery (RAS) can benefit patients by reducing the risk of conversion to open surgery, reducing intraoperative blood loss, improving cosmesis, improving postoperative morbidity, allowing a quicker return to normal bowel function and shorter hospital stays [2], all whilst providing comparable oncological outcomes. For the seated surgeon, RAS provides a number of advantages over open and laparoscopic surgery including improved surgeon comfort. Additionally, RAS provides three-dimensional visualisation of a magnified operative field, with surgeon-led camera control. Surgical precision is improved through increased articulation of robotic instruments, and via improved anatomical access into the confined pelvic region [3]. Furthermore, RAS provides access to advanced technology such as Firefly® camera technology, artificial intelligence enabled staplers, and Integrated Table Motion.

E. Rudge · I. Shaikh (✉)
Sir Thomas Browne Colorectal Surgery Department, Norfolk and Norwich Hospital, Norfolk, UK
e-mail: irshad.shaikh@nnuh.nhs.uk

© The Author(s), under exclusive license to Springer Nature Switzerland AG 2022
P. Coyne and J. Khan (eds.), *Robotic Colorectal Surgery*,
https://doi.org/10.1007/978-3-031-15198-9_1

To make the most of these advantages, there are several major factors that must be addressed, and optimised, in order to achieve successful RAS. These include a good understanding of the procedure, standardised surgical skills and training, flawless teamwork with experienced bedside assistance, and most importantly, optimal patient positioning and robotic port placement. Although this chapter mainly discusses port placement, patient positioning and port placement are arguably inextricably linked. Thus, the main goal of optimal patient positioning and port placement is to ensure and maintain the safety of the patient, avoiding compression injuries, allowing maximum mobility of the robotic arms, and facilitating a smooth and efficient surgery [3]. We would strongly encourage a single docking technique for any particular operation as this not only reduces operative time, but also helps to limit operative steps and their associated variables. Optimal port placement is extremely important for single docking technique.

RAS, using the Intuitive da Vinci® robot system, allows the many colorectal procedures to be carried out, including total colectomy, left and right hemicolectomy, sigmoid colectomy, abdominoperineal resection, low anterior resection and rectopexy. This chapter will discuss and detail our suggested port positions for two colorectal procedures: anterior resection and right hemicolectomy. The other colorectal procedures listed above will use similar port placement to these two described procedures with some variations depending on the type of da Vinci® system used.

Equipment Required

Robot: There are several different types of surgical robot available. Within this chapter port positioning pertaining to Intuitive's da Vinci® robot will be described. Three da Vinci® robot models are currently available: the Si, X and Xi. The Si robot is an older system and, thus, not used as much as the more advanced X and Xi versions. The X has some fourth- generation capabilities, however, it is the Xi system which comes with several advanced features, including the additional benefit of Integrated Table Motion (ITM), meaning that port-positioning is perhaps less pivotal in this newer generation robot compared to its counterparts. There is an option of Flex and patient clearance facilities further enhancing the versatility.

Ports: All standard ports are 8 mm in Si/ X/Xi systems. If the use of a stapler is required, then a larger 12 mm robotic port is used to transmit the device. At the Norfolk and Norwich Hospital (NNUH), we have devised a method to try and reduce the number of 12 mm ports placed and, thus, reduce the number of post-operative complications such as acute or delayed port-site hernias. This involves using an Alexis port placed in the supra-pubic region, via a Pfannenstiel incision, or in the umbilicus, to transmit the robotic stapler [2]. It is the surgeon's preference as to whether a 5 or 12 mm port is used for the assistant port, which we place in the right or left lumbar region, (approximately 5–6 cm away from the robotic ports). Avoiding the use of a 12 mm port reduces the chance of a port-site hernia forming, however, a 12 mm port is perhaps more useful than a 5 mm, as it can be used to insert swabs into the abdominal cavity, and to transmit a 10 mm Hem-o-lok® for vessel clipping. More recently, we have started using the laparoscopic port (at either the umbilicus or in the suprapubic region) to transmit swabs and 10 mm Hem-o-loks®. This has enabled us to use a 5 mm assistant port to reduce morbidity. If a 12 mm assistant port is to be used, then it is important that the fascia is formally closed. Our assistant port (either 5 mm or 12 mm) also facilitates a smoke evacuation system (see below). The da Vinci® ports and trocars come as reusable or disposable. The trocars come as blunt or sharp, and choice of trocar is dependent on the surgeon's preference.

Smoke evacuation system: We use the Conmed Airseal® System, although several systems are available. A smoke evacuation system helps maintain a more stable pneumoperitoneum, allowing operations to be carried out at lower intra-abdominal pressures, which can help to reduce post-operative pain. It also provides good visibility requiring less camera lens cleaning, whilst maintaining intra-abdominal pressure regardless of whether suction is applied, or if a gas leak occurs. As a result, using a smoke evacuation system enables the surgeon to operate within a clearer field, as gas is constantly removed, filtered, and recirculated back to the AirSeal® port. Use of this system can help reduce operative time [4]. As discussed above, the Airseal® port also serves as the assistant port, aiding suction/irrigation, vessel ligation, and retraction.

Alexis Wound Protector/Retractor: Use of this device provides 360° of circumferential, atraumatic retraction. It can help reduce pain, post-operative analgesia requirements (due to uniform stretch) and surgical site infections. Additionally, it comes with a cap which enables the surgeon to redock, or laparoscope, without needing to close the wound.

Marking Pen: To increase precision of port position, robotic surgeons often like to draw out the proposed port positions using a purple surgical marker pen. This allows them to appraise the port sites before committing to an incision, and to make any adjustments as necessary. This can be done over a sterile sheet such as an Ioban to reduce marking the patient's abdomen.

Instrumentation: The most common instruments used in robotic colorectal surgery include a bipolar fenestrated grasper, Cadier grasper, curved scissors, large needle driver, Maryland bipolar forceps, monopolar hook diathermy, tip-up grasper, robotic clip applicator (which comes in a variety of sizes), robotic suction/irrigation, and robotic vessel sealers, including SynchroSeal. In our practice, we commonly use the Cadier grasper, the fenestrated bipolar grasper and the scissors, supplemented by a vessel sealer as required. A set of basic laparoscopic instruments, including graspers, Johann's forceps, Hem-o-lok® clip applicator, and suction/irrigation are required.

Procedural Steps

The patient is anaesthetised and positioned in a modified Lloyd Davies position on a vacuum bean bag mattress. Shoulder supports and a pelvic strap can also be used to secure the patient in position. If using a da Vinci® Xi, the Integrated Table Motion (ITM) is set up to achieve a Trendelenburg position of up to 33° (in practice, 20–25° will suffice), with side-to-side tilt as required. If using an Si or X system, with no ITM available, then table tilt is measured by experience, with enough tilt placed on the operating table to position the small bowel away from the area of proposed dissection for optimal exposure. The robotic arms are robust and insensate. Each arm moves within its own field, and pivots around a central point called the remote centre. Therefore, it is important to protect the patient's face, along with the endotracheal tube, against these heavy robotic arms. An L-shaped, padded metal bar can be placed over the patient's chest to help to avoid injury caused by forceful movement of the arms, and to prevent displacement of the endotracheal tube. The ideal height of the L-bar is 2–3 cm above the patient's nose. The patient is prepped and draped, with the optional use of an Ioban™ Antimicrobial Incise Drape.

Pneumoperitoneum creation and initial entry: Pneumoperitoneum is performed as per the surgeon's choice. Techniques include: open insertion of the first port, Visiport blunt dissection, or use of a Veress needle. Our preferred initial entry for **left-sided resections** requires a Pfannenstiel incision (5–6 cm in length) for pneumoperitoneum, with care taken to ensure that bladder injury is avoided. An Alexis retractor is then inserted, and the cap placed securely on top (Fig. 1.1i). The Pfannenstiel/Alexis port site acts as the specimen extraction site later on. Additionally, a port can be placed via the Alexis and connected to a smoke evacuation system, instead of using the assistant port.

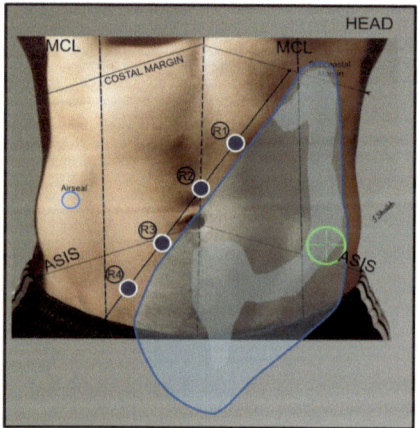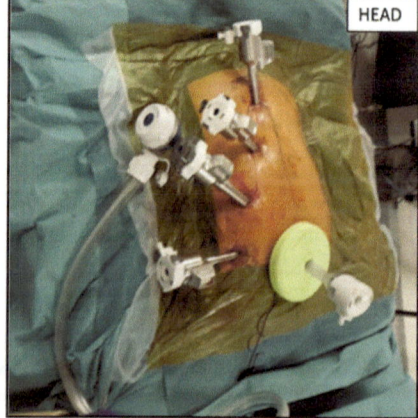

Fig. 1.1 i, ii Port placement for left-sided procedures for the Xi system; R3 is usually a 12 mm port for stapler insertion. *Note:* for the X system, the robotic arm configuration is 4123 (3 being at RIF, with R2 a 12 mm port for stapler insertion). Ports should be 3–4 cm away from bony points

Our initial entry for **right-sided resections** is via a vertical supra-umbilical incision (Fig. 1.2ii).

The port inserted at this point is connected to gas (prior to the gas tubing be switched over to the assistant port smoke evacuation system) and is used as a camera port, facilitating robotic port positioning and, later, as an additional assistant port. This port is also extended in a vertical direction to facilitate extraction of the resected colon when extra-corporeal anastomosis is carried out. If intracorporeal anastomosis is selected, and an oblique port placement approach has been used, then we also extract the specimen via an extended umbilical excision. However, if a transverse supraumbilical port positioning approach has been adopted, then we join two of the suprapubic port-sites to create the extraction site (Fig. 1.3ii). This approach is increasingly becoming our preferred option for right hemicolectomies involving complete mesocolic excision.

A diagnostic laparoscopy is performed by inserting the camera via the initial access port to assess for adhesions, to check that safe placement of robotic ports is possible, and to confirm surgical feasibility. A surgical marker pen is used to plan out the port positions. Port positioning depends on the type of the procedure, patient body habitus and any previous abdominal surgery. An empty trocar is used to create a circular indentation on the patient's skin, which guides the subsequent incision across its radius. This ensures a snug fit of the port within the abdominal wall, which is essential in preventing gas leakage. The ports are inserted under direct vision (using the robotic endoscope via the initial access port), either using blunt or sharp robotic (8 mm or 12 mm) ports. An AirSeal® assistant port (5 mm or 12 mm) is placed in the right or left lumbar region, depending on the side of the planned colonic resection. Left-sided resections will require a right-sided lumbar assistant port, and right-sided resections a left-sided lumbar port. These lumbar assistant ports need to be positioned approximately 5–6 cm away from the robotic ports to avoid external clashing. The da Vinci® robotic ports have three black markings at the distal end of

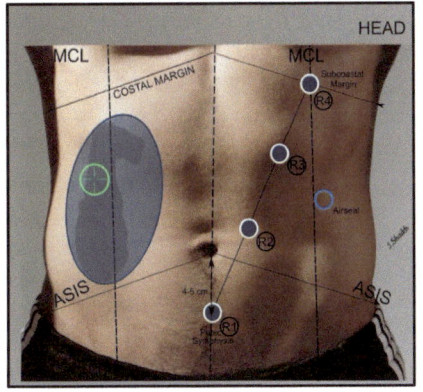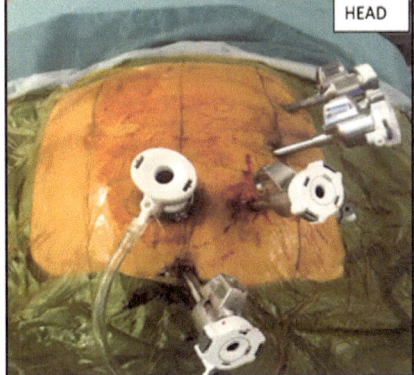

Fig. 1.2 i, ii Port placement for right-sided procedures with oblique approach. For intracorporeal stapling, R3 can be converted to a 12 mm port

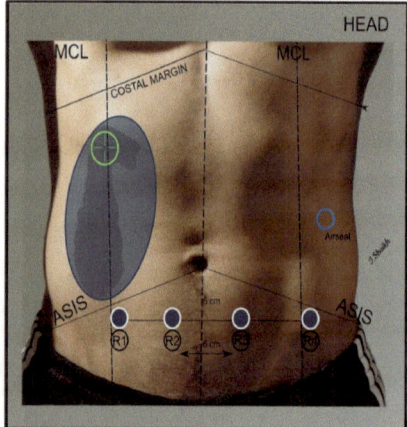 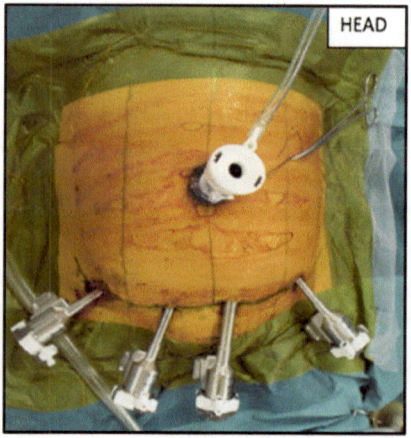

Fig. 1.3 i, ii Port placement for right-sided procedures with transverse approach. R3 can be converted to a stapling 12 mm port.

the trocar. It is important that the thick, middle mark (known as the remote centre) is positioned in line with the posterior rectus sheath to avoid injury to the abdominal wall, as it is around this point that the robotic arm will rotate. Positioning the port in this way helps to minimise tissue injury and, thus, reduce postoperative pain. The thin, proximal line is positioned at the level of the skin.

Type of Procedure

Port positions vary according to patient, procedure and surgeon. Good port positions serve to optimise views, allow maximum instrument reach, and help to minimise external arm clashing. Detailed below are suggested port positioning methods for left and right sided colorectal procedures. Port positioning can differ between Si, X and Xi systems. Port positioning, along with pre-docking arm configuration, needs to be more accurate using the Si and X systems. Due to its additional features, such as the 'Flex' and 'patient clearance' options, the Xi system has a greater degree of manoeuvrability and, therefore, port-positioning and robotic arm configuration is less of a consideration. Surgeons will also need to decide whether they wish to operate with two 'left-sided' arms, or two 'right-sided'. If necessary, however, this can be changed intraoperatively by "port hopping".

Using the da Vinci® X system, our preferred option for left-sided resections is a robotic arm arrangement of 4,1,2 and 3, with port 2 set up as the camera port, and port 3 as the most inferolateral port for left-sided resections. The Xi system has an arm arrangement of 1,2,3,4, with port 3 or 4 set up as the camera port, and port 4 as the most inferolateral port. With both X and Xi systems the operating surgeon will normally be in control of two 'left hands' and one 'right hand'. However, some surgeons prefer to have two 'right hand' instruments, which means that the camera is placed in the arm 1 position with the X system, and in the arm 2 position with the Xi system. For right-sided colectomies, our preferred option is 1,2,3,4 for both X and Xi systems.

Left sided resections

Under direct vision, using the robotic endoscope freehand via the Alexis port, the robotic camera port is inserted, with close attention to the following:

- The camera should be in line with the target anatomy.
- The camera should be at 10–20 cm distance from the target anatomy.
- The camera should be in line with the centre column of the patient cart.

The optimal distance between each of the four robotic ports should be 6–8 cm. All ports should be at least 3 cm away from bony prominences. For anterior resection, using a surgical marker pen, the left and right costal margins and the left and right anterior superior iliac spines (ASIS) are defined. The left mid-clavicular line, which is approximately 8 cm away from the midline, is drawn on. An oblique line is then drawn from the right femoral head, towards the left upper quadrant, to join the junction of the mid-clavicular line and costal margin. All four ports should then be placed on this oblique line (Fig. 1.1i). An assistant port is placed laterally on the patient's right, at least 5–6 cm away from the oblique port line. We find that making the angle of the oblique line slightly more obtuse allows better access to the splenic flexure. Thus, the most superior port adopts a midline position to facilitate easier splenic flexure mobilisation and tension-free anastomoses in patients with low rectal cancers (Fig. 1.1ii).

For segmental colectomy, i.e. splenic flexure cancers, the port positioning line can be taken one step further and arranged in a vertical setup, along the midclavicular line, as there is less need for access to the pelvis (Figs. 1.4i, ii).

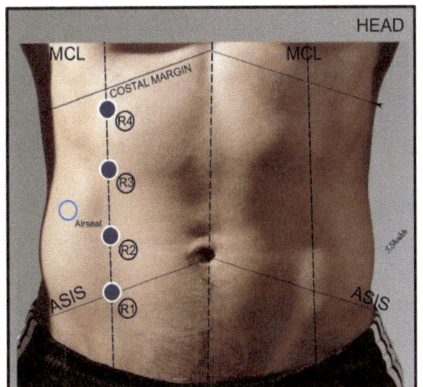
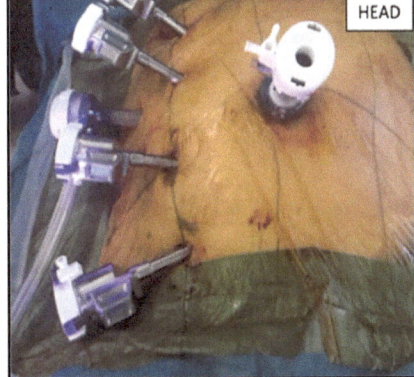

Fig. 1.4 i, ii Port placement for segmental colectomy i.e. splenic flexure

Right sided resections (standard, or using complete mesocolic excision approach (supra- or infra-ileal))

As mentioned above, two different approaches are described; oblique and transverse. Transverse suprapubic ports result in better cosmesis, with two of the ports combined to make one extraction site. Additionally, there is a reduced incidence of incisional hernia and wound infection with a Pfannenstiel style transverse extraction site [5].

Oblique approach: The setup is similar to left sided resections, with linear port placement in an oblique line. However, we use a more acute port positioning line, so that the most inferior port (port 1) lies in the midline (Figs. 1.2i, ii). Additionally, the robot approach is from the patient's right, and the 12 mm assistant port lies on the patient's left. If an umbilical port is used for pneumoperitoneum, then it can also be used as an additional assistant port, with a 5 mm flank assistant port used. Many surgeons, however, prefer a Veress needle technique—in this situation, an umbilical port is not required and, therefore, a lateral 12 mm assistant port is placed in order to allow introduction of swabs, needles etc.

Transverse approach: This setup involves supra-pubic port placement. The four robotic ports are placed transversely in the suprapubic area, 3 cm away from bony prominences and 5 cm from the symphysis pubis (Fig. 1.3i, ii). A distance of at least 6 cm between each port is required to avoid external clashing of the arms. The assistant port (5 or 12 mm) is positioned in the left flank. In addition, the umbilical port can be used to insert swabs or suture needles. If an intracorporeal anastomosis is planned, the R3 port tends to be a 12 mm port to allow passage of the robotic stapler.

Dealing with Scars and Stomas

The presence of abdominal scars should alert surgeons to the possibility of adhesions and the associated danger of nearby small bowel. The position of a peri-stomal port has to be selected carefully, with slight medial or lateral adjustment if there is a stoma in close proximity. There should be awareness of the presence of a parastomal hernia and the risk of bowel injury during placement of trocars in patients with previous stomas. If there is concern about the possibility of intra-abdominal adhesions, pneumoperitoneum can be created using the lateral assistant port to provide entry into the abdominal cavity under direct vision.

Steps Required for Docking

Once the ports have been inserted in the desired arrangement, the robot can then be docked. The operating table, including table tilt, should be positioned according to surgeon preference before docking of the robotic arms. The Xi system has an inbuilt camera targeting function which automatically adjusts the robotic arms to find the optimal position for a given procedure. However, the X system requires a guided setup aided by the use of a laser beam. The Si system is manually arranged, with the basic principles, such as distance from operating area to camera and the distance between robotic arms, needing to be observed as discussed above. Once the robot arms are docked to the ports, and the instruments inserted, patient position should remain unchanged. This is particularly pertinent for the Si and X systems. There is more manoeuvrability with the Xi system. Once the patient cart is positioned over the patient, patient cart breaks are applied. The camera arm is docked first, followed by the instrument arms. Finally, the system setup is checked.

Docking will be covered fully within Chap. 2.

Top Tips for Robotic Operative Success

- A preoperative check, intraoperative conduct and post-operative care all need to be considered to achieve an optimal outcome.
- High quality communication between the surgeon on the console and the surgical assistant is paramount.
- A skilled assistant should be able to control multiple instruments through the assistant port at the same time, for example, in situations which require assistant retraction and suction/irrigation.
- Awareness of how to resolve intra-operative arm collisions is important. Initial accurate port position helps to avoid intra-operative collisions and, thus, it is paramount to get the port positioning correct from the start. The Xi system provides a Flex option, as well as a patient clearance option. Because this is not available using the X or Si systems, undocking and redocking may be required, especially if ports are not placed correctly, or an extreme body habitus forces compromised port placement.
- Awareness of when to convert to laparoscopic or open surgery if the operation is failing to progress.
- Awareness of guided tool change—this is very useful for rapid change of instruments.
- The port position for total colectomy/panproctocolectomy differs based on the robot system used. With the X system, dual-docking is needed, along with repositioning of the bowel, to complete the operation. With the Xi system dual-docking may also be needed. However, with the option of Flex to adjust the joints, by rotating the boom, retargeting and through Intergrated Table Motion, a single docking technique can be used. These Xi system options can be used either in combination or in isolation.
- Our preferred approach for total colectomy/panproctocolectomy requires suprapubic port placement, which allows access to the right, transverse, and most of the left colon. Once the majority of bowel has been mobilised, we redock the robot with the addition of two 8 mm ports on the right side of the abdomen, to complete the left side of the operation. Some authors describe port placement diagonally across the umbilicus, and rotation of the boom is used to complete the operation in all quadrants.

- The port position for robotic abdominoperineal resection is like anterior resection except that arm 1 is placed further towards the right upper quadrant.

Checklist

- Pre-operative review of all investigations, along with cancer staging, is essential.
- Awareness of any previous abdominal operations.
- Check that all required robotic instruments are available.
- Ensure the correct choice of patient positioning for Si and X systems, especially for higher BMI patients, and consider the use of an additional port.

Acknowledgements Many thanks to Farhan Shaikh for his construction of the operative diagrams. Some diagrams taken from: https://pixabay.com/images/id-1685810/.

References

1. Pai A, et al. Robotic colorectal surgery for Neoplasia. Surg Clin North Am. 2017;97(3):561–72.
2. Cuk P, et al. Improved perioperative outcomes and reduced inflammatory stress response in malignant robot-assisted colorectal resections: a retrospective cohort study of 298 patients. World J Surg Oncol. 2021;19(1):155.
3. Chang C, et al. Patient positioning and port placement for robot-assisted surgery. J Endourol. 2014;28(6):631–8.
4. Patel DVAB. Laparoscopic Gastrointestinal surgery during COVID-19 pandemic: single-center experience. J Laparoendoscopic Adv Surg Techniq. 31(4).
5. DeSouza A, et al. Incisional hernia, midline versus low transverse incision: what is the ideal incision for specimen extraction and hand-assisted laparoscopy? Surg Endosc. 2011;25(4):1031–6.

Chapter 2
Robotic Docking

Charles Evans

Abstract The initial robotic set up and robot docking are critical components to successfully performing robotic colorectal surgery. There are 7 key principles and steps to this process: (1) Theatre set up (2) Patient positioning, (3) Port placement, (4) Patient cart docking (5) Targeting (6) Manual arm adjustment (7) Robotic instrument introduction. Familiarisation of the robotic equipment, a standardised practice with adherence to the key principles of robotic set up and docking, will ensure the process can be safely and efficiently performed as well as enabling the best access for robotic surgery to be undertaken. This chapter describes the optimum theatre set to perform robotic colorectal surgery combined with the author's recommendations, tips and tricks for patient set up, creation of pneumoperitoneum and robotic port placement for the common robotic colorectal cases.

Keywords Robotic docking · Port placement · Surgical ergonomics · Theatre safety

Introduction

The introduction of robotic surgery to colorectal practice offers significant benefit to the surgeon; improved 3D vision, articulating instruments and better ergonomics. However, the technologies involved result in significant changes to the operating room. The presence of large, new equipment results in a more complicated theatre set up with additional surgical team roles. This is combined with changes to the surgical approach of the surgeon. A new port placement strategy is necessary to enable the optimum range of instrument access intra abdominally whilst minimising external robotic arm collision. At the commencement of a robotic program this can initially feel daunting; especially in the context of attempting to perform a complex colorectal operation. However, familiarisation of the robotic equipment, a standardised practice

C. Evans (✉)
Consultant Colorectal Surgeon, University Hospitals of Coventry and Warwickshire NHS Trust, University Hospital, Clifford Bridge Rd, Coventry CV2 2DX, UK
e-mail: charles.evans2@nhs.net

with adherence to key principles of robotic set up and docking, will ensure the process can be safely and efficiently performed as well as enabling the best access for robotic surgery to be undertaken.

Robotic set up and docking can be broken down into a series of key steps and processes:

(1) Theatre set up
(2) Patient positioning
(3) Port placement
(4) Patient cart docking
(5) Targeting
(6) Manual arm adjustment
(7) Robotic instrument introduction.

Theatre Set Up

There is remarkable variability in the design and layout of the operating room (OR). Ideally robotic surgery should take place in a theatre of significant space to easily accommodate all components of the robotic surgical device including surgeon console, patient cart and vision cart (Fig. 2.1). Positioning these three components must ensure optimum patient safety; allowing clear communication between the surgeon, the bedside surgical assistant, and the anaesthetist whilst also enabling docking and undocking the robot to take place freely. The patient cart is of considerable size and in the case of the DaVinci Xi robot significant height and weight. (There are occasions in which it has been necessary to reinforce the theatre floor before the Xi robot can be installed). The main operating lights within the theatre must be able to be raised up and out of the way to allow the patient cart to reach over the patient. Certain operating lights have a deep central boom which can cause obstruction and clash with the boom of the cart and thus in some theatres it may be necessary to position the patient off to one side rather than being directly below the operating lights. Similarly, some theatres have laminar flow systems with rigid panels coming down from the theatre ceiling around the operating table which obstruct the patient cart from being moved in to reach the patient. Rigid panels may need to be replaced with flexible ones or removed prior to starting a robotic program.

Before determining the position of the robot in theatre, the OR dimensions and sites for anaesthetic machine set up should be identified as these are the fixed components around which the planning will be made. The surgeon console position should ideally allow for a direct line of vision between the surgeon and the scrubbed surgical assistant to ensure optimum communication (Fig. 2.2). The console position should also allow the surgeon to be in an undisturbed part of the theatre cart with minimal distraction from theatre staff requiring entry and exit to the theatre.

The patient cart position is dependent upon the operation being performed and the related necessary surgical workspace. The general principle is that the patient cart will be positioned on the ipsilateral side of the body as the surgical workspace

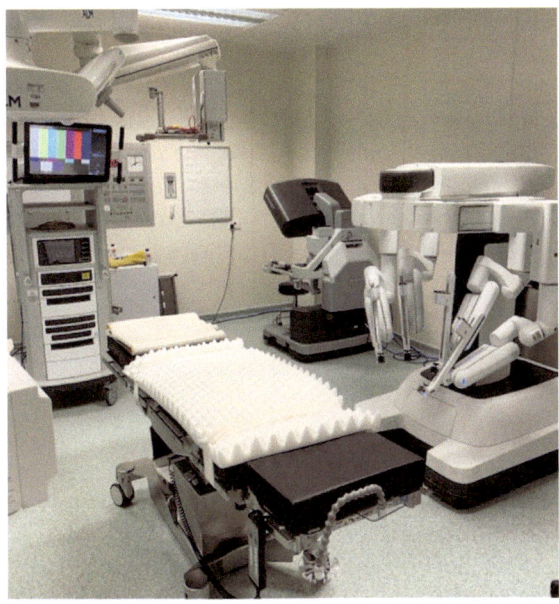

Fig. 2.1 Key components of Da Vinci Xi System: Surgeon console, Patient cart and Vision stack

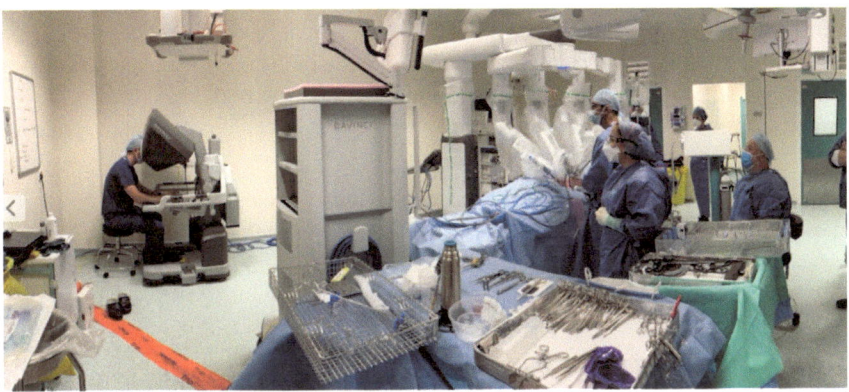

Fig. 2.2 Theatre set up: Surgeon has clear line of communication to bed side assistant, with vision cart screen easily accessible for assistant

(right side of patient for an operation on the right colon, left side of patient for left colon/rectal operations). However, the robotic arms of the Xi robot rotate off a central boom allowing them to be spun around the patient. This allows the patient cart to be remain on a single side of the body no matter where the robotic ports are placed and which side of the body is being operated on, and thus facilitating multi quadrant access to the abdomen and pelvis. If the X system is being used it should be identified which side the surgeon would prefer his second assisting hand to be, (operating with either two right-handed instruments or two left-handed instruments) as the 4th robotic arm will need to swing around to the correct side of the patient cart before docking.

The vision cart is then placed so there is access to the 2-D operative screen for the bed side surgical assistant and leads from the energy devices, diathermy and camera can be attached tension free to the robotic instruments. For most colorectal operations, the vision cart is placed at the patients' feet or just to the side of the feet pending on the theatre size.

Patient Positioning

It helps to have a standardised set up for patient positioning when performing robotic colorectal operations (Fig. 2.3). The positioning requires appropriate access to the patient, including the anus and rectum for pelvic surgery, whilst ensuring the patient is safely secure and protected when the operating table is tilted to aid intraabdominal exposure to organs. Patients are routinely placed in the modified Lloyd Davis position with legs placed within adjustable fins/leg stirrups abducted to 15°. Surgery on the colon can be performed in a standard supine position, however the authors would recommend that all patients are placed in the Lloyd Davis position to ensure patient stability on the operating table, easier access to the patient for the surgical assistant plus it continues a standardisation of the patient pathway. To reduce the risk of deep vein thrombosis all patients should have hydraulic Flowtrons placed but calf compression stockings removed as the combination of both combined with long pelvic surgery has been linked with the development of calf compartment syndrome.

Fig. 2.3 Llyod Davis position recommended for robotic colorectal procedures with arms wrapped and hydraulic flowtrons placed

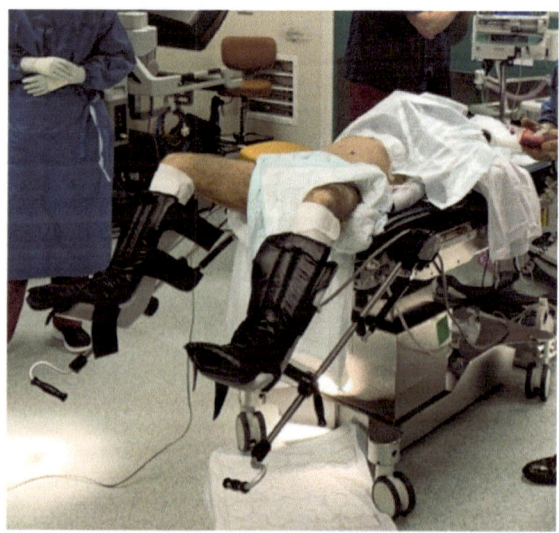

To stop the patients sliding on the theatre table when positioned the arms are wrapped at the side and the patient is placed on an anti-slip mat. Chest straps can also be placed. Previous use of shoulder supports to prevent slipping has become less popular due to reports of brachial nerve injuries combined with the reduced need for extreme patient positioning when undertaking robotic procedures. All patients should have a urinary catheter with an orogastric tube only required to decompress the stomach if it was insufflated at the time of intubation.

To allow access to the surgical field and enable the small bowel and omentum to be kept out of the way, the operating table is tilted. When operating on the left colon and rectum patients are placed 15° head down (Trendelenburg) with a right lateral tilt (right side down) 10–15°. Whereas when operating on the right colon and transverse colon the patients are placed in neutral or mild head up (Reverse Trendelenburg) of 5–10° with left lateral tilt (10–15°).

It is important to note that once the robot is docked it is not possible to readjust the patient position without undocking the robotic arms. Thus, to avoid frustrating time delays and a disjointed procedure it is preferable to ensure patient position and exposure is as optimum as possible prior to docking the robot. An alternative option is to use Hillrom's surgical operating table TS7000dVb. This has been specially developed to work with the Da Vinic Xi system. Using Integrated Table Motion the operating table is wirelessly connected with the Xi system, coordinating movement of the robotic arms as changes are made to table position and thus avoids any traumatic injury to the patient. This facilitates operative flow and enables more free changes to surgical access which are frequently required in multiquadrant surgery. Similarly, many institutions advocate the use of intraoperative patient -supine relief during longer cases (once a patient has been operated on for over 4 h in a steep Trendelenburg position there is a need to have a break and correct the physiological impact of the position with the patient returned to a neutral stance for at least a 30-min period). This can be undertaken without the need for undocking the robot if the Ts7000dVb table is us.

Port Placement

Robotic port placement has been modified with the use 4th generation Da Vinci robots. This is a result of the updated design of the robotic arms which are less bulky and have improved mechanics and articulation plus the camera is no longer restricted to one specific endoscopic port. The placement of the robotic ports is determined by some key principles:

(i)   Robotic arms work optimally when ports are placed in in a line perpendicular to the target anatomy.
(ii) To avoid external clashing of the robotic arms, ports should be 6–10 cm apart depending on patient body habitus (8 cm recommended in most cases).
(iii) Ports should be at least 2 cm away from bony structures to avoid injury.
(iv) Assistant port should be at least 7 cm away from the robotic ports and not placed between any robotic ports and the target anatomy.

It steps of port placement and positioning is covered within Chap. 1 in detail but in short involves:

(1) Creation of pneumoperitoneum—entry to abdominal cavity and creation of pneumoperitoneum has classically been performed by General surgeons using the Hasson open technique with open cut down at the umbilicus. However robotic ports are often not ideally placed at the umbilicus so alternative strategies are frequently employed including: use of Verres needle, use of optical trochar, open cut down at port site or planned specimen extraction site with Alexis + cap (or glove) then placed within wound to create airtight seal. The technique chosen is governed by surgeon preference and previous experience. The authors of this chapter would recommend open cut down using pfannensteil incision followed by placement of a small alexis + cap if requiring extraction site during the operation such as anterior resection or right hemicolectomy plus intra corporeal anastomosis (Fig. 2.4). If no extraction is required alternatives include optical trochar or a Verres needle.

(2) Marking of Bony Landmarks (costal margin + anterior superior iliac spine (ASIS)), midline and mid clavicular points (8 cm from midline to costal margin) once pneumopertoneum is created.

(3) The surgical workspace and target anatomy are then determined with a line drawn across the abdomen running perpendicular to this site. For example, when performing an anterior resection involving surgery from up in the splenic flexure all the way round and down into the pelvis a line is drawn running from the left mid clavicular point on the left costal margin down towards the head of the right femur (Fig. 2.5 (i)) whilst for a right hemicolectomy or a sub total colectomy a line is drawn running horizontally across the lower abdomen

Fig. 2.4 Pfannensteil incision with Alexis placed plus cap to initiate pneumoperitoneum at start of robotic procedure

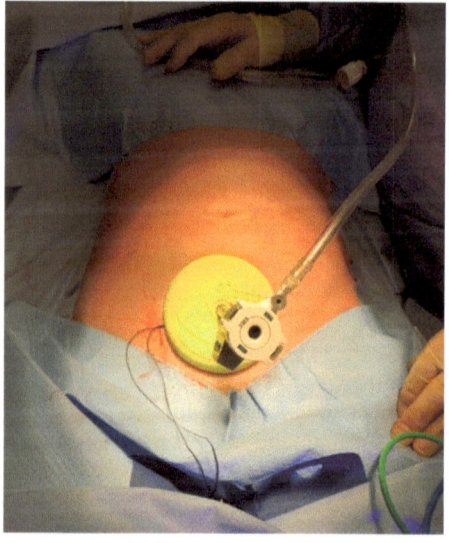

(Fig. 2.5(ii)). The actual sites of the 4 robotic ports are then marked along this line ensuring there is 6- 10 cm between them and that no one are within 2 cm of a bony structure. If a robotic stapler is going to be used it should be decided which port this provide optimum access for the stapler as this will need to be a 12 mm port as opposed to the standard 8 mm ports. The final port to be marked is the assistant port which needs to enable optimum access to assist within the case but also be the required 7 cm from any robotic port to avoid collision.

(4)   The ports are then placed at the marked sites with entry to the abdominal cavity ideally under direct endoscopic vision. Skin incisions for the ports are made to the optimum size by marking the skin beforehand with an empty port trocar. The depth of trocar insertion is determined by a thick black line marked on

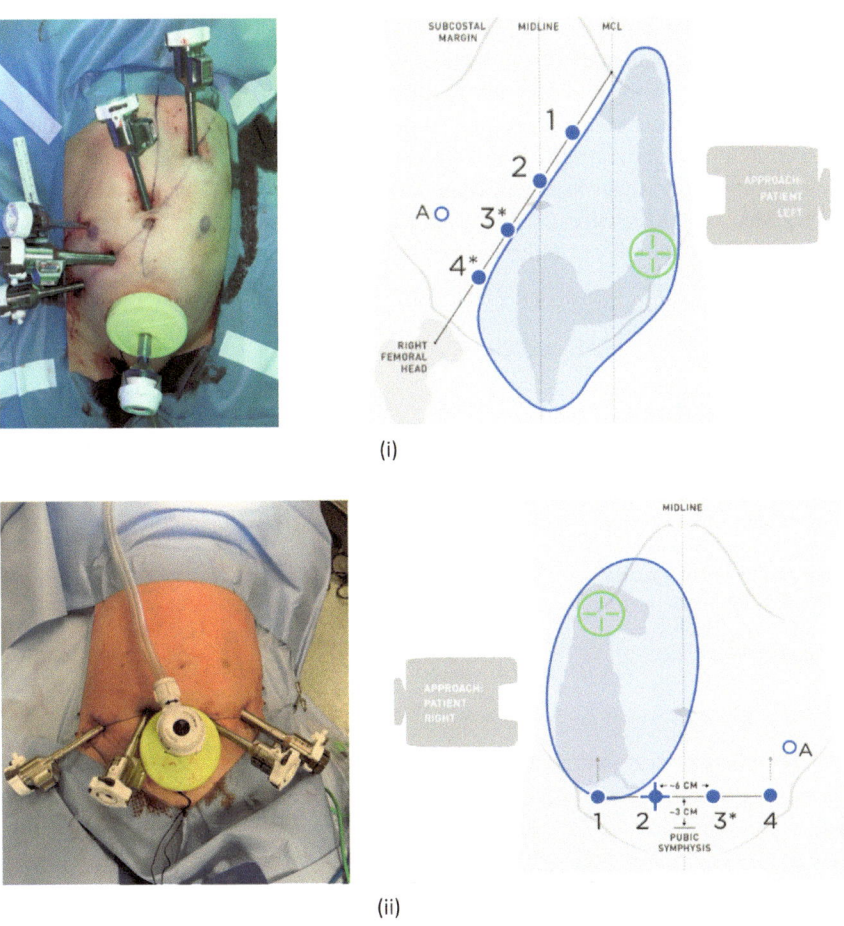

(i)

(ii)

Fig. 2.5 i Robotic ports plus assistant port for anterior resection (in line perpendicular to target anatomy set at ASIS, **ii** Robotic ports plus assistant port for right hemicolectomy (in line perpendicular to target anatomy set at hepatic flexure

the cannula. This thick black line should be at the level of the abdominal wall muscle. Once docked to the robotic arms the port pivots on an axis around the black line and thus trauma to the abdominal wall is minimised. The assistant port is usually the one used for insufflation of the abdominal cavity to maintain the pneumoperitoneum. The size of the assistant port will depend on if it will be used for deployment of laparoscopic Hem-O-Lok clips– (preferred by some surgeons as able to use larger size Hem-O-Lok's), laparoscopic staplers or for insertion of swabs or needles as these will not be passed down a 5 mm laparoscopic port.

Prior to patient cart docking it is recommended that the small bowel is mobilised out of the way of the target anatomy laparoscopically. This is possible robotically but generally it is easily done laparoscopically and avoids inadvertent iatrogenic damage to the bowel as a result of its handling in big movements robotically without tactical feedback.

Owing to the challenges of colorectal surgery and the fact operations are frequently multi-quadrant it may be necessary to adapt some of the principles stated above to facilitate better access. For example, some surgeons performing a robotic anterior resection will undertake splenic flexure mobilisation with the target anatomy in the left upper quadrant and then will retarget towards the pelvis when performing the Total Mesorectal Excision (TME). This requires a modification of port placement with an additional robotic arm placed in the RUQ (Fig. 2.6).

Fig. 2.6 Alternative port positions for anterior resection with original arm one port replaced with ports at two sites (1a and 1b) enabling broader access to target anatomy in LUQ for mobilisation of the splenic flexure when using 1a followed by broader access the pelvis for ports when retargeting in the pelvis using arm 1b

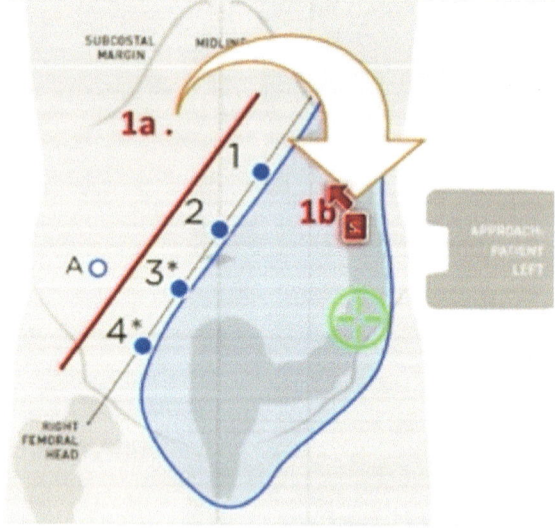

Patient Cart Docking

Once the patient has all ports inserted and is correctly positioned the robotic patient cart can now be docked. The cart needs to be checked it is correctly set for docking. The Xi cart has an automated Deploy for Docking system. Using a touch screen, the side of the patient the cart is coming from plus the part of the body to be operated on is selected. On pressing and holding the Deploy for docking button the boom automatically rotates and pivots to optimise access to the patient whilst simultaneously readying it to be driven to the patient. Once set the cart can be walked towards the operating table. As the cart is moved a laser line projects down from the boom. The laser line is directed to within 5 cm of the port which has been determined the endoscopic port (port 2 if two right arms are to be used or port 3 if two left arms are to be used). The cart can be driven in at any angle to the operating table but due to its size of it base it is easier to get overlying boom close to the ports when walked in directly side on or end on to the table. However, the boom cannot be rotated 180° opposite the base due to issues with the stability of the cart. Therefore, it is recommended the cart is generally placed on the same side of the patient as the side of the procedure: left side for a left side procedure etc. If multi-quadrant surgery is being performed such as a panproctocolectomy it is possible to keep the cart on one side of the patient but rotate the boom fully around by walking the cart in at a slight angle to the operating table so that the arms are never the full 180° opposite to the base (Fig. 2.7). However if the cart remains on the opposite side to the pathology this can hamper the ability of the assistant who is cramped for space to work.

If using the X system, it is necessary to check the arm 4 has been moved to the correct side of the cart to enable the surgeon to operate with either two left or two

Fig. 2.7 Xi Patient cart on the left side of the patient with arms rotated enable access to operate the right side of the body

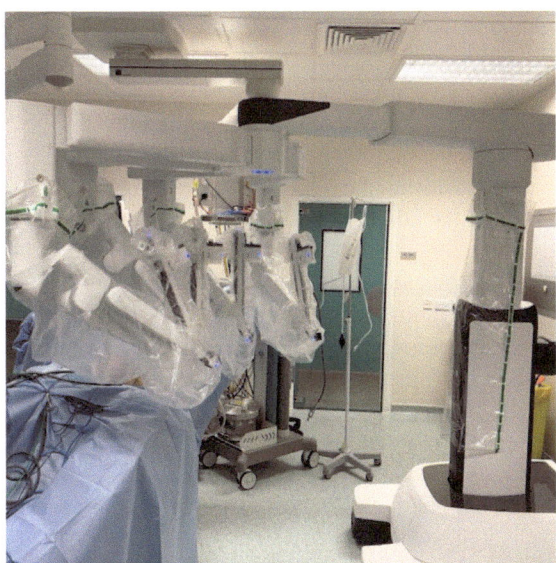

right instruments (Fig. 2.8i, ii). The setup joint of Arm 2 must then be angled away from arm 4 to avoid arm collision. The setup joint of arm 2 should then be adjusted to ensure the arrow on this joint is anywhere within the solid band (the sweet spot) (Fig. 2.8iii). Finally arm 2 must be aligned so that the port clutch and setup structure are in a straight line with the main column of the cart (Fig. 2.8iv). All arms are then raised to ensure clearance of the patient when the cart is walked into the operating table. When the throttle on the patient cart is turned on a laser line projects directly out from under arm 2. As the cart is walked towards the operating table the laser line is used to guide the cart in such a way that the laser line intersects the target anatomy and heads towards the initial endoscope port (perpendicular to the line of robotic ports). Arm 2 is then docked to the endoscope port. If correctly positioned the cart column, setup structure joints, port clutch and target anatomy are all in a straight line. The setup joint is still within the 'sweet spot' pointing away from arm 4. Once confirmed the remaining arms can be docked.

Targeting

To ensure the optimum alignment of the robotic arms on the Da Vinic Xi device the surgeon is asked to performing targeting. This involves the surgeon docking the robotic arm to be used as the endoscope port. The camera is then loaded into the arm and brought into the abdominal cavity. Manually the surgeon will then point the camera at the point within the abdomen or pelvis which has been determined the centre of the surgical workspace. Holding on to the camera port the surgeon will then press the targeting button on the camera which will lead to the boom of the patient cart rotating and pivoting the robotic arms so that they will be exactly in align with direction the camera is facing. The port should be stabilised while this is performed to stop it moving within the abdomen. The purpose of this is to optimise the robotic arm placement and thus enabling the greatest range of instruments internally with as minimal clashing of the arms externally. At the end of targeting, it is important to check the endoscope arm is parallel to the laser line on the boom as this aligns the arm with the target anatomy (Fig. 2.9). Any movements of the endoscope arm through the adjust flex joint can be done manually whilst pressing the port clutch button.

The placement of the camera targeting will depend upon the operation being performed and the patient anatomy, however generally for a robotic right hemicolectomy the camera a will be targeting will be towards the patient's hepatic flexure facilitating instrument access from down in the right iliac fossa and the caecum/terminal ileum all the way up and around to the transverse colon and middle colic vessels. If an extended right hemicolectomy or subtotal colectomy is being undertaken targeting towards the middle transverse colon and the middle colic vessels recommended up. For a left hemicolectomy it would be recommended to target on the spleen and the splenic flexure. With any sigmoid or rectal operation requiring mobilisation of the splenic flexure targeting towards the left iliac fossa heading towards the left ASIS is

Fig. 2.8 **i** X cart set up to
allow operation of 2 left
instruments, **ii** X cart set up
to allow operation of 2 right
instruments, **iii** X cart arm 2
setup joint with solid band
within which the arrow is
required the 'sweet spot',
8(iv) Alignment of arm 2
port clutch and setup
structure with cart column

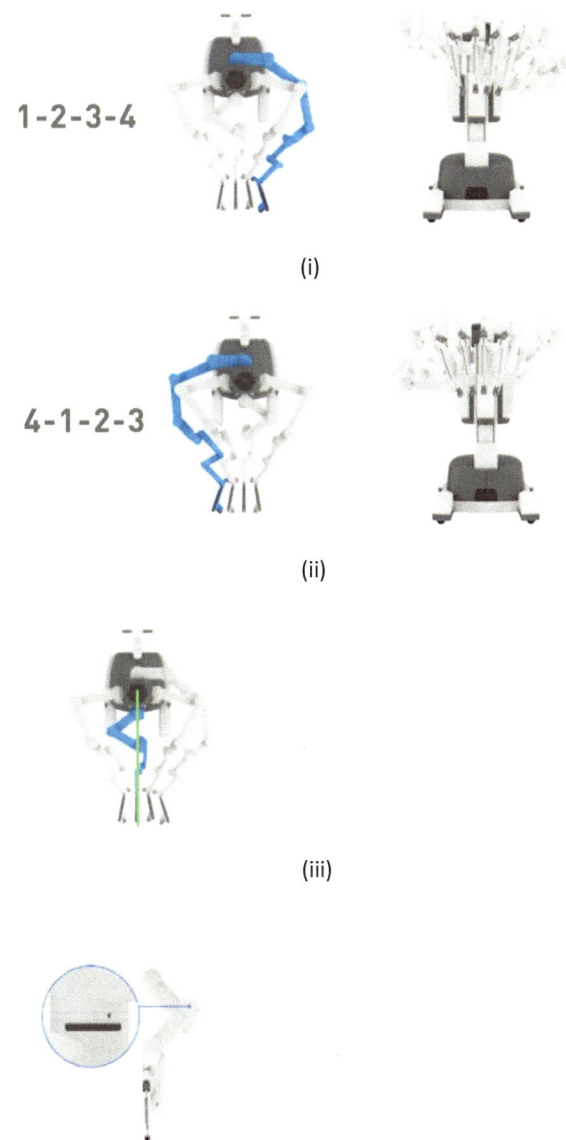

recommended enables access both up to the splenic flexure and also down into the
pelvis to mobilise the rectum. If it is solely the rectum being operated on such as in
a proctectomy or rectopexy it is possible to target more directly into the pelvis, optimising instrument access within the pelvis whilst reducing more proximal colonic
access.

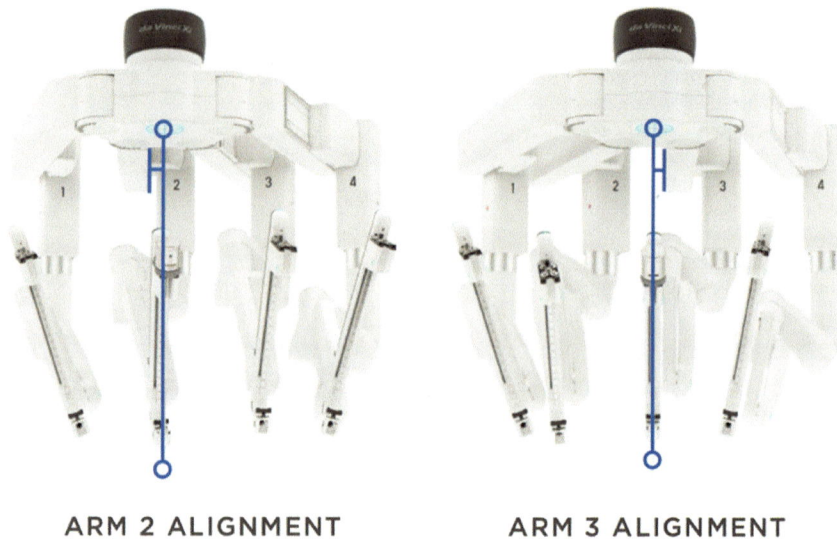

ARM 2 ALIGNMENT   ARM 3 ALIGNMENT

Fig. 2.9 Xi patient cart endoscope arm alignment with boom laser to ensure alignment with target anatomy

Targeting is performed at the beginning of the procedure to enable the best instrument access for the procedure being performed. However, it may be necessary to retarget during the operation. This is recommended when multi quadrant surgery is being performed such as a panproctocolectomy when one or even two retargets are required to target on the right side of the colon, the left side and then in the pelvis.

Once targeting of the patient cart has been performed the other robotic arms are docked. This is done based on orientation and alignment with the camera arm that was set during targeting.

Manual Arm Adjustment

All the arms require an appropriate distance between them. Ideally there should be approximately a hands breath between each arm at each articulating joint. If the joints are too close together there will be clashing of arms externally as the instruments move internally. Similarly, if the joints are too far apart this restricts the internal movements of the robotic instruments. The port clutch is then used to manually move the arms and ensure there is balanced equal space between them all. The Xi also has an additional patient clearance button on the arms to rotate the joints whilst maintaining the arm position to provide additional space between the arm joints and also between the arms and the patient or other sterile objects (Fig. 2.10).

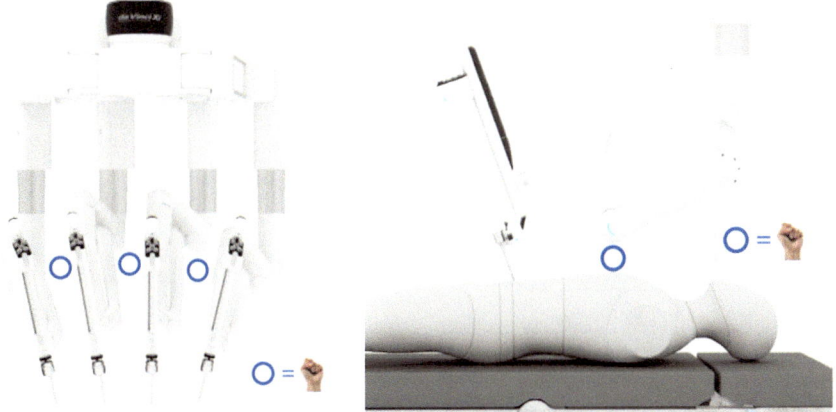

Fig. 2.10 Xi clearance between robotic arms and the patient

(7) Robotic instrument introduction

Once the surgeon is happy the robotic arms have been successfully docked with adequate clearance the robotic instruments can be loaded on the arms. It is recommended that all instruments are introduced to the abdominal cavity under direct vision as there is a risk of iatrogenic injury with inadvertent damage caused as the instruments are passed in blindly without adequate tactile feedback. Observing instrument entry can be done with the robotic camera loaded onto the endoscope port. However, this often leads to clashing of robotic arms as the endoscope needs to look back on itself to the other robotic ports. To avoid this, it is recommended that the bed side assistant to holds the camera manually through the assistant port facilitating far easier access to view the robotic ports as the instruments are entered. Once all instruments have been placed in close proximity towards the target anatomy the endoscope can then be inserted in the endoscopic robotic arm and directed towards them. With the camera and all instruments loaded and safely in view on screen, the cart optimally docked with the patient safely positioned it is now possible for the surgeon to commence robotic operating.

Top Tips

1. Plan your theatre layout—a picture board can be sued to optimise equipment positions, facilitate communication and ensure optimal usage of space.
2. Select and plan your port positions to ensure ease of docking.
3. Target to the workspace required and consider whether single or dual targeting is needed.
4. Put all instruments in under direct vision to avoid iatrogenic injury.
5. Do a check of all joints/arms/instruments prior to leaving the table to reduce the chance of having to re-scrub to make adjustments.

Chapter 3
Preventing Instrument Clashing in Multi-quadrant Surgery

Neena Randhawa

Abstract Despite robotic surgery's relatively quick acceptance for a wide range of surgeries, adoption and performance difficulties persist. Collisions are most prevalent in poorly arranged workspaces. Every case should start with meticulous preparation. This aims to discuss some of the common problems and provide troubleshooting tips and methods for dealing with often encountered surgical difficulties.

Keywords Da Vinci Xi · Robotic colorectal surgery · Robotic instruments · Ports · Flex joints · Port hopping · Table motion

1. Accurate distance between the ports

   Old dV systems required the external arms to be spaced out to maximise the working field. This is opposite to the current Xi system which requires FLEX joints to positioned no more than one fist-width (Blue arrow) (Fig. 3.1). This is sufficient spacing between the arms to allow parallel movements whilst avoiding collision. This is ideal for multi-quadrant surgery where arms can move without collision between the arms and the instruments.

   As the surgery progresses away from the targeted area, it may help to reposition the flex joints back to the neutral position.

   Adjusting flex joints on the arms to be parallel to each other prevents front end interference (Fig. 3.1b).

2. Patient clearance joints

   The efficiency of Xi system is appreciated by adjusting the patient clearance joints. Increasing the patient clearance moves the arm joint axially and thereby rotating it away from the patient and adjacent arms. This helps create more space between the arms. This is particularly useful in thin patients in multi-quadrant surgery.

N. Randhawa (✉)
Newcastle Upon Tyne Hospitals NHS Foundation Trust, Tyne, UK
e-mail: neena.randhawa@nhs.net

Fig. 3.1 **a** Gap between the
flex joints (blue arrow), **b**
Adjusting flex joints

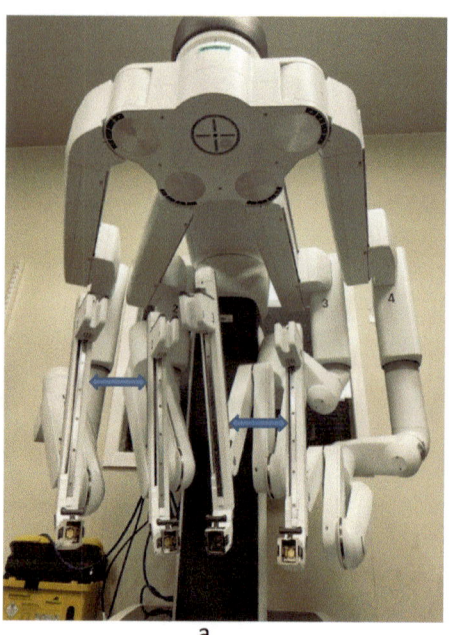

a

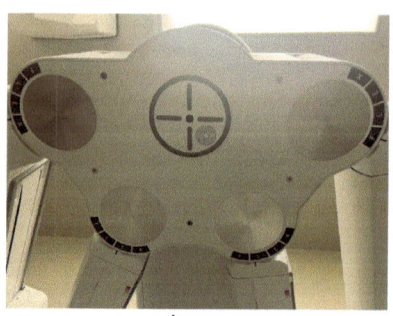

b

Adjusting patient clearance joints will prevent back end interference (Fig. 3.2).

3. Port hopping

Camera for the Xi system is suitable for 8mm ports which provides flexibility of using any port for better visualisation of the anatomy (Fig. 3.3). This offers flexibility of switching instruments to provide better access. Also, camera view can be altered by the surgeon from the console minimise the need for the assistant to remove and re-insert the camera.

4. Dual Docking

In circumstances where operative field lies outside the reach of the flex joints, there are two options for overcoming this. First option is to manually move the arm towards the new target. In multi-quadrant surgery such as subtotal colectomy

Fig. 3.2 Adjusting patient clearance joints

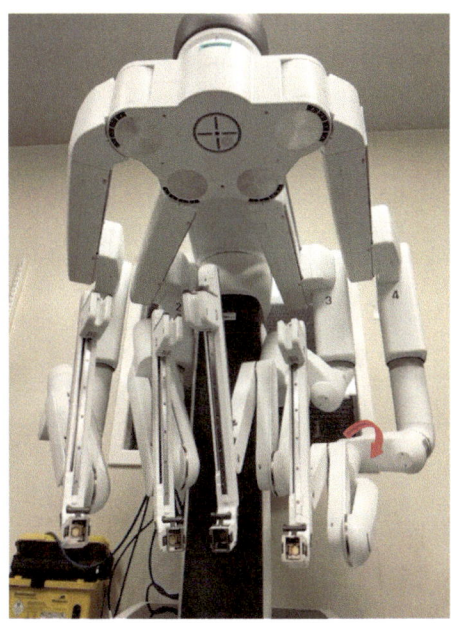

Fig. 3.3 Port Hopping

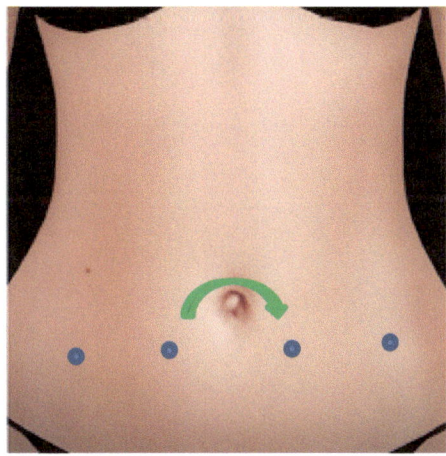

or panproctocolectomy, it will be easier to undock, re-orientate the entire boom and perform the retargeting.

5. Table-motion

   Pairing the table helps position patient intra-operatively without the need to undock the arms and instruments.

6. Change Vantage Point

Port hopping can help visualise instruments and anatomy. If anatomy is still difficult to view then camera angle can be changed from 30° down to 30° up from the Surgeon's console.

7. Use of trained assistant/Surgical care practitioner—this will be covered in detail in Chap. 4 but an experienced assistant—skilled in both laparoscopic assisting and the nuances of the robot is vital for safe procedures and will make the case run much more smoothly.

8. Zoom—using the ability to zoom in means you can keep the camera further back-this helps to reduce smoke/plume fogging the scope and also means the camera will clash less internally with the abdomen.

9. Flexing—this enables the surgeon to reach laterally in the line of the ports. It opens the arms and therefore reduces arm-arm interference. It involves moving the arm closest to the anatomy first e.g. splenic flexure. Adjust the flex to the maximum and then adjust the other arms to their maximum—this will allow extra reach but will need readjustment as you start to work away from the area again. This key manoeuvre is most useful for the splenic flexure and has the advantage of avoiding dual docking.

Disclaimer Author's experience is limited to Intuitive System so these tips may not apply to other robotic platforms.

Chapter 4
Robotic Ergonomics: Different Systems—CMR Versius Robot System

Jeremy R. Huddy and Henry S. Tilney

Abstract CMR Surgical is a medical technology company based in Cambridgeshire, United Kingdom and founded in 2014. The Versius Surgical System is a novel modular teleoperated robotic surgical system that was first used in clinical practice in 2019. It is the first surgical robotic system developed in the United Kingdom to be used in clinical practice and end users were involved in its design and development from the outset (Morton et al., Surg Endosc 35(5):2169–2177, [1]). Initially, used in India the robotic system has now been implemented at several NHS hospitals with uptake increasing around the world with centres in France, Italy, Germany and Australia.

Keywords Robotic surgery · Versius · Cambridge medical robotics

Overview of System

The surgeon interacts with the system through hand controllers attached to an open heads-up display with an immersive high-definition 3D screen that can be placed in a sitting or standing position (Fig. 4.1). The open design permits communication with the theatre team verbally and visually as well as allowing the operating surgeon to monitor the patient and bedside units (Fig. 4.2). The assistant, scrub nurse and other theatre personnel follow the operative feed through a two-dimensional auxiliary screen. Icons are overlaid on the surgical feed that demonstrate active bedside units,

J. R. Huddy · H. S. Tilney
Department of Colorectal Surgery, Frimley Health NHS Foundation Trust, Camberley, UK
e-mail: jeremy.huddy@nhs.net

Department of Surgery and Cancer, Imperial College London, London, UK

H. S. Tilney (✉)
Department of Colorectal Surgery, Frimley Park Hospital, Portsmouth Rd, Frimley, Camberley GU16 7UJ, UK
e-mail: henry.tilney@nhs.net

what instruments are attached and warning alarms. Bedside controls are available on each arm to stop the procedure in the event of safety concerns.

Five colour coded bedside units complete the system that are moved around the patient independently of each other. One of these is a visualisation arm and holds a fine control stable 3D laparoscope that enhances depth perception. The other four bedside units are instrument arms and at present can control bipolar graspers, Maryland tissue forceps, needle holders (Fig. 4.3a), hook diathermy and scissors (Fig. 4.3b).

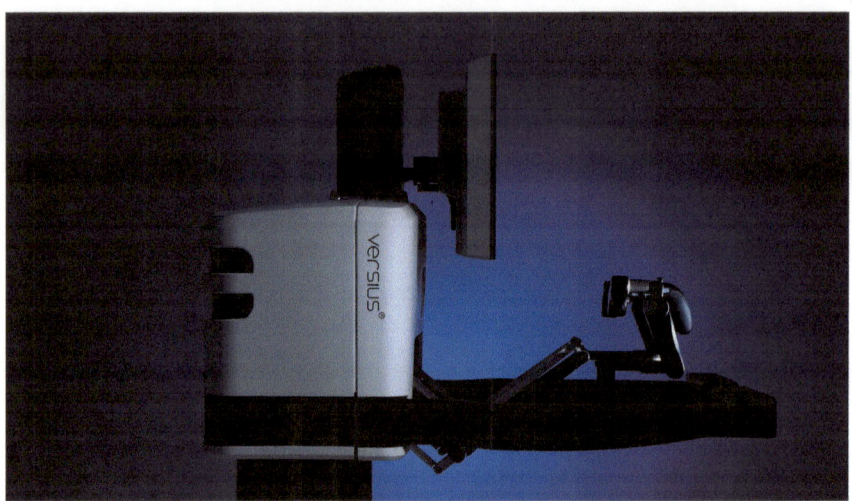

Fig. 4.1 Versius open surgeon console

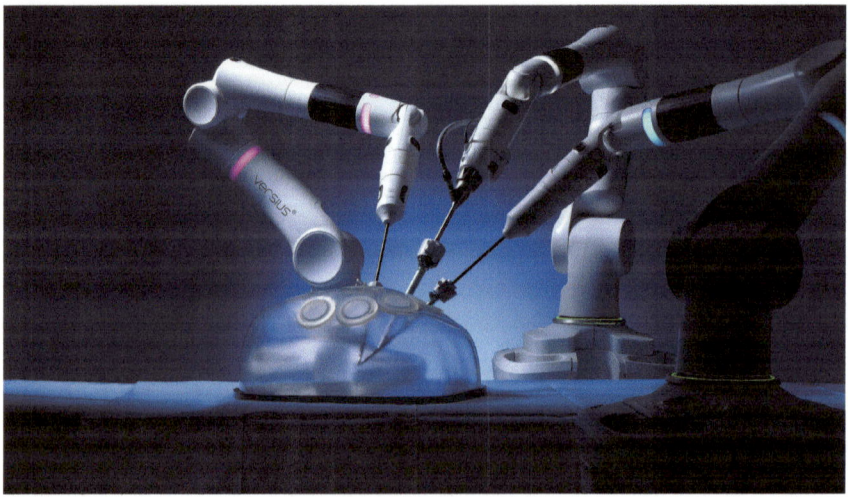

Fig. 4.2 Dry-box demonstration of Versius camera and 2 operative arms

These instruments can be easily and quickly exchanged during procedures using an 'instrument exchange' feature. The bedside units are able to flex at the elbow and shoulder and have fully articulated wrists and are inserted using existing disposable 5 mm ports. Bedside units can be moved repeatedly during surgical procedures allowing a high degree of flexibility mirroring that of standard laparoscopic surgery.

(a)

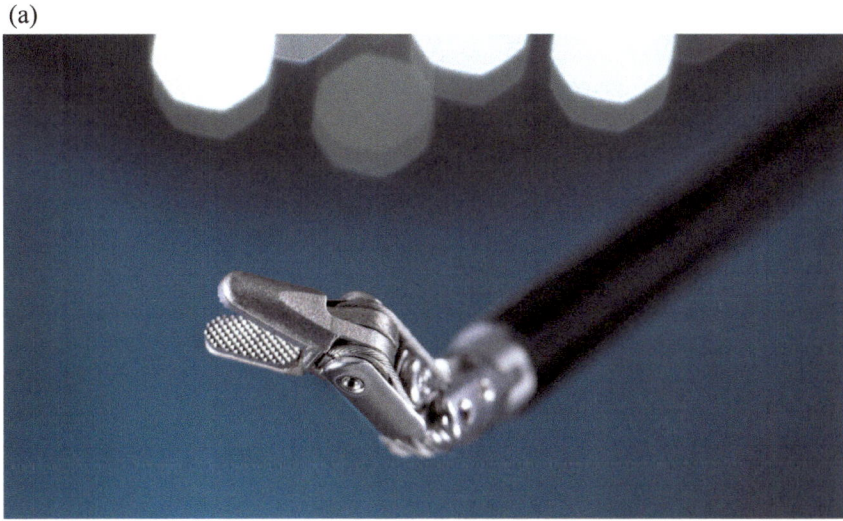

(b)

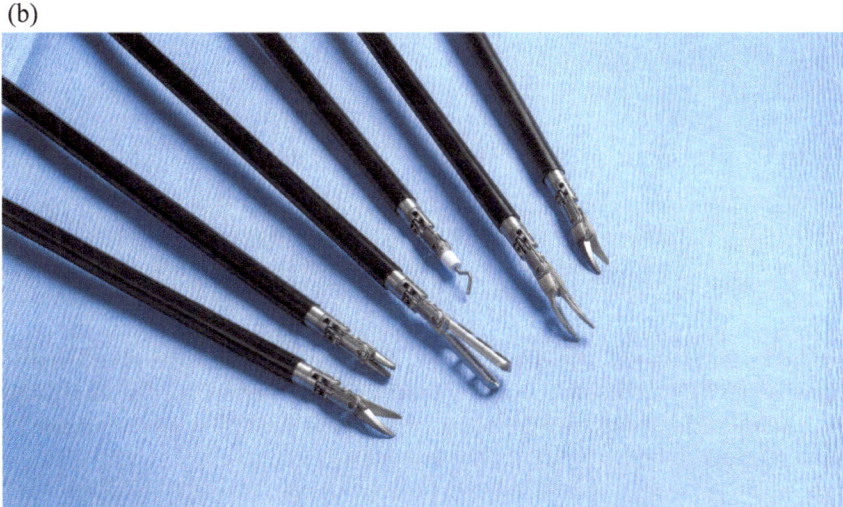

Fig. 4.3 **a** Wristed 5 mm robotic needle driver, **b** Current suite of Versius instruments

Training

CMR Surgical have an established training programme for the Versius robot and adopt a theatre team-based approach. Robotic surgery teams are made up of four members: an operating surgeon, a surgical assistant, scrub nurse and circulating nurse. All new Versius teams undertake an initial training programme that comprises four stages:

1. Online modules (all team members): thirteen online modules with assessments are taken that introduce individuals to the robot, its set-up, functioning and alerts.
2. Versius training simulator (operating surgeon): the Versius simulator has 15 tasks that progress from simple tasks such as movement, using diathermy and switching arms to complex tasks such as suturing a gastrointestinal anastomosis. Feedback from each task is collated on a smartphone app to monitor progress. A minimum of 5 h and 45 min of simulator time is required before progressing to the technical course.
3. A three-day technical training course is undertaken as a team. This course is unique in encouraging the theatre team to train together in view of the human factors and communication skills that are required to safely utilise robotic technology. The course includes hands-on training in setting up the robot, responding to alarms and cleaning the robot. Cadavers are used for procedural training that is tailored to the speciality of the team.
4. Finally, following an in-hospital dry run of the Versius set up process, at least the first five cases undertaken by each team are proctored by an experienced Versius surgeon. A Versius specific training the trainers course is currently in development to support the development of preceptors.

Data Capture

At the time of writing clinical data relating to the Versius is limited. Small case studies have demonstrated feasibility for both colorectal [2, 3] and gynaecological surgery.

Following each operation, the robotic system accumulates data from the procedure. This data, as well as operative videos, are collated on the surgeon's smartphone app through a QR code. Data is also collated by CMR surgical to allow prospective real-world safety and clinical performance data collection to be kept in a registry of all operations performed and patient outcomes.

Set-Up for Procedures

The low profile of the individual bed-side units allows for a greater flexibility of use of the system compared to other robotic systems. Smaller theatres can accommodate the system (during the coronavirus pandemic we were able to resite the system into a relatively small day case theatre in a COVID-secure isolated theatre suite with no problems). Being lighter there is no need to check for reinforcement of the floors, and the units can be fitted in around existing theatre infrastructure such as ceiling hung electrical and gas supplies.

Standard surgical ports are used with set up mirroring laparoscopic surgery. Applied Medical (California, United States) 5 mm and 10 mm balloon ports have been validated for the robotic system and are used for all robotic arms. The positioning of bedside units varies by procedure and is flexible allowing for individual patient characteristics. Bedside units are easily moved during procedures to move from one anatomical region to another and to avoid arm clashing. Once a bedside unit has been placed alongside a patient the height can be adjusted and each arm requires orientation and calibration through a rapid port training process undertaken by a scrubbed member of the team. During procedures individual arms can be moved adjusted outside the patient to avoid arm clashing internally without affecting the internal movement of instruments.

An advantage when moving from laparoscopic to Versius surgery is that the system is designed to enhance the laparoscopic approach, by adding articulated instruments, motion control and 3-d visualisation, rather than requiring an entirely new set-up and port placement plan. As such the preparation and set-up is essentially a refinement of the positions the surgeon would use in their laparoscopic practice. Some minor modification is required to accommodate for the system, however, and it is good practice to check the instrument reach between the intended target organ and the proposed port site by comparing it to the length of the robotic instrument outside of the patient before inserting the port. The outside shape of the arms can be set initially to allow maximum manoeuvrability during surgery. This entails ensuring that joints are gently angled at the outset which affords an optimal range on intra-abdominal movement.

Certain alterations are sometimes required to set-up to minimise clashing. For example, if the visualisation (camera) arm impedes the free movement of operative arms then it can help to use a 30° scope in the 'up' orientation as this means the visualisation arm can be set much higher than for the 'zero' or '30-down' scope, making an external clash much less likely. A current safety requirement of the system also dictates what is known as the '5 cm rule' whereby the instrument tips must be at least 5 cm within the abdomen before they can be used. To allow for this, especially in individuals with small abdominal cavities, it is sometimes necessary to position the instrument access ports further away from the target anatomy than might otherwise be the case.

The placement of bedside arms is flexible, and some adaptation is made for individual patient factors. However, typical port placement and robotic bedside unit positions for colorectal procedures are demonstrated in Fig. 4.4a, b.

Viewpoint of a unit with two systems, strengths and weaknesses, selection of system (Table 4.1).

Fig. 4.4 a Suggested port placements for left-sided colorectal resection, **b** Suggested port placements for right sided colonic resection

(a)

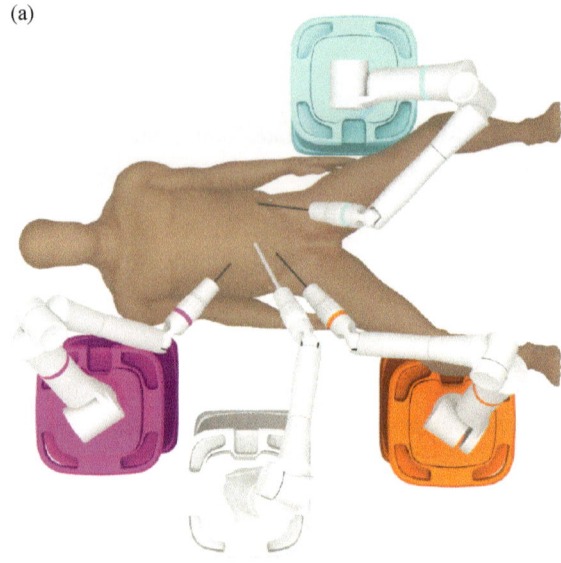

(b)

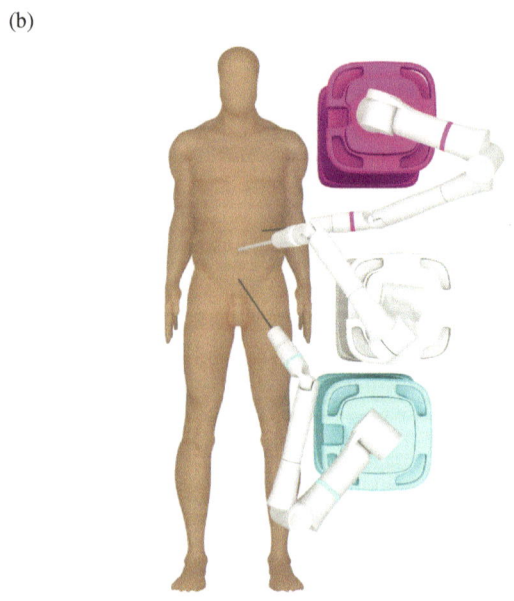

Table 4.1 Comparison of features

	DaVinci	Versius
Display	Seated, Immersive 3D	Seated/Standing Open 3D
Interface	Finger Loops	Joysticks
Mobility	✔	✔✔✔
Number of arms	$1 + 3$	$1 + 5$
Available Instruments	Extensive	Limited at present
Robotic energy devices	✔	✗
Robotic staplers	✔	✗
Other available features	Dual Console for training Integrated table motion Single Port Robot	

At our institution we use adjacent theatres to house both the CMR Versius robot and the Intuitive Da Vinci surgical robot. The Da Vinci robot has been used for colorectal surgical procedures since 2008 and the Versius robot since 2020. Our default position is to offer a robotic resection for all rectal resections. New robotic systems coming to the market will inevitably improve access to the advantages of robotic surgery for patients, increase training opportunities for surgeons and drive innovation in the next generation of robotic systems.

We usually perform a hybrid procedure for rectal cancer surgery using the Da Vinci with a laparoscopic medial to lateral splenic flexure mobilisation and inferior mesenteric artery dissection before docking the robot to undertake the TME dissection. This allows training in laparoscopic surgery and avoids the need to redock the robot to operate in different regions of the abdomen as we currently use the Da Vinci Si system.

The Versius robot has now been used for right hemicolectomy, sigmoid colectomy and low anterior resection with TME dissection to the pelvic floor (Fig. 4.5). As all users remain on the learning curve, careful patient selection is undertaken for Versius cases, and to ensure safety and reasonable operating times we would always advocate consideration of a hybrid approach for those starting out with this system. The current lack of advanced energy devices also means that in all colorectal cases a scrubbed assistant with a port available for the application of clips or advanced energy is a key safety requirement. However, early opportunities demonstrated by Versius include the ease in which the robot can be moved between theatres or even hospital sites, reduction in size of theatre required and flexibility in port positioning and setup.

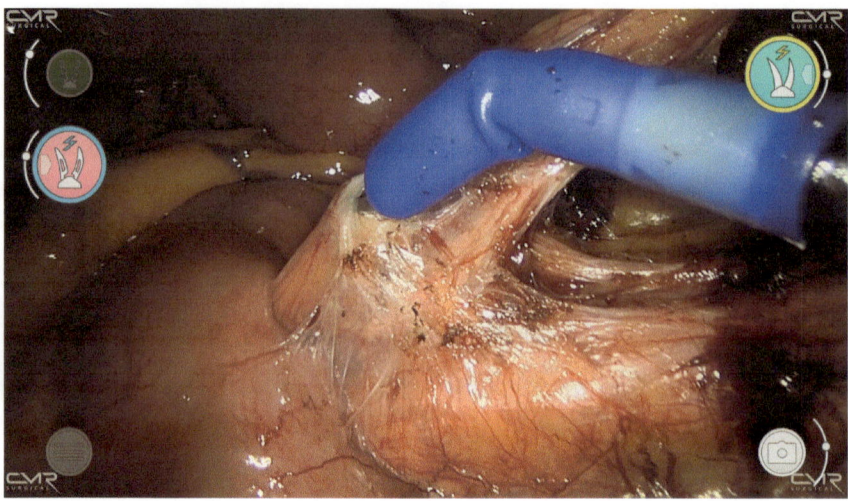

Fig. 4.5 Operative view of Versius robotic IMA dissection during low anterior resection for cancer

References

1. Morton J, Hardwick RH, Tilney HS, Gudgeon AM, Jah A, Stevens L, Marecik S, Slack M. Preclinical evaluation of the versius surgical system, a new robot-assisted surgical device for use in minimal access general and colorectal procedures. Surg Endosc. 2021;35(5):2169–2177. https://doi.org/10.1007/s00464-020-07622-4. Epub 2020 May 13. PMID: 32405893; PMCID: PMC8057987.
2. Puntambekar SP, Goel A, Chandak S, Chitale M, Hivre M, Chahal H, Rajesh KN, Manerikar K. Feasibility of robotic radical hysterectomy (RRH) with a new robotic system. Experience at Galaxy Care Laparoscopy Institute. J Robot Surg. 2020. https://doi.org/10.1007/s11701-020-01127-x. Epub ahead of print. PMID: 32710253.
3. Collins D, Paterson HM, Skipworth RJE, Speake D. Implementation of the Versius robotic surgical system for colorectal cancer surgery: First clinical experience. Colorectal Dis. 2021. https://doi.org/10.1111/codi.15568. Epub ahead of print. PMID: 33544433.

Chapter 5
Colorectal Surgery with the Senhance Digital Laparoscopic Platform

Ibrahim Darwich⊙ and Dietmar Stephan

Abstract Surgical robotics has been on the rise since the turn of the century. Due to the high costs of this advancement as well as the still missing clear clinical benefit, the market penetration of this technology has been relatively modest. Expiring patents of the currently worldwide leading robotic surgical system has led as expected to the introduction of a suite of similar systems by competing manufacturers. This might lead to a drop in the cost of this technology in the near future. To improve the clinical outcome however, new technologies might be useful. Real time overlay and fluorescence enhanced imaging, artificial intelligence and partial automation of defined surgical tasks may someday achieve this benchmark. The manufacturers of the Senhance digital laparoscopic platform have adopted this path. In this chapter we discuss some of the main features of the Senhance surgical system and its engagement in colorectal procedures. We also provide an overview of the current literature and we shed a light on the future perspectives.

Keywords Senhance · Robotic surgery · Digital laparoscopy · Colorectal surgery

Introduction

Since the introduction of robotic surgery in the 1990s, there has been an impressive advancement at the level of widening the surgical spectrum utilizing this technology while upgrades were being added to existing platforms and a multitude of new systems were being introduced [1, 2].

There is a common perception among surgeons that robotics delivers superior surgical quality. A large number of non-randomized prospective and retrospective trials assessed the clinical outcome following robotic assisted surgery compared to standard laparoscopy. Some of these studies assumed a benefit for the patient in terms

I. Darwich (✉) · D. Stephan
Department of Surgery, St. Marienkrankenhaus Siegen, Kampenstr. 51, 57072 Siegen, Germany
e-mail: ibrahim@darwich.net

D. Stephan
e-mail: dietmar.stephan@stephan-siegen.de

© The Author(s), under exclusive license to Springer Nature Switzerland AG 2022   39
P. Coyne and J. Khan (eds.), *Robotic Colorectal Surgery*,
https://doi.org/10.1007/978-3-031-15198-9_5

of autonomic nerve preservation and reduction of the estimated blood loss as well as the conversion-to-open rate [3, 4]. A recently published systemic review failed to confirm these results [5]. Similarly, randomized trials were not able to show a clear clinical benefit of surgical robotics on any level [6, 7].

In general, articulation has been up till now the most striking feature of robotic surgery. Taking the above mentioned lack of clear clinical benefit into account, there is serious hope that the integration of artificial intelligence (AI) into Robotics might bring about the awaited change [8].

Compared to standard Laparoscopy however, robotic surgery still does not enjoy the same market penetration. This is probably explained by the high acquisition, maintenance and running costs of a surgical robotic system [9]. The da Vinci® surgical robotic system (Intuitive Surgical, Sunnyvale, CA, USA) was until recently practically the only player on the ground. This monopoly ended however with the introduction and approval of the Senhance digital laparoscopic platform (TransEnterix Inc., Morrisville, North Carolina) in 2016 [10].

In 2017 our institute acquired the Senhance digital laparoscopic platform (Asensus, formerly TransEnterix Inc., Morrisville, North Carolina). The main drive behind choosing this platform was the fact that it resembled standard laparoscopy not only in terms of trocar placement but also due to the ability to utilize conventional laparoscopic trocars (5, 10 and 12 mm) and reusable instruments which obviously means a reduction in running costs. The Senhance platform also enjoyed unique novel technological features which included haptic feedback coupled to the controllers, an eye-tracking device to navigate the camera as well as the ability to use articulated 5- and 10-mm instruments and straight 5- and 3-mm instruments [11–14]. In the recent past, system upgrades included a 4 K monitor, advanced energy, integration of ICG Fluorescence (Novadaq®) and the first version of the ISU (Intelligent Surgical Unit) as the AI integration platform.

In its years of activity at our institute, the Senhance robotic platform was used to perform hundreds of surgical procedures including colorectal resections for both benign and malignant indications, hernia repair, cholecystectomies, fundoplications, adrenalectomies and hysterectomies. In this chapter we share our expertise with the reader in using the Senhance system in colorectal surgery. We provide a detailed description of the general peri- and intraoperative setup while emphasizing more on a standardized guide for performing colorectal procedures. We discuss also tips and tricks in case of trouble shooting.

General Technical Aspects in Colorectal Procedures

Positioning of the Patient

In general, a bean bag positioner is used with adequate padding of the shoulders, elbows and the lower extremities, both padded arms being tucked at the patient's

side. This is particularly important during colorectal surgery due to frequent repositioning of the operation table in order to perform different steps of the procedure like
colon flexure mobilization or skeletonizing the mesenteric vessels. Typical positions
include the Trendelenburg and reverse Trendelenburg positions as well as the right
and left tilted positions.

Trocar Placement

A minimum distance of 8–10 cm between the trocars is helpful to prevent collision
between the robotic arms. In adults with short stature (e.g., some racial-ethnic groups)
or in pediatric surgery, this distance is not mandatory due to the smaller operation field
which leads to smaller movements outside of the patient. While the configuration
of trocar placement is similar to that used in standard laparoscopy for the respective
surgical procedure, the trocars should be placed an additional 3–4 cm away from
the zone of dissection as a rule of thumb to avoid a too steep position of the robotic
instruments. Since conventional laparoscopic trocars of 5 mm or 10 mm size are
utilized, conversion to standard laparoscopy is possible at any stage of the procedure.

Setting the Robotic Arms

The Senhance platform consists of a surgeon's open console and a maximum of 4
manipulator arms, each mounted on a single cart. All instruments, the scope included,
are compatible with all arms and can be docked interchangeably as such. The pitch
and yaw as well as the in–out movements of the end instrument's shaft are delivered
by motorized vertical and horizontal telescopic extensions on the cart. The pitch is
delivered by the vertical extension while the yaw as well as the in–out movements
are executed by the horizontal one. This horizontal extension is mounted on an axis
with rotating capability. Another motorized machine controls the axial shaft rotation
and the grasping function of the end effector. Each telescopic extension has a marked
midpoint intended to designate the optimal starting position when this marking is
present at the rim of the vent (Fig. 5.1). Extended visualization and maximal range
of mobility are achieved when this optimal starting position is taken into account
[11]. The carts are brought in a pre-designated position characteristic for the trocar
placement during the respective procedure.

Coupling of the End Instruments with the Robotic Arms

Once the carts and the arms are placed in the pre-designated positions according to
the planned trocar placement and after adjusting the arms' telescopic extensions for

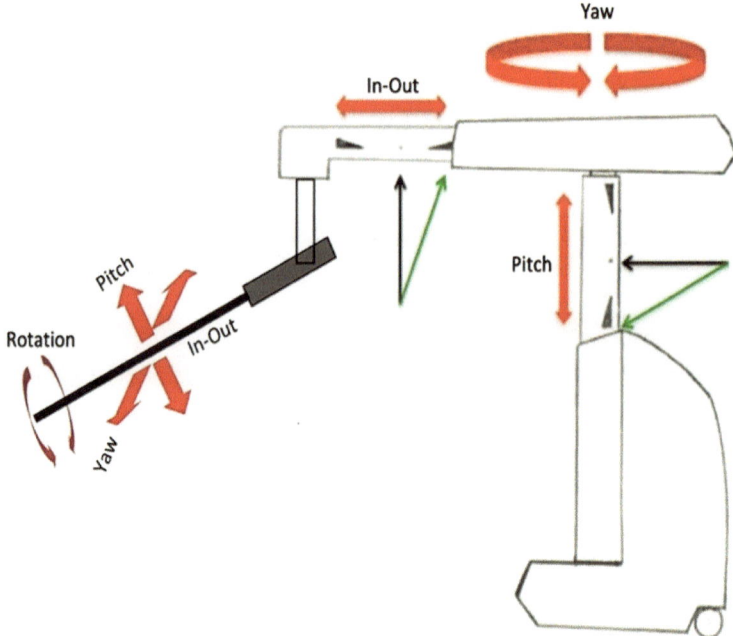

Fig. 5.1 A schematic representation summarizing the movement spectrum of the robotic arm and the manner of transferring this movement to the end instrument. The green arrows are pointing to the optimal starting position of the marked midpoint on the telescopic extension

maximal range of mobility, the endoscope, fitted into its robotic adapter, is brought manually into the abdomen via the trocar. Coupling with the robotic arm follows. Electromechanical calibration of the "fulcrum point" is then initiated. The instruments are brought manually in a similar fashion into the abdomen under endoscopic vision and are then coupled with the robotic arms before calibration of the fulcrum point is performed. The joint of the robotic arm should be rotated to match the position and orientation of the arm (right and left, dominant and non-dominant) of an imaginary surgeon who would stand at the operation table to perform the same planned procedure (Fig. 5.2). If the joint is rotated in an opposite direction, paradoxical instrument movement would result.

The Number of Robotic Arms to Be Engaged

In principle, 4 robotic arms can be simultaneously used for a procedure. One arm drives the endoscope, one drives the dissecting instrument and another one drives the forceps. A fourth arm can be additionally engaged to grasp tissue so as to offer countertraction (only three arms have been approved by the FDA in the Unites States).

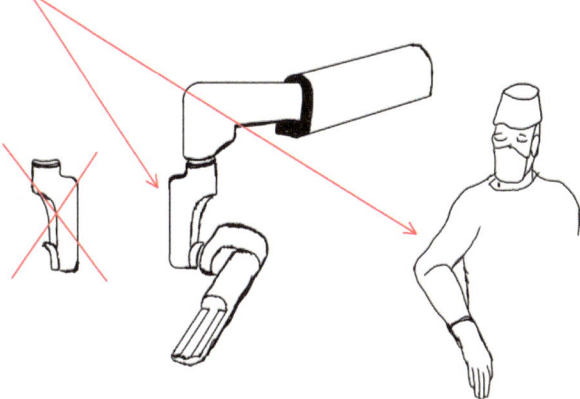

Fig. 5.2 The joint of the robotic arm is rotated here to match the direction and position of the elbow of the surgeon. An opposite setting of the joint should be avoided like shown in this figure

The Lineup of Instruments

A wide range of 5 mm (and 3 mm) instruments is available with the Senhance robotic system. This includes graspers, Maryland dissectors, scissors, a hook and an ultrasonic energy device for vessel sealing. Both modes of cautery, monopolar and bipolar can be used. A 5 mm bipolar grasper and a 5 mm needle holder are also available with articulation. These have been successfully tested in a clinical trial [13] and are currently in the process of CE certification and FDA approval. It is possible to freeze the articulation in a defined position or to set it to floating mode.

Surgery with Senhance

Colorectal Surgery

A roadmap describing sigmoid colectomy performed with the Senhance robotic system for diverticular disease was published by our working group in 2019 [11].

Sigmoid colectomy with the Senhance robotic system is performed in our department for diverticular disease according to the internal standard which dictates a close to the colon dissection in order to preserve the inferior mesenteric artery (IMA) in adherence with the German S2K guidelines. Current evidence suggests a lower rate of anastomotic leaks as well as a lower risk of defecation disorders when the IMA preserved [11].

4 Senhance arms are used to perform the procedure

In general, a so called "star configuration" can be used to perform any colorectal procedure. This configuration provides enhanced reachability of the entire bowel without the need of changing the position of the manipulator arms. This means that only the instruments, scope included, are used interchangeably with the arms without having to reposition the latter (Fig. 5.3).

Alternatively, an array of three carts is positioned on the right side of the patient with a fourth arm being positioned on the left side. This configuration is designed

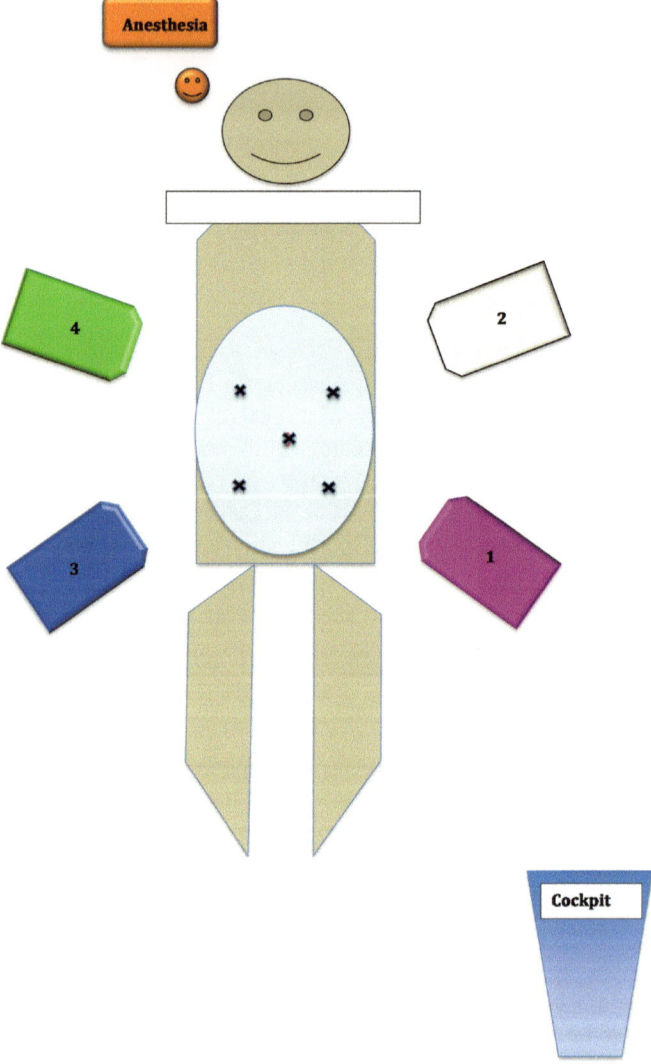

Fig. 5.3 Star configuration

in such a way so as to avoid repeated re-positioning of the carts and thus be able to perform the whole procedure with a single docking in case of a sigmoid colectomy (Fig. 5.4). An opposite configuration with an array of three carts on the left side of the patient and one cart on the right is used for right hemicolectomy.

A Senhance assisted sigmoid colectomy for diverticulitis is performed in three steps. The first step consists of division of the left-sided gastrocolic as well as the splenic ligaments to take down the splenic flexure. Lateral dissection along the peritoneal reflection follows in the second step. In the final third step, close to the colon skeletonization is performed. A 4-trocar technique is utilized, three robotic trocars and one for the assistant. Trocar placement and sizes as well as the instruments used per trocar are described in details in Fig. 5.4.

Similar configurations are used in oncological colectomies. If a medial-to-lateral approach is planned, it is generally recommended to adopt the configuration described in Step 2 of Fig. 5.4 in order to be able to skeletonize the mesenteric vessels. The order of the steps depends on the location of the cancer.

Tips and Tricks in Case of Trouble-Shooting

Limited Motion and Exceeding Force

Every Robot has a limited range of movement and as such, it cannot be as flexible as a human outside the pre-defined field of motion. Correct positioning and careful setting of the robotic arm prevents limited motion and provides the surgeon with the maximum range of enhanced dexterity. Once the telescopic extension has reached its maximum or minimum length, the range of movement of the robotic arm becomes limited. This issue can be solved simply by adjusting the starting position so that both midpoints of the telescopic extension are located at the rim of the vents (Fig. 5.1). Sometimes, the position of the cart itself must also be optimized in order to make this possible. Yet, we occasionally observed situations in our experience in which the instruments and the endoscope come in in a such steep position into the abdomen so that limited motion is practically unavoidable. This was mainly an issue when central dissection at the level of inferior mesenteric artery was attempted in an obese patient. In some cases, the trocar placement tended to be too close to the field of dissection. In such a situation, two options might be helpful:

1. temporary conversion to normal laparoscopy to overcome the difficulty and returning to robotic afterwards [11].
2. changing the trocar positions to a more favorable one.

Exceeding force is a safety feature that depends on the haptic feedback sensors. If the applied pressure on the instrument exceeds a defined limit, e.g., by stretching tissue too strongly or by pushing the instrument against a bony structure, a notification of "exceeding force" appears on the screen. The robot stops working automatically.

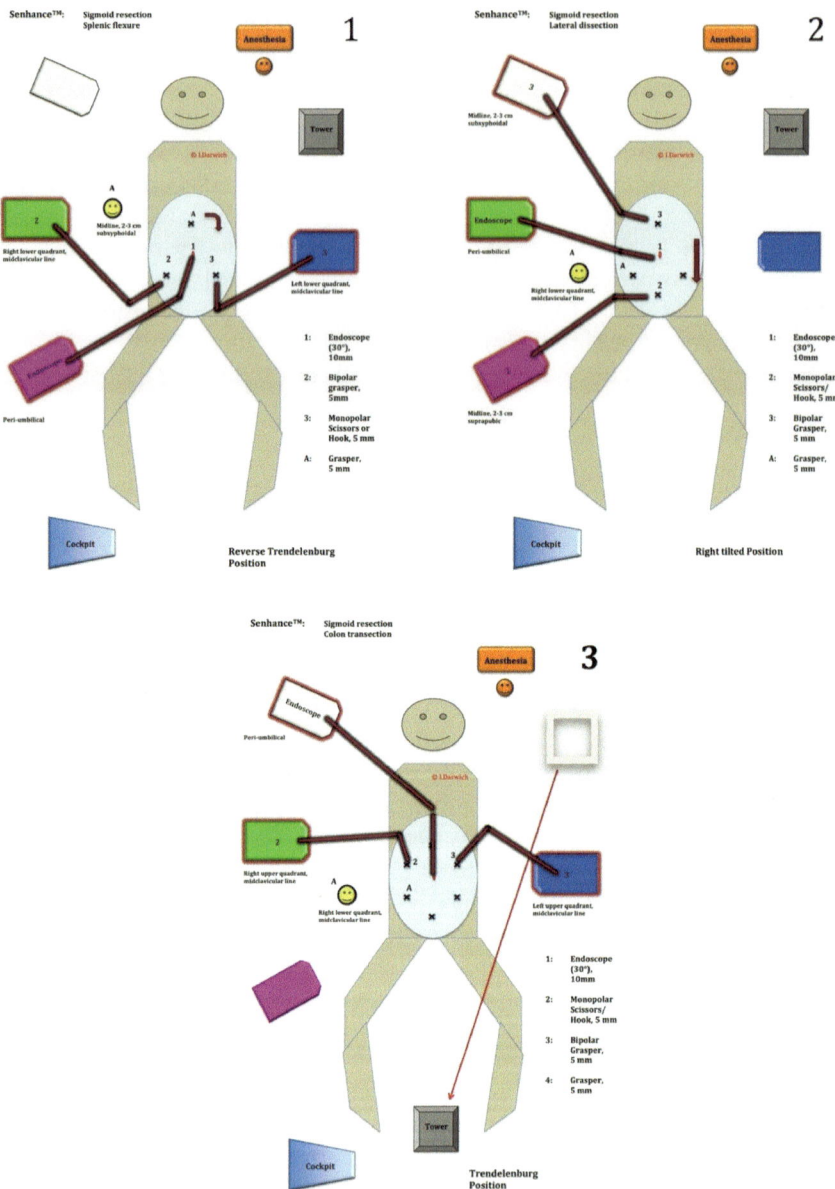

Fig. 5.4 The three steps of sigmoid colectomy for diverticular disease using the Senhance robotic system: (1) taking down the splenic flexure, (2) lateral dissection, (3) close to the colon skeletonization

This same situation may arise as a result of arm collision which should be anticipated and avoided by the assisting surgeon present at the table. The assistant at the table can easily restart the system by canceling the fulcrum point. The robotic arm is then repositioned before setting the new fulcrum point.

4-years Senhance

Just recently our working group published the Transenterix European Patient Registry for robotic assisted laparoscopic procedures in which results from more than three years coming from 5 different centers in Europe were demonstrated [10]. The overall complication rate in 871 patients was 5.5% (2.8% severe). No mortalities were recorded. 33% of the patients had received inguinal hernia repair, 20% had a radical prostatectomy, 18% a cholecystectomy, 7% a total hysterectomy and rest 22% varied between different colorectal and gynecological procedures. Conversion to standard laparoscopy amounted to 3.7% whereas the conversion to open rate was 1.6%. Those results came very similar to previous relatively large case series coming from single centers around the globe [15–17]. They also demonstrate the wide spectrum of procedures that can be performed with this robotic platform.

Furthermore, short docking times ranging between 6–8 min as well as the ability to convert to standard laparoscopy with relative ease have been a common observation in the published data until now.

There is however room for improvement surrounding the Senhance robotic system that has to be addressed.

The Limited Articulation

With exception of the articulated 10 mm and 5 mm bipolar forceps as well as the articulated 10 mm and 5 mm needle holder, all of the instruments available with the Senhance robotic system are straight. This has been, in the past and currently, a disadvantage of the system [18]. In our experience, especially an articulating monopolar dissection instrument would be very helpful especially when performing oncologic colorectal resection in relatively obese patients. This is realized at the latest when central lymphadenectomy is attempted at the level of the mesenteric vessels. Of course, this is expected to change as more upgrades with increased number of articulation instruments are due to be added to the system. All articulating instruments in surgical robotics are at least partially designed as single-use instruments since the articulating part cannot be safely re-sterilized. The advantage of using reusable instruments is therefore limited to straight instruments.

Senhance as a Digital Laparoscopic Platform: An Expert Opinion

The Senhance robotic system provides a form of advanced digital laparoscopy in terms of ergonomics, an eye tracking camera control system and axial rotation of the shaft of straight instruments in addition to articulation in a limited number of instruments. Surgeons who intend to perform procedures with the Senhance robot need, in our opinion, to possess an advanced level of experience in standard laparoscopy. It is of course not easy to define a general number of laparoscopic procedures needed to achieve advanced laparoscopic experience, since experience and learning curves are rather measured in terms of defined procedures [19]. But in general, we do not advise surgeons with no experience in laparoscopy to shift immediately to operating with the Senhance robotic system.

Surgeons are required to obtain a certificate of training, issued by Asensus before they are officially licensed to perform surgical procedures with the Senhance robotic system. Furthermore, these surgeons are advised to perform robotic procedures under high volume conditions in order to achieve a sufficient routine in engaging the robot.

Routine is also achieved more quickly if a specific and constant team of personnel is assigned for robotic surgery. It is also highly beneficial for the whole staff to be present in the operation theatre during preoperative and perioperative preparation as well as during the draping and docking process. This improves the workflow and increases its efficiency.

The integration of AI in robotics might constitute a decisive approach to bring about a significant benefit of robotic surgery in terms of clinical outcome. With the Integration of ISU (Intelligence Surgical Unit) in the Senhance® System, Asensus has begun the path to Performance Guided Surgery. More and more extensive support from AI (e.g., real-time structure detection and measurement in the endoscopic screen, overlay of MRI, etc.) will further improve and make robotic colorectal surgery safer. Of course, clinical studies will be needed to support this expert claim.

5 Top Tips

1. Keep a minimum distance of 8–10 cm between two trocars to avoid arm collision
2. The trocars should be placed an additional 3–4 cm away from the zone of dissection, compared to standard laparoscopy
3. A bean bag positioner and adequate padding is imperative
4. The midpoints of the telescopic extensions should be set at the rim of the vents during the docking process to allow for extended visualization as well as maximal range of arm mobility
5. The joint of the robotic arm should be correctly rotated (Fig. 5.2).

Checklist

– Correct positioning of the patient and the arm carts before any instruments are brought into the abdomen is important
– The procedure is performed according to a predefined standard operating procedure (Roadmap)
– In our experience, starting with taking down of the splenic flexure then moving on to lateral mobilization and followed by close-to-the-colon dissection avoids unnecessary re-dockings in sigmoid colectomy for diverticular disease. Oncologic resection is usually started with the medial-to-lateral approach, central division of the mesenteric vessels and lymphadenectomy.

References

1. Sackier JM, Wang Y. Robotically assisted laparoscopic surgery. From concept to development Surg Endosc. 1994;8(1):63–6.
2. Longmore SK, Naik G, Gargiulo GD. Laparoscopic robotic surgery: current perspective and future directions. Robotics. 2020;9(2):42.
3. Wang G, Wang Z, Jiang Z, Liu J, Zhao J, Li J. Male urinary and sexual function after robotic pelvic autonomic nerve-preserving surgery for rectal cancer. Int J Med Robot. 2017;13(1).
4. Trastulli S, Farinella E, Cirocchi R, Cavaliere D, Avenia N, Sciannameo F, et al. Robotic resection compared with laparoscopic rectal resection for cancer: systematic review and meta-analysis of short-term outcome. Colorectal Dis. 2012;14(4):e134–56.
5. Dhanani NH, Olavarria OA, Bernardi K, Lyons NB, Holihan JL, Loor M, et al. The evidence behind robot-assisted abdominopelvic surgery a systematic review. Ann Intern Med. 2021.
6. Prete FP, Pezzolla A, Prete F, Testini M, Marzaioli R, Patriti A, et al. Robotic versus laparoscopic minimally invasive surgery for rectal cancer: a systematic review and meta-analysis of randomized controlled trials. Ann Surg. 2018;267(6):1034–46.
7. Jayne D, Pigazzi A, Marshall H, Croft J, Corrigan N, Copeland J, et al. Effect of robotic-assisted vs conventional laparoscopic surgery on risk of conversion to open laparotomy among patients undergoing resection for rectal cancer: the ROLARR randomized clinical trial. JAMA. 2017;318(16):1569–80.
8. Panesar S, Cagle Y, Chander D, Morey J, Fernandez-Miranda J, Kliot M. Artificial intelligence and the future of surgical robotics. Annals Surg. 2019;270(2).
9. Childers CP, Maggard-Gibbons M. Estimation of the acquisition and operating costs for robotic surgery. JAMA. 2018;320(8):835–6.
10. Stephan D, Darwich I, Willeke F. The TransEnterix European Patient Registry for Robotic-Assisted Laparoscopic Procedures in Urology, Abdominal, Thoracic, and Gynecologic Surgery ("TRUST"). Surg Technol Int. 2021;38.
11. Darwich I, Stephan D, Klöckner-Lang M, Scheidt M, Friedberg R, Willeke F. A roadmap for robotic-assisted sigmoid resection in diverticular disease using a Senhance™ surgical robotic system: results and technical aspects. J Robot Surgery. 2019.
12. Schmitz R, Willeke F, Barr J, Scheidt M, Saelzer H, Darwich I, et al. Robotic Inguinal Hernia Repair (TAPP) first experience with the new Senhance robotic system. Surg Technol Int. 2019;34:243–9.
13. Stephan D, Darwich I, Willeke F. First clinical use of 5 mm articulating Instruments with the Senhance® robotic system. Surg Technol Int. 2020;37:63–7.

14. Montlouis-Calixte J, Ripamonti B, Barabino G, Corsini T, Chauleur C. Senhance 3-mm robot-assisted surgery: experience on first 14 patients in France. J Robot Surg. 2019;13(5):643–7.
15. Samalavicius NE, Janusonis V, Siaulys R, Jasėnas M, Deduchovas O, Venckus R, et al. Robotic surgery using Senhance(®) robotic platform: single center experience with first 100 cases. J Robot Surg. 2020;14(2):371–6.
16. Siaulys R, Klimasauskiene V, Janusonis V, Ezerskiene V, Dulskas A, Samalavicius NE. Robotic gynaecological surgery using Senhance(R) robotic platform: single centre experience with 100 cases. J Gynecol Obstet Hum Reprod. 2021;50(1): 102031.
17. Lin CC, Huang SC, Lin HH, Chang SC, Chen WS, Jiang JK. An early experience with the Senhance surgical robotic system in colorectal surgery: a single-institute study. Int J Med Robot. 2021;17(2): e2206.
18. Koukourikis P, Rha KH. Robotic surgical systems in urology: what is currently available? Investig Clin Urol. 2021;62(1):14–22.
19. Tekkis PP, Senagore AJ, Delaney CP, Fazio VW. Evaluation of the learning curve in laparoscopic colorectal surgery: comparison of right-sided and left-sided resections. Ann Surg. 2005;242(1):83–91.

Chapter 6
Robotic Surgery: Role of the Surgical Care Practitioner

Nikki Bredin

Abstract Successful implementation of a robotic surgical programme relies on many factors, one of which is the presence of excellent bedside assistants, who not only have to be competent surgical assistants, but also have a strong working knowledge of the robotic equipment and procedures. A Surgical Care Practitioner, as part of the robotic surgical team, can not only provide this assistance but also help with training, allow surgical trainees to get console experience, and more.

Keywords Robotic surgery · Surgical care practitioner · Medical associate professions · Surgical assistance/assisting

About SCPs

The Surgical Care Practitioner, or SCP, is one of the available roles in the new breed of medical associate professions; non-medically qualified practitioners who fill the gap created by an increasing patient population and a shortage of junior doctors in order to provide quality, accessible care. SCPs are usually operating department practitioners or nurses with a theatre background who have completed extra training to enhance their skills and scope of practice to include not only intra-operative assistance and basic surgical skills, but pre-operative and post-operative tasks including (but not limited to) assessing patients in clinic, taking consent, writing operation notes, wound management and discharge planning [1]. They are invaluable members of the extended surgical team, often working in one specific surgical specialty, providing support to the clinicians and a link to the theatre staff in order to facilitate safe and effective perioperative care. It is also a great career choice for those who have ambition, but don't necessarily have management aspirations; an option to upskill clinically as opposed to clerically.

It's not an easy road however. To become an SCP requires hard work and dedication. Eligibility for training requires 1–2 years of experience as a registered healthcare

N. Bredin (✉)
Newcastle Hospitals NHS Foundation Trust, Newcastle upon Tyne, UK
e-mail: nikki.bredin@nhs.net

© The Author(s), under exclusive license to Springer Nature Switzerland AG 2022
P. Coyne and J. Khan (eds.), *Robotic Colorectal Surgery*,
https://doi.org/10.1007/978-3-031-15198-9_6

51

professional and evidence of being able to study at Masters level in order to qualify for a place. The 2 year MSc is assessed academically via essays and exams, and practically via clinical portfolios and workplace based assessments of the same type used for surgical trainees [2].

The role of the SCP is a challenging, but ultimately very rewarding one, with a variety of routes and specific job roles to fulfil once qualified. One such role is as part of a robotic programme, as a Robotic Surgery Coordinator. In this role, the SCP provides surgical assistance, expertise concerning the robotic system of choice, support with organising lists and provision of equipment, and training for both surgeons and theatre staff.

The obvious question is, why is an SCP needed for this role? Surgical trainees often provide assistance—it is an opportunity to learn and gain operating experience. Furthermore, the company providing the robotic equipment provides training that can be cascaded to all theatre staff from a dedicated few core team members. The above is certainly true, but the benefits the SCP brings to the table make them far more than just an alternative filler of these roles.

Expert Assistance

Unlike surgeons-in-training, a SCP would be a permanent member of the robotic team within a surgical specialty. An established SCP will have a wealth of knowledge and experience with the robotic system and the procedures performed with it that will only grow over time. Specialty trainees and registrars rotate, and are only in a particular post for a certain amount of time [3]. They also have other responsibilities far beyond the smooth running of the robotic service. Relying on surgical trainees for assistance means training a new batch of doctors, possibly from scratch, every rotation. Training which might only consist of online assessment and one, or possibly two evening sessions with the company rep. This means that the level of assistance will never be consistent. Surgical trainees might be more than capable of assisting laparoscopically, but they won't have the familiarity with the robot that the consultants or even the theatre staff possess, and so are less likely to be able to set up the system effectively, or troubleshoot instrument clashes, without the consultant's help. A robotic SCP on the other hand, will have this knowledge in abundance, and with training, can become as good an assistant as a surgical trainee, if not a better assistant. This is because the robotic service is their only focus. Some surgical trainees might be extremely interested in the robot and the benefits it can bring to patients; they might even have aspirations to become robotic surgeons themselves. But they have other duties and responsibilities to both their patients and their learning and, unless they're somehow lucky enough to work in a centre with a multitude of robots, limited opportunities to be involved in robotic lists.

Training

There is an argument that if opportunities are so limited, then the SCP is effectively taking those away from the surgical trainees [4], especially those who come to a robotic centre specifically for that experience. This is not the case. Robotic surgery differs dramatically from traditional open or even laparoscopic surgery in that the scope for learning the surgical techniques is very limited from the bedside. Optimal port placement, targeting the anatomy and instrument insertion can all be taught while from this position, and every budding robotic surgeon should have these skills. But when the robot is docked, the learning opportunities diminish to assisting when required and observing the procedure on the 2-D vision cart screen. During open or laparoscopic procedures, the operating surgeon/consultant can easily swap positions with the assisting trainee and let them undertake some of the steps of the surgery, or act as assistant while the trainee performs the procedure and offer help and guidance as required. During robotic procedures this approach is neither safe nor feasible. However, with an SCP as part of the robotic surgical team, there is an available, competent assistant who frees the surgical trainee from the bedside while the robot is docked, allowing them an opportunity to gain console experience.

Whether specifically interested in robotics or not, most registrars and surgical trainees who work in a specialty that offers robotic procedures will be rotated into a robotic list at some point and will need training on the equipment in order to safely assist. An SCP is an obvious choice to facilitate that training and organise sessions in collaboration with the reps to provide both generic and specialty- or procedure-specific knowledge and extra support to any trainees who require it [5].

Of equal importance is the training of the theatre staff regarding the new equipment and procedures. An SCP can facilitate this as well, providing the theatre team with the knowledge required to support the robotic service and acting as the link between the surgeons and the staff.

Future Goals

The presence of an SCP also benefits the consultants in a more direct way, as they can take to the console with assurance that they have a reliable assistant at the table and won't have to keep scrubbing in and out every time there's an issue. In time, and depending on the procedure, the consultant might not even have to scrub in at all. The scope of an SCP's practice extends beyond assistance to initial laparoscopic port insertion as well as skin closure. This, coupled with the knowledge required to position and dock the robot means there is the potential to have everything set up ready for the consultant to go straight to the console.

Robotics may be the exciting future of surgery, but providing a worthwhile and efficient service requires a competent, multidisciplinary team of surgical and theatre staff, with the SCP as the link between them.

Tips for Robotic SCP's

Having (hopefully) made a good case for how SCPs can benefit robotic surgery, what if you are an SCP just starting out as part of one such robotic programme? Here's a few tips.

Communicate effectively. The surgeon has their head in the console and doesn't know what is happening at the table unless you tell them. It may feel awkward at first to narrate your every move, but it is essential for patient safety.

Get comfortable, Or at least as comfortable as possible. The ergonomic benefits of the surgeon console unfortunately do not extend to the bedside assistant. Robotic procedures are often long, and access to the assistant port isn't always the most straightforward depending on the movements of the arms. Don't be afraid to sit down, and if you're straining to look at a screen, don't suffer in silence. Ask the theatre staff to move them. But don't lean on the scrub practitioner's trolley. They don't like that.

Tell the consultant how they can help you. A benefit to robotics is the camera is fixed to one of the arms and controlled by the surgeon, allowing for a stable picture and less pressure on the assistant. However, not being in control means you can't follow your own instruments in when using graspers or suction etc. If you have any concerns about the proximity of internal structures to your instruments, get the surgeon to show you where you are. Or ask to take control of the camera yourself briefly.

Experience with laparoscopic assistance is invaluable. The operating surgeon is controlling wristed instruments with a greater range of motion than the human hand while looking at a 3-D image. The assistant, on the other hand, will be using standard laparoscopic instruments and visualising the operating field via a 2-D screen; so will encounter all the same difficulties with depth perception and inversion of movement that comes with laparoscopic surgery, and will be doing it while also trying to navigate around 4 moving robotic arms.

Last but not least, make friends with your scrub practitioner. As previously mentioned, robotic cases are often long, and you'll probably be there a while!

References

1. Wicker P, Dalby S. Rapid perioperative care. Chichester: Wiley Blackwell; 2016.
2. Royal college of surgeons of England. The curriculum framework for the surgical care practitioner [Internet]; 2014. Last Accessed: http://accreditation.rcseng.ac.uk/pdf/SCP%20Curriculum%20Framework%202014.pdf
3. Quick J. The role of the surgical care practitioner within the surgical team. BJN. 2013;22(13):759–65.
4. Freudmann M. Surgical care practitioners are having a detrimental effect on surgical training. BMJ. 2006;333: s97.
5. Hall S, Quick J, Hall AW. The perfect surgical assistant: Calm, confident, competent and courageous. J Periop Practice. 2016;26(9):201–4.

Part II
Rectum

Chapter 7
Robotic High Anterior Resection

Eleanor Rudge and Irshad Shaikh

Abstract High Anterior Resection (HAR) is removal of the sigmoid colon, including the blood supply and associated lymph glands, with or without the upper part of the rectum. Indications include malignant and benign pathology, and within elective and emergency settings. Robotic Assisted Surgery (RAS) allows precise embryological plane dissection, with complete mesocolic excision of the left side of the bowel. It also facilitates splenic flexure mobilisation, which can be a challenging part of left sided colonic resections.

Keywords Robotic assisted surgery · High anterior resection · Sigmoid colectomy

Introduction

High Anterior Resection (HAR) is removal of the sigmoid colon, including the blood supply and associated lymph glands, with or without the upper part of the rectum. Indications include colorectal carcinoma, endoscopically unresectable adenomatous polyps, inflammatory bowel disease, sigmoid volvulus, ischaemic colitis/stricture and diverticular disease (with its associated strictures and fistulae). As with other colorectal procedures, Robotic Assisted Surgery (RAS) has also gained popularity for performing HAR. RAS allows precise embryological plane dissection, with complete mesocolic excision of the left side of the bowel, autonomy of camera control and an excellent 3D visual field. In our experience, it also facilitates splenic flexure mobilisation, which can be a challenging part of left sided colonic resections.

RAS is most commonly used for elective surgery, however, an emergency setting might not be viewed as a contraindication for robotic surgery provided there has been effective training of the operating surgical team, along with sensible patient selection [1]. Any surgery which is delivered by a laparoscopic approach can be performed using a robotic platform.

E. Rudge · I. Shaikh (✉)
Sir Thomas Browne Colorectal Surgery Department, Norfolk and Norwich Hospital, Norfolk, UK
e-mail: irshad.shaikh@nnuh.nhs.uk

© The Author(s), under exclusive license to Springer Nature Switzerland AG 2022   57
P. Coyne and J. Khan (eds.), *Robotic Colorectal Surgery*,
https://doi.org/10.1007/978-3-031-15198-9_7

Absolute contraindications for a robotic HAR would include patients who are unable to tolerate pneumoperitoneum and Trendelenburg positioning, for example, those with cardiorespiratory disease, or those with haemodynamic instability, including emergency patients with haemorrhage, where the probability of conversion to open surgery is expected to be high. Relative contraindications include bowel obstruction (due to reduced intra-abdominal working space), extensive adhesions, and locally advanced cancer with retroperitoneal involvement, where tactile sensation is needed to aid successful oncological clearance.

Equipment Required

Robot: There are several different types of surgical robots available, including active, semi-active and master-assistant systems. Within this chapter, HAR pertaining to Intuitive's da Vinci® robot will be described.

Ports: All standard ports are 8 mm in Si/ X/Xi systems. If the use of a stapler is required, then a larger 12 mm robotic port is used to transmit the device. At the Norfolk and Norwich Hospital (NNUH), we have devised a method to try and reduce the number of 12 mm ports placed and, thus, reduce the number of post-operative complications such as acute or delayed port-site hernias. To achieve this, an Alexis port is placed in the supra-pubic region, via a Pfannenstiel incision, or in the umbilicus, to transmit the robotic stapler [2].

It is the surgeon's preference as to whether a 5 or 12 mm port is used for the laterally placed assistant port. As above, avoiding a 12 mm port reduces the chance of a port-site hernia forming, however, a 12 mm port is perhaps more useful than a 5 mm, as it can be used to insert swabs into the abdominal cavity, and to transmit a 10 mm Hem-o-lok® for vessel clipping. More recently, we have started using the laparoscopic port (at either the umbilicus or suprapubic region) to transmit swabs and 10 mm Hem-o-loks®. This has enabled us to use a 5 mm assistant port to reduce morbidity. If a 12 mm assistant port is to be used, then it is important that the fascia is formally closed. Our assistant port (either 5 mm or 12 mm) also facilitates a smoke evacuation system. We use the Conmed *Airseal® System*. The da Vinci® ports and trocars come as reusable or disposable. The trocars come as blunt or sharp, and choice of trocar is dependent on surgeon's preference.

Instrumentation: The most common instruments used in robotic colorectal surgery include a bipolar fenestrated grasper, Cadier grasper, curved scissors, large needle driver, Maryland bipolar forceps, monopolar hook diathermy, tip-up grasper, robotic clip applicator (which comes in a variety of sizes), robotic suction/irrigation, and robotic vessel sealers, including Synchroseal. In our practice, we commonly use the Cadier grasper, the fenestrated bipolar grasper and the scissors, supplemented by a vessel sealer as required. A set of basic laparoscopic instruments, including graspers, Johann's forceps, Hem-o-lok® clip applicator, and suction/irrigation are required.

Smoke evacuation system: Several systems are available. We use the Conmed *Airseal*® *System*, which helps maintain a more stable pneumoperitoneum, allowing operations to be carried out at lower intra-abdominal pressures, and providing good-quality visibility.

Stapler: We use a powered CDH circular stapler (Ethicon Inc., Somerville, NJ, USA), normally of 29 mm diameter, for the colorectal anastomosis. However, depending on the size of the patient's large bowel, smaller and larger sizes may be required. We use a purse-string applicator and double ended Prolene stitch for the extra-corporal component of the procedure, which deals with preparing the descending colon for anastomosis to the rectum. There are other circular stapling devices available, and it remains the surgeon's preference and experience when it comes to choosing the right size and manufacturer.

Alexis Wound Protector/Retractor: Use of this device provides 360° of circumferential, atraumatic retraction.

Hem-o-lok®*clips*: Our practice is to apply three Hem-o-lok® clips (two placed proximally, and one placed distally—see Fig. 7.2a) on vessels, so that two clips stay with the stump of the divided vessel. Using the robotic clip applicator allows clips to be applied from multiple angles, augmented by the 3D console views. However, for straightforward inferior mesenteric artery clipping, laparoscopic clip applicators can be used.

Adjuncts to anastomosis:

- **Indocyanine green (ICG) dye**: identifies good vascularisation of the rectum required to achieve a well perfused anastomosis.

  - ICG is administered intravenously and is cleared by the liver, with a half-life of around 3–4 minutes.
  - It becomes fluorescent once excited by infra-red light and this fluorescence is detected using a specifically designed camera.
  - We dilute 25 mg of ICG with 5 ml water, and we administer 1–1.5 ml doses, up to 2 or 3 times.

- **Flexible or rigid sigmoidoscopy:** if the anastomosis is low, we check the join under direct vision, as this technique is associated with a reduced rate of postoperative anastomotic leak and staple-line bleeding [3]. We also use sigmoidoscopy to perform an underwater air leak test.

Procedure

Setup

The patient is prepped and draped, with the optional use of an 3 M™ Ioban™ Antimicrobial Incise Drape. Pneumoperitoneum is performed as per the surgeon's choice.

Techniques include open insertion of the first port, Visiport blunt dissection, or use of a Veress needle. Our preferred initial entry for left sided resections requires a Pfannenstiel incision (5–6 cm in length) for pneumoperitoneum, with care taken to ensure that bladder injury is avoided. An Alexis retractor is then inserted, the cap placed securely on top, and a port placed via the Alexis and connected to gas (AirSeal® System) insufflation. The Pfannenstiel/Alexis port site acts as the specimen extraction site later on (see chapter on Robotic Port Positioning).

The optimal distance between each of the four robotic ports should be 6–8 cm. All ports should be at least 3 cm away from bony prominences. Using a surgical marker pen, the left and right costal margins and the left and right anterior superior iliac spines (ASIS) are defined. The left mid-clavicular line, which is approximately 8–10 cm away from the midline (depending on body habitus), is then drawn on. An oblique line is constructed from the right femoral head, towards the left upper quadrant, to join the junction of the mid-clavicular line and costal margin. Under direct vision, using the robotic endoscope freehand via the Alexis port, all four ports should then be placed on this oblique line (Fig. 7.1a and b). An assistant port is placed laterally on the patient's right, at least 5–6 cm away from the oblique port line.

Before docking the robot, position the omentum over the top of the liver, and carefully move small bowel safely out of the way (usually on to the right side of the abdominal cavity) using laparoscopic instruments. Still using the robotic endoscope freehand via the Alexis port, the robotic camera port is inserted, with close attention to the following:

- The camera should be in line with the target anatomy.
- The camera should be at 10–20 cm distance from the target anatomy.
- The camera should be in line with the centre column of the patient cart.

(a)   **(b)**

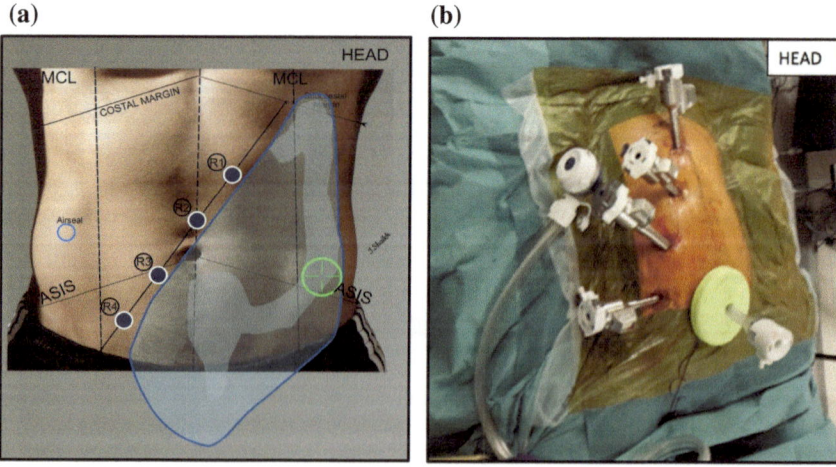

Fig. 7.1 a and **b**: Port placement for high anterior resection

Our preferred approach is a single docking technique, however, patient body habitus or location of tumours can mean that double docking is required, or retargeting if the Xi system is being used. However, need for this can be minimised by using Integrated Table Motion. We perform a medial to lateral dissection, hence, the left colon is dissected medially, towards the side wall and splenic flexure. We always aim to mobilise the splenic flexure for HAR, as it gives the option to divide the descending colon more proximally, whilst maintaining good vascularity. Routine mobilisation of the splenic flexure also provides a training opportunity for surgical trainees.

The dissection plane is entered above the sacral promontory. Whilst we recognise that the left ureter is commonly searched for, we don't routinely look for it as we find that the robot gives a 3D view showing a clear embryological plane dissection, allowing us to chase the IMA to the aorta and safely clip. Of course, when there is retroperitoneal inflammation, i.e. with perforated diverticular disease, retroperitoneal fibrosis, or with previous left sided surgery, we would certainly recommend identification of the ureters. We also appreciate that, for cases which have pre-operatively identified a risk to one or both ureters i.e. re-operative surgery/cancer close to ureter or previously perforated sigmoid colon, it may well be prudent to use ureteric stents. On the other hand, we are aware of complications of ureteric stent insertion, such as transient haematuria, post-operative urinary tract infection and hydronephrosis. On occasions, this will add to theatre time. In the future, we speculate that recent improvements in technology, such as injection of dye, will routinely guide intraoperative navigation of vital retroperitoneal structures.

Modular Approach to HAR

There are six modules involved with the completion of HAR:

MODULE 1: Identification of the inferior mesenteric artery and securing it at its origin.
MODULE 2: Medial to lateral dissection.
MODULE 3: Dissection of the inferior mesenteric vein, mobilisation of the splenic flexure using a medial to lateral approach, and lateral dissection to complete the mobilisation.
MODULE 4: Dissection and preparation of the rectosigmoid junction and upper rectum for stapling.
MODULE 5: Delivery of the specimen and preparation of the left colon for anastomosis.
MODULE 6: Anastomosis of the colon and rectum.

MODULE 1: The Inferior Mesenteric Artery (IMA) pedicle is identified, along with the left colic artery. Our practice is to take the IMA at the origin. This can either be flush on the aorta (Fig. 7.2a), if the surgeon is confident not to cause aortic or nerve injury, or 1–2 cm distal to the aorta (Fig. 7.2b).

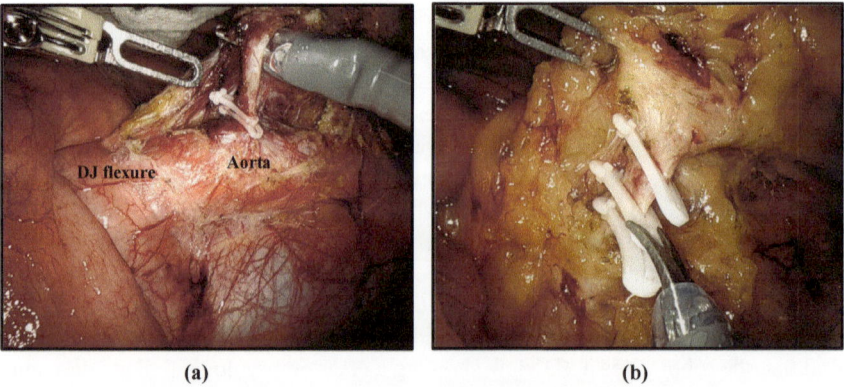

Fig. 7.2 a Taking the IMA flush to the aorta. **b** Taking the IMA 1–2 cm distal to the origin

This allows subsequent dissection of the Inferior Mesenteric Vein (IMV) in the medial to lateral direction. However, surgeons may decide to preserve the left colic artery and take the IMA more distally, known as high ligation. This can be a good strategy in situations of poor vascularity and, in oncological terms, this technique does not appear to impact surgical outcomes. Similarly, the position of the pathology may influence which vessel is taken, and where along its length. For example, if the pathology in question is just distal to the splenic flexure, the left colic (Fig. 7.3), and not the IMA, might be taken.

We use this approach for segmental colectomy. In confirmed benign pathology within the sigmoid or rectum, the IMA might be taken even higher (distal to left colic artery), or even preserved altogether (IMA-preserving HAR). Our practice is to apply three Hem-o-lok® clips (two placed proximally, and one placed distally) on vessels, so that two clips stay with stump of the divided vessel. With new and advanced bipolar energy devices, such as the da Vinci® SynchroSeal, vessels up

Fig. 7.3 IMA with left colic heading superiorly

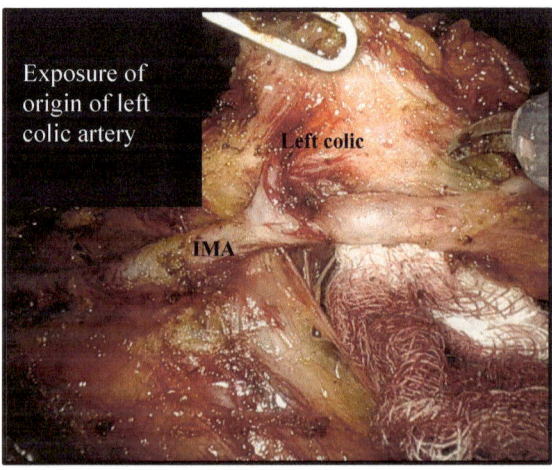

to 7 mm can be divided without clipping. Nevertheless, it is our practice to apply clips for any named major vessel. Sometimes, due to retroperitoneal inflammation or difficult dissection of the IMA, finding the correct planes can be challenging. In these situations, the surgeon may choose to dissect the IMV first and join the planes towards the IMA. Indeed, some surgeons prefer dissection of the IMV first, and it is a well described approach.

MODULE 2: Once the pedicle is secured, medial to lateral dissection is continued over Gerota's fascia, with the lateral limit being the abdominal side wall (Fig. 7.4). Immediately superolaterally to the IMA, the peritoneum is relatively thin. Due to the lack of haptics within robotic surgery, care must be taken not to enter breach the peritoneum and go out of plane. If this happens, it is best to go back to the IMA origin and dissect towards the IMV, or even to start at the pelvic brim within a clear plane.

This dissection usually finishes after complete mobilisation of sigmoid colon, descending colon and rectosigmoid junction. It is worth noting that, from time to time, surgeons may enter incorrect planes. This is often signified by bleeding and needs to be corrected quickly. In low BMI patients it is easy to dissect posterior to the retroperitoneal structures such as the ureters and gonadal vessels, and so care needs to be taken to avoid this.

MODULE 3: Careful dissection along the duodenojejunal flexure leads to IMV insertion into the splenic vein. The IMV is identified and taken with Hem o lok® clips, usually about 1 cm before its point of entry into the posterior pancreatic space, where it joins the splenic vein (Fig. 7.5).

In low BMI patients, care must be taken not to dissect the pancreas posteriorly, to avoid damage to retro-pancreatic structures. Once the IMV is divided, it is important to stay above the pancreas, extending the peritoneal incision towards the transverse mesocolon. In some patients, an accessory vessel traversing towards the left colic artery is encountered and may need to be divided to obtain tension free mobilisation

Fig. 7.4 Medial to lateral dissection—note the white line on the left between Gerota's fascia and the mesocolon

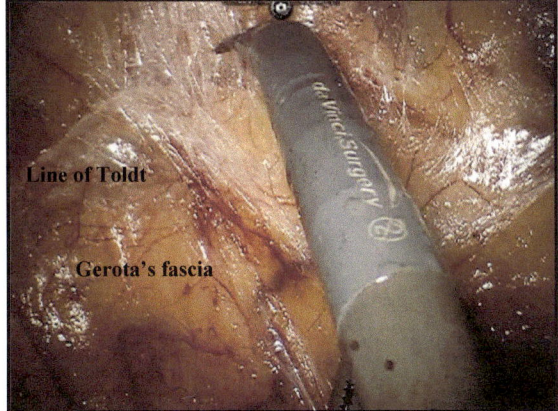

Fig. 7.5 Taking the IMV

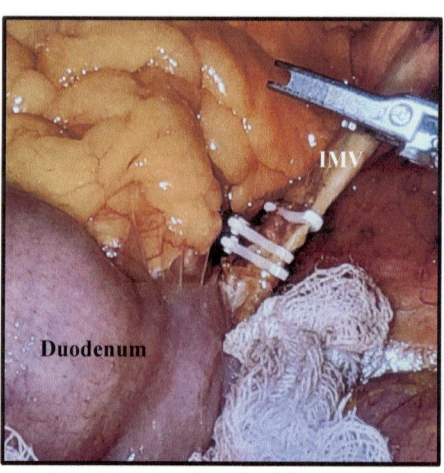

of the splenic flexure. Maintaining careful dissection above the pancreas, the lesser sac is then entered (Fig. 7.6). In our practice we often keep a swab placed over the pancreas at the time of dissection of the lesser sac. This allows easy identification of structures and helps us to avoid accidently entering an incorrect plane, which can lead to damage to the pancreatic tail. Usually there is a tough fascial layer between the pancreas and transverse mesocolon, known as the pancreatico-colonic fascia (Fig. 7.7). Detaching this will help in freeing up the transverse colon mesentery. The approach to this line of fusion is shown in Figs. 7.8 and 7.9.

The dissection then continues along the inferior margin of the pancreas and towards the lateral abdominal wall, joining up with the earlier dissection from over the top of Gerota's fascia.

Fig. 7.6 Entering and defining the lesser sac

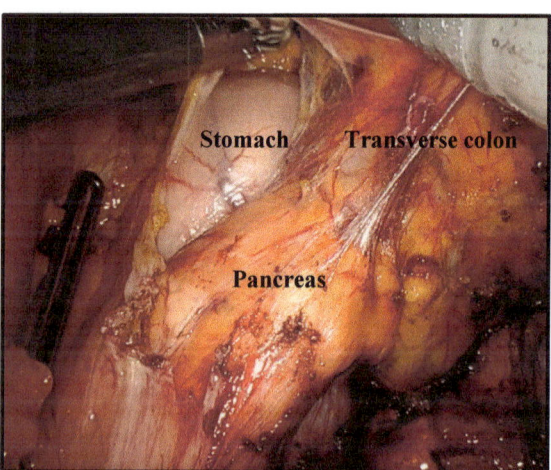

Fig. 7.7 Sagittal view of organs in relation to pancreatico-colonic fascia in the anatomical position

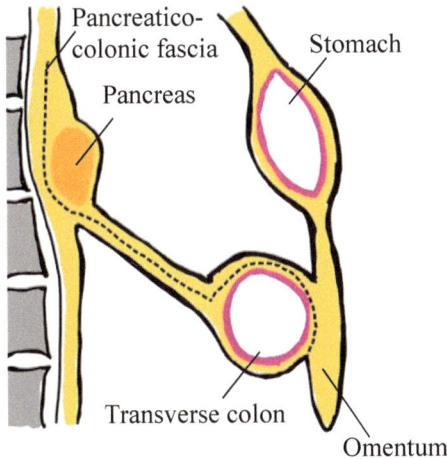

Fig. 7.8 Sagittal view of organs in relation to pancreatico-colonic fascia in the intra-operative position, with transverse colon retracted superiorly

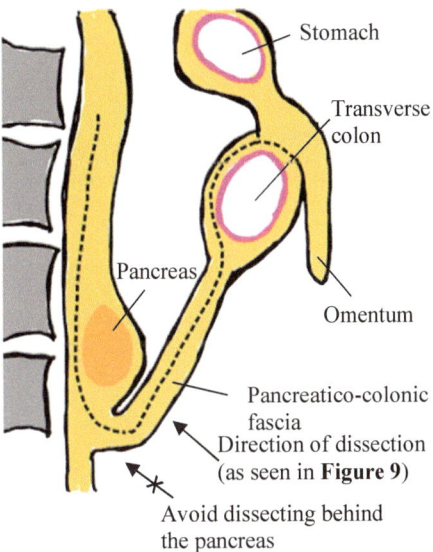

Lateral dissection of the descending colon is then performed (Fig. 7.10), with completion of splenic flexure mobilisation from the supracolic compartment down to the upper rectum, with care not to undermine Gerota's fascia, and to preserve both ureters and the hypogastric plexus. It is important to be aware of the varying nature, and number, of adhesions between the greater omentum and splenic flexure. Often, omental fat is plastered onto the transverse or descending colonic mesentery. Without due caution, marginal artery damage can occur. If this happens, extensive mobilisation of the transverse colon is required to gain an adequate length for the colonic conduit to achieve a tension-free anastomosis.

Fig. 7.9 Dividing the pancreatico-colonic fascia

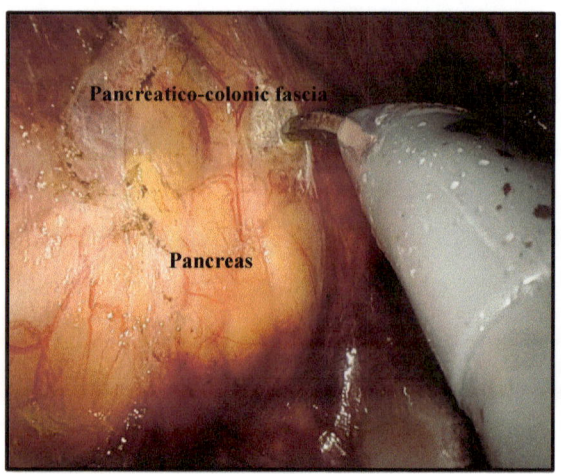

Fig. 7.10 Lateral dissection of descending colon

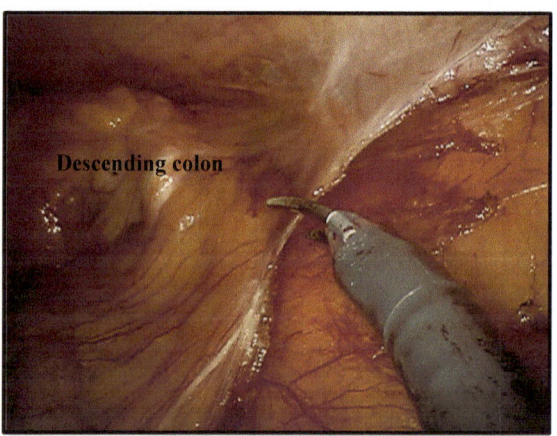

MODULE 4: Partial or Total Mesocolic Excision (TME) plane may need to be entered, depending on the position of the pathology and the resection margin required. After a 360° mobilisation of the rectosigmoid, the rectum is then thinned out. Usually, two to three vessels are encountered, which can vary in size. For the superior rectal artery, we prefer clip application, however, the vessel sealer would also be a suitable option to secure haemostasis. At this point, Indocyanine green (ICG) fluorescence can be used to check for good vascularisation of the rectum to achieve a well-perfused anastomosis (Fig. 7.11). The upper rectum is stapled off with a Sureform 60 mm stapler. This robotic stapler allows monitoring of tissue compression before and after firing, and it can make automatic adjustments to optimise the quality of the staple line. Additionally, it has 120° of articulation available, which allows for an easier staple, with less stress placed on the tissues (Fig. 7.12). We aim to staple off the rectum with one staple firing and, in our practice, we find that this is possible in

approximately 75 to 80% of cases. Occasionally, the uterus may need to be hitched up in female patients to gain a clear view of the rectum. The specimen is then extracted through the Pfannenstiel or umbilical Alexis port site.

MODULE 5: The large bowel mesentery is prepared along the IMA, and a purse-string applicator, with a double-ended Prolene stitch, applied above the pathology whilst ensuring that there is good oncological clearance. In our practice, we look for evidence of good bleeding from the marginal artery to ensure adequate vascularity to the anastomosis. A fresh scalpel is then used to excise the specimen, and a powered CDH circular cutting stapler anvil (usually of size 29 mm, however, a 25 mm or a 33 mm can be used if the bowel is particularly small or large respectively) is introduced into the cut end of the of the descending colon. Both needles are then cut off and the Prolene tied firmly around the anvil. Excess fat can be carefully stripped off at this point. The descending colon, with anvil inserted and secured, is then dropped back inside the abdominal cavity.

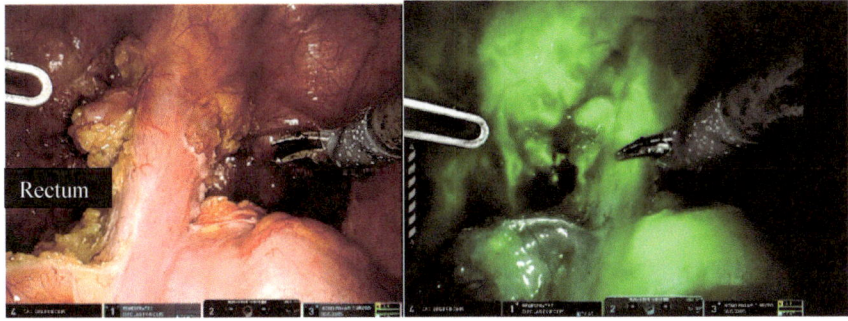

Fig. 7.11 ICG test to confirm the perfusion

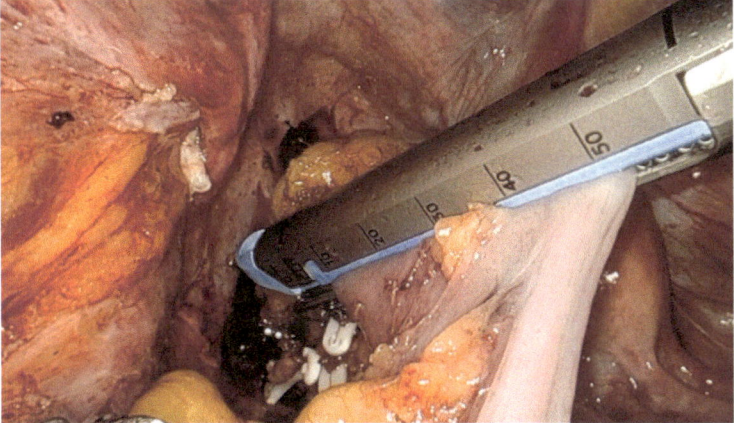

Fig. 7.12 Sureform stapler application to upper rectum

MODULE 6: We prefer to perform an end-to-side anastomosis between the end of the descending colon and the side of the rectum, taking great care to confirm an untwisted orientation of the colon. We find that an end-to-side approach helps to avoid cross stapling of the anastomosis. However, we appreciate there are other well-established techniques, including end-to-end anastomosis, with the spike of the gun pierced through the middle of the staple line, and end-to-corner anastomosis. Additionally, the robot allows straight forward robotic suturing to reinforce the anastomosis if there are any concerns about the integrity of the staple line. We use a powered CDH circular cutting stapler. However, non-powered staplers, or other appropriate brands, are equally valid depending on surgeon preference. We check the doughnuts for completion, but don't routinely send for histopathological analysis.

A leak test is then performed by filling the pelvis with water, compressing the descending colon, and insufflating the rectum via bladder syringe, rigid or flexible sigmoidoscopy. A recent meta-analysis found that this technique is associated with a reduced rate of postoperative anastomotic leak and staple line bleeding [3]. We routinely use rigid sigmoidoscopy, with flexible sigmoidoscopy on standby, to check the anastomotic staple line under direct vision. Flexible sigmoidoscopy gives superior views when there is concern regarding the integrity of the anastomosis, or a staple-line bleed. We tend to insert an abdominal drain and secure with a silk stitch. We appreciate that drain insertion in HAR is slightly contentious and may not be common practice in every colorectal department, however, we find that it helps to identify post-operative bleeding and allows drainage of residual wash fluid. The drain is placed in arm 3 port in the da Vinci X, and in arm 4 port in the Xi. The drain usually comes out in 1–2 days. Transversus abdominus plane (TAP) blocks are then placed under direct vision using a red needle and high volume 0.2% Ropivicaine which has a concentration of 2 mg/ml. The maximum safe dose is 3-4 mg/kg. Therefore, for a patient weighing 80 kg, we use 120-160 ml. The Pfannenstiel, or periumbilical, incision is closed using two loop PDS sutures. The skin is closed with 3/0 Monocryl and sealed with Liquiband glue.

Top Tips for Robotic Operative Success

- Careful skin marking and placement of ports ensure that internal and external clashing of the robotic instruments and arms is minimised, ensuring a more fluid procedure.
- Routine splenic flexure mobilisation helps to hone skills and allows a much easier procedural step when required.
- Look for marginal artery bleeding to ensure good blood supply to the anastomosis.
- Consider performing a Hartmann's Procedure in high risk patients, especially those requiring ongoing treatment i.e. chemotherapy.
- Defunctioning ileostomy is not routinely performed, however, if there are intra-operative complications or adverse patient factors (high BMI, smoker), this may be a a safer option.

- In polyp cancers, ensure identification of the tattoo so that the resection specimen contains the pathology in question.
- Use rigid/flexible sigmoidoscopy to visualise the anastomosis.
- It is vitally important to have an accurate understanding of the tumour location. This requires careful review of the pre-operative CT scan and colonoscopy. Information needs to be assimilated, amalgamated, and digested. This is especially important in cases of cancer reported to be within the proximal sigmoid colon. If the pathology is found to be more proximal, for example, in the descending colon, a change of strategy may need to be adopted to ensure adequate length for a tension free anastomosis, and segmental colectomy may need to be considered instead.

Acknowledgements   Many thanks to Farhan Shaikh for his construction of the operative diagrams. Some diagrams taken from: https://pixabay.com/images/id-1685810/

References

1. de'Angelis N, et al. Robotic surgery in emergency setting: 2021 WSES position paper. World J Emerg Surg. 2022; **17**(1):4.
2. Holzgang M, et al. Economizing on a 12 mm port incision site: modification of robotic bowel stapling technique in Da Vinci X/Xi left colonic resections-the modified Norfolk and Norwich robotic stapling technique. J Robot Surg. 2022.
3. Aly M, et al. Does intra-operative flexible endoscopy reduce anastomotic complications following left-sided colonic resections? A systematic review and meta-analysis. Colorectal Dis. 2019;21(12):1354–63.

Chapter 8
Rectal Surgery: Low Anterior Resection

Patricio Bernardo Lynn and Julio Garcia-Aguilar

Abstract Robotic surgery is the preferred minimally invasive approach for rectal cancer at Memorial Sloan Kettering Cancer Center. In this chapter, we describe our proposed technique for low anterior resection in a step-by-step fashion.

Keywords Rectal cancer · Surgery · Robotic surgery · Surgical technique

Introduction

Treatment of rectal cancer involves a multidisciplinary approach, including surgery, chemotherapy, and radiotherapy. The surgical management of rectal cancer can be technically challenging because of the anatomic constraints of the pelvis and the surrounding critical structures [1].

The advent of laparoscopy provided surgeons with a new tool to better operate in the pelvis, with better visualization and easy maneuverability. However, laparoscopy has limitations, including a limited range of motion and two-dimensional imaging.

Robotic surgery emerged to facilitate and overcome the limitations of conventional laparoscopic surgery and has become the preferred Minimally Invasive (MI) approach at Memorial Sloan Kettering Cancer Center for rectal procedures.

The technique we describe is the one we use for cancer patients and follows the principles of Total Mesorectal Excision, with sharp dissection between the embryological planes and central vascular ligation of the pedicles. The robot's enhanced visualization and precise Endo-wrist movements allow a safe and appropriate mesocolic excision and dissection.

We use the Da Vinci XI system with a dual operative console, enabling an integrated teaching and supervising environment without compromising operative and patient outcomes.

P. B. Lynn
Surgery Department, NYU Langone Health, NY New York, USA

J. Garcia-Aguilar (✉)
Colorectal Surgery Service, Memorial Sloan-Kettering Cancer Center, NY New York, USA
e-mail: garciaaj@mskcc.org

71

Patient Position

The patient is placed in a modified lithotomy position with both arms secured alongside the body and padded at pressure points to prevent injuries. Both lower extremities are placed in stirrups adequately padded. The Knees should be flexed at 45° and positioned in line with the contralateral shoulder. A foam mattress is placed directly under the patient, who is secured to the table at the chest level using a strap. These measures are enough to prevent the sliding of the patient during the procedure.

For this operation, we use a dual docking approach with the robotic platform on the patient's left side. During the first docking, the vascular pedicles are centrally ligated, the splenic flexure is taken down, and the left/sigmoid colon is fully mobilized. The second docking is targeted to the pelvis and is when Total Mesorectal Excision and pelvic dissection are performed.

Equipment

- 30° scope.
- Monopolar scissors.
- Fenestrated Bipolar grasper.
- Vessel Sealer.
- Prograsp forceps.
- Laparoscopic Suction/irrigation device.
- Air/Seal trocar.
- Laparoscopic fenestrated grasper.
- Robotic linear stapler (60 mm green load).

Port Placement and Docking

Trocar placement is described in Fig. 8.1. As previously said, we use a dual docking technique with the robotic platform on the patient's left side. During the first docking, targeting is performed to the left flank, the vascular pedicles are centrally ligated, the splenic flexure is taken down, and the left/sigmoid colon is fully mobilized (Fig. 8.2). The second docking is targeted to the pelvis and is when Total Mesorectal Excision and pelvic dissection are performed (Fig. 8.3).

In patients with no previous abdominal surgeries, we prefer to start the pneumoperitoneum with a Verres Needle in the left upper quadrant (2 cm from the costal margin in the mid-clavicular line). In the case of previous laparotomies, when the technique mentioned above might not be safe, a cut-down in the supraumbilical area or wherever the abdomen is scar-free is attempted. The 8 mm robotic trocar used for

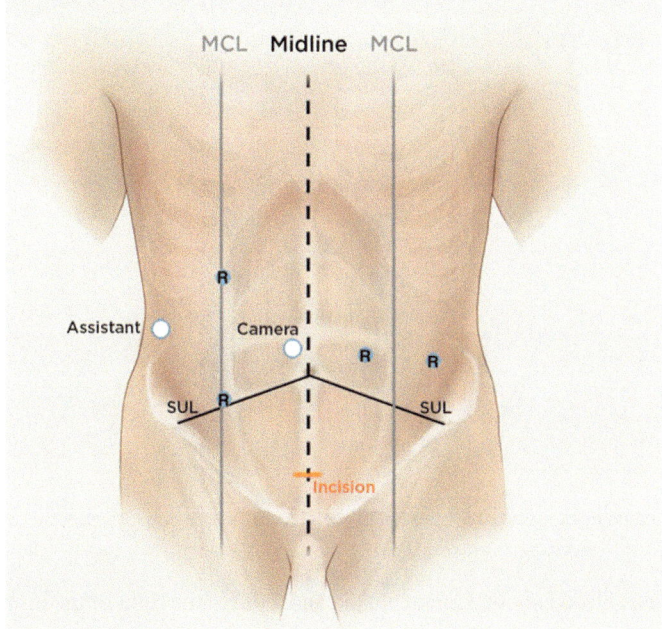

Fig. 8.1 Trocar positioning

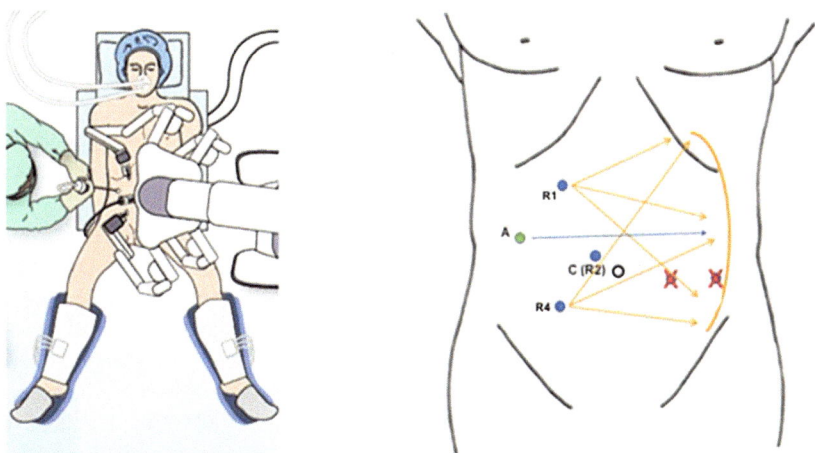

Fig. 8.2 First docking and ports used for the first part of the operation. A = assistant trocar, C = Camera, R = robotic arm

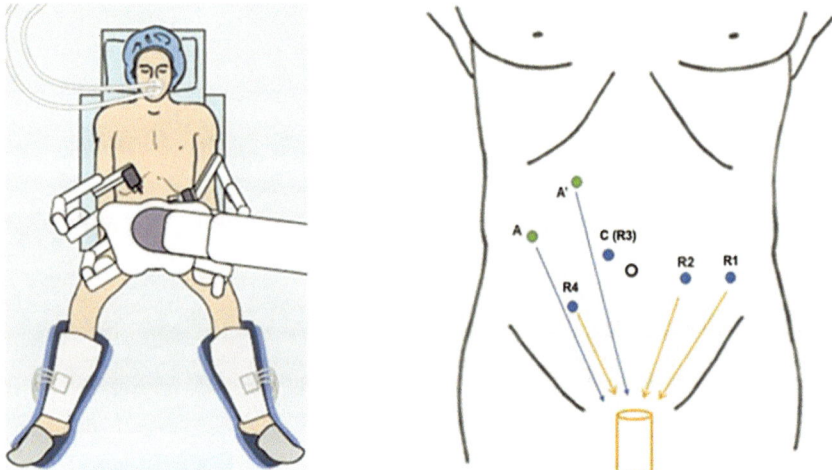

Fig. 8.3 Second docking (used for total mesorectal excision and pelvic dissection)

the camera is placed about 3 cm cephalad and 2 cm to the right of the umbilicus; this facilitates pedicle visualization. During the pelvic dissection, the camera will remain in this position.

An 8 mm robotic trocar is placed in the right upper quadrant in the mid-clavicular line 3 cm below the costal margin; this will be used for robotic arm #1 with a fenestrated/bipolar grasper for the left hand during the first docking. For the pelvic dissection, this trocar becomes an additional auxiliary port through which the bedside assistant can introduce a grasper or suction. A 12 mm trocar is placed in the mid-clavicular line in the right lower quadrant, a little below the umbilicus. This is used for robotic arm #4 holding the monopolar scissors for dissection in both docking times and the robotic stapler once the rectum is fully mobilized.

Another two 8 mm robotic trocars are placed in the LLQ in a horizontal line about 2–3 cm below the level of the camera port, one hand apart from the camera and each other. These will be used only during the pelvic time of the operation; the medial one is used for robotic arm #2 holding the bipolar grasper, the lateral one will be used with robotic arm #1 with a Prograsp forceps and will be used for retraction/exposure. An accessory 6 mm Air Seal trocar is placed in the right flank around the anterior axillary line at the level of the trocar used for the camera; the bedside assistant will use this for suction and eventual retraction.

Operative Technique

The pneumoperitoneum is established, the 8 mm camera port is placed, and an exploration of the abdominal cavity is undertaken to detect adhesions and assess resectability. The rest of the trocars are placed under direct vision.

Before robot docking, the patient is rotated right 20–30° and placed in Trende-lenburg position (30°). If present, adhesions are taken down. The greater omentum is retracted cephalad, exposing the transverse colon. Small bowel loops are placed in the right-upper quadrant exposing the left/sigmoid colon with its mesocolon, the first jejunal loop, and the inferior mesenteric vein (IVM).

Robot docking is then performed, targeting a point between the IVM and inferior mesenteric artery (IMA), and the robotic arms are connected to the trocars.

We prefer a medial to lateral approach for splenic flexure take-down and left colon mobilization. Dissection starts below the IVM in the plane between the mesocolon and the Gerota's fascia (Fig. 8.4). Following this plane laterally and then inferiorly, the IMA will be encountered.

Dissection of the IMA is facilitated by incising the peritoneum at the base of the sigmoid mesocolon above the right iliac artery and below the arch of the superior rectal vessels. The left ureter and gonadal vessels are identified and protected during this step. After performing this, the mesocolon is lifted and stretched; the IMA will be within the remaining attachments of the mesocolon to the retroperitoneum (Fig. 8.5). The vessel is dissected with monopolar scissors and sectioned 2 cm from its origin with the vessel sealer device. Lymph nodes in the origin of the vessel should be dissected and included with the specimen.

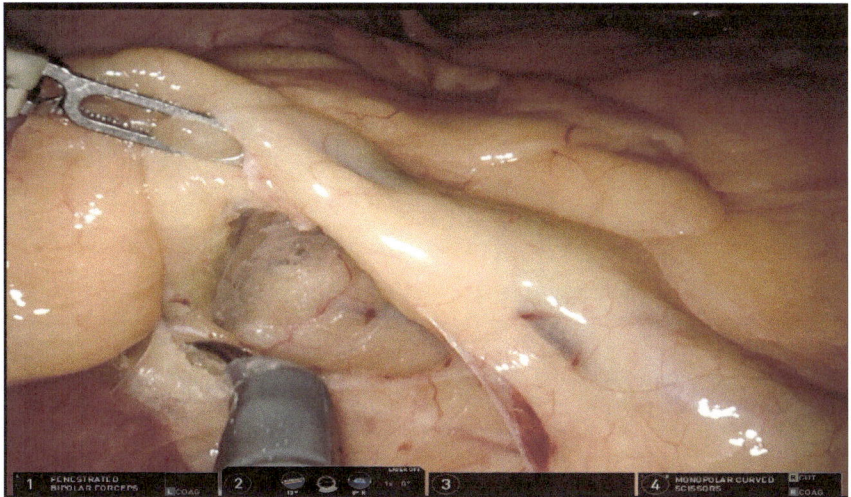

Fig. 8.4 Identification of the dissection plane below the Inferior Mesenteric Vein

(a)

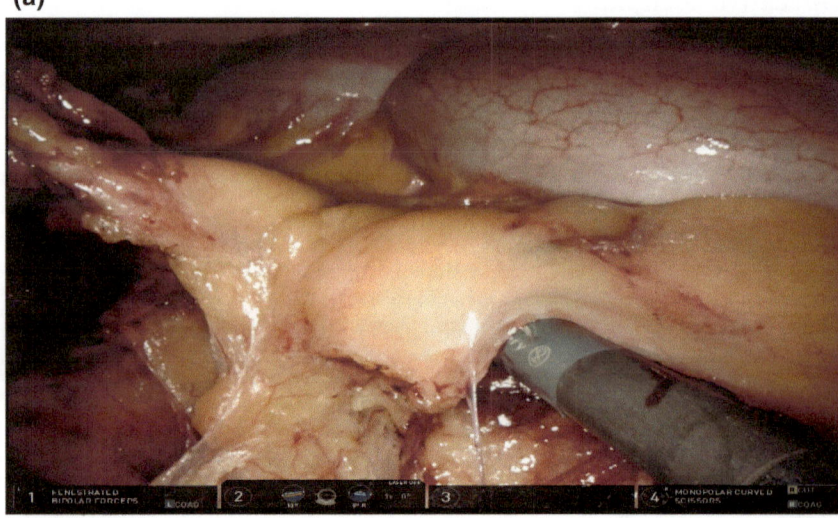

(b)

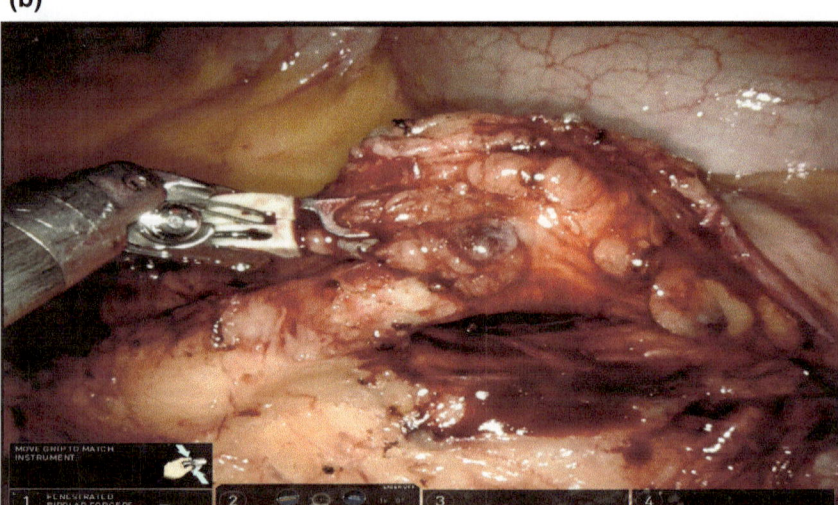

Fig. 8.5 Exposure and dissection of Inferior Mesenteric artery (**a** and **b**)

The mesocolon is mobilized laterally and cephalad until the inferior border of the pancreas is found (Fig. 8.6). At this point, the IVM is transected with the vessel sealer device.

For splenic flexure mobilization, we prefer an infra-mesocolic medial to lateral approach [2]. This dissection is carried over the pancreas from medial to lateral with the monopolar scissors, and the lesser sac is accessed at this point (Fig. 8.7).

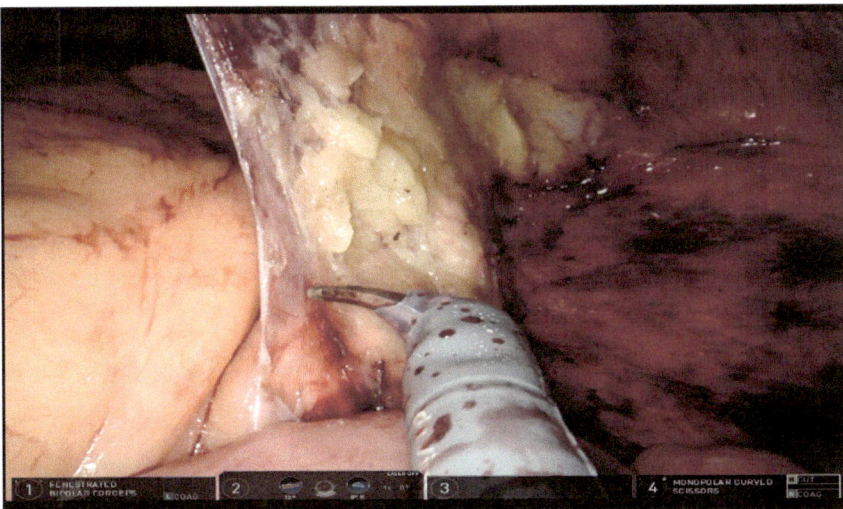

Fig. 8.6 Identification of the inferior border of the pancreas

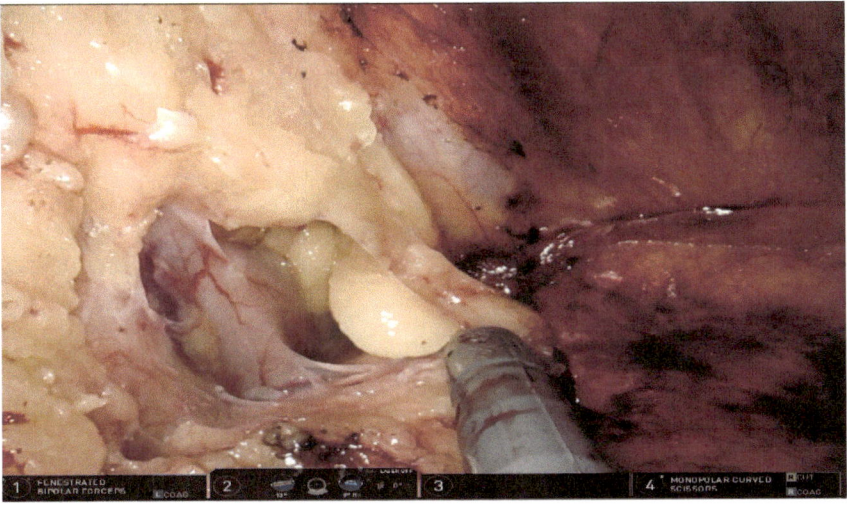

Fig. 8.7 Access to the lesser sac above the pancreas and below the mesocolon, infra-mesocolic medial approach for splenic flexure mobilization.

Following the anterior surface of the pancreas, toward its tail and the hilum of the spleen, the splenocolic ligament is transected from medial to lateral. The left side of the transverse mesocolon is completely mobilized. Lateral attachments of the ascending colon to the abdominal wall are taken down from caudal to cranial and left to right.

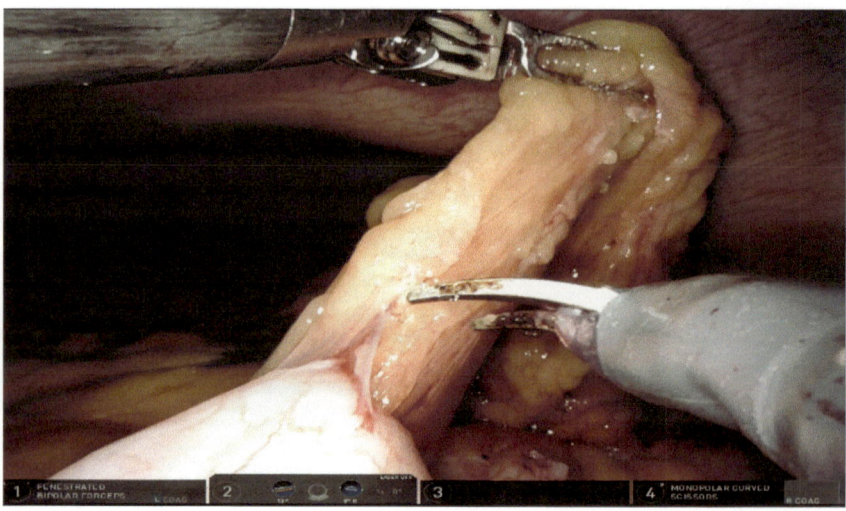

Fig. 8.8 Omentum dissection from the transverse colon

Next, the omentum is completely detached from the left transverse colon, in this case from lateral to medial (this can generally be performed with the monopolar scissors, Fig. 8.8). Once the splenic flexure is taken down, medial attachments of the colon to the stomach are released, and the avascular part of the mesocolon close to the Treitz is partially transected; these maneuvers elongate the mesocolon facilitating its reach into the pelvis.

At this point, the attention is placed on the rectal dissection. The robot is undocked, the patient is leveled and repositioned on a 25° Trendelenburg. The robot is re-docked, and targeting is performed aiming at the pubic symphysis. The camera is placed in arm #3, arm #2 is moved to the medial left flank trocar, and a fenestrated bipolar grasper is placed through it. Arm #1 will be used with a fenestrated grasper, and arm #4 keeps the monopolar scissors. Of note, the right upper quadrant robotic trocar can be used as a second assistant port by the bedside assistant (Fig. 8.3).

The upper rectum is grabbed with arm #1 grasper and pulled anteriorly to the abdominal wall; arm #2 is used for traction and counter-traction.

Rectal dissection starts at the right, opening the lateral pelvic peritoneum; for this step, the bedside assistant can stretch the peritoneum providing adequate tension for correct plane identification (Fig. 8.9).

Immediately after this, dissection continues posteriorly following the areolar tissue that separates the mesorectum from the pelvic fascia (Fig. 8.10). This dissection between the pelvic and mesorectal fascias follows a series of principles; adequate traction with the left hand (exposing the areolar tissue and avoiding grasping the mesorectum, which might result in bleeding); sharp dissection with monopolar scissors close to the rectum (the correct plane is generally closer to the rectum than what it seems at first sight) and gentle pushes from time to time to expose the right plane.

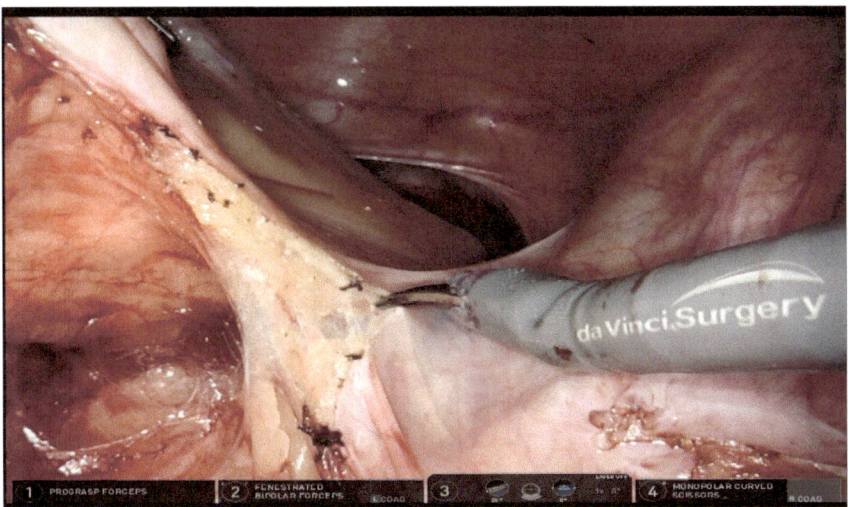

Fig. 8.9 Access to the Mesorectal plane, "the Holy plane of Rectal Surgery"

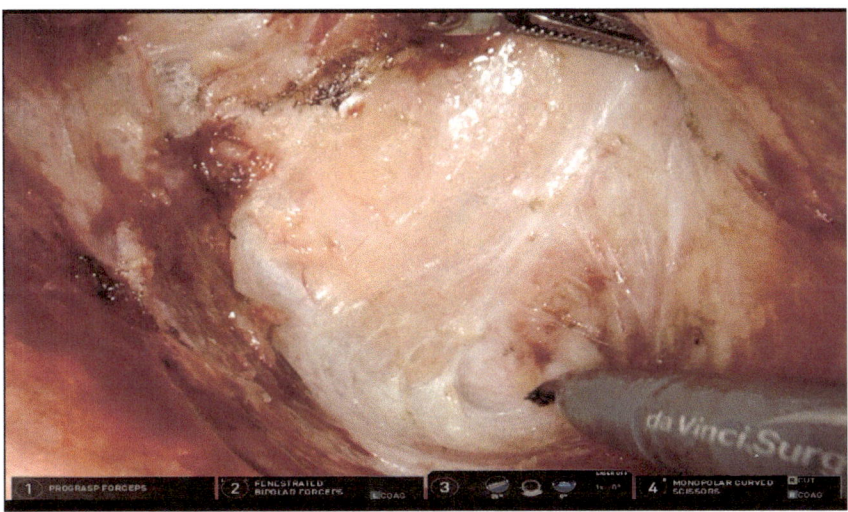

Fig. 8.10 Posterior mesorectal dissection

The dissection progresses deep into the pelvis up to the coxys; this plane is used as a reference to guide lateral dissections on the right and left (Fig. 8.11).

Traction and counter-traction are again critical to expose the plane and avoid nerve injuries. The anterior dissection starts a few millimeters above the peritoneal reflection, following the avascular plane, posterior to the Denonviliers fascia (Fig. 8.12). Robotic arm #1 is used to retract the seminal vesicles/prostate or cervix/vagina anteriorly.

To facilitate distal rectal dissection and rectal transaction, a previously cut to 10 cm vaginal packing sponge, is introduced and tied around the distal rectum (rectal hanging maneuver, Fig. 8.13). Dissection is carried on until the levator muscles are encountered (Fig. 8.14).

The distal transection point is confirmed with an intraoperative flexible sigmoidoscopy, ensuring a safe distal margin. The 60 mm robotic stapler is introduced through the 12 mm port used for arm #4. The rectum is transected vertically from anterior to posterior; in this case, two loads were needed to transect the rectum (Fig. 8.15) completely.

The mesocolon of the descending colon is transected intracorporeally with the vessel sealer device, starting proximally to the transected IMA aiming to the distal descending colon.

The vaginal tape around the rectum is grasped with laparoscopic forceps, and a Pfanestiel incision is then performed. The specimen is extracted through the incision covered with a wound protector device, and the descending colon is transected at the level of the mesocolon's dissection performed intracorporeally. The specimen is then passed to an auxiliary table.

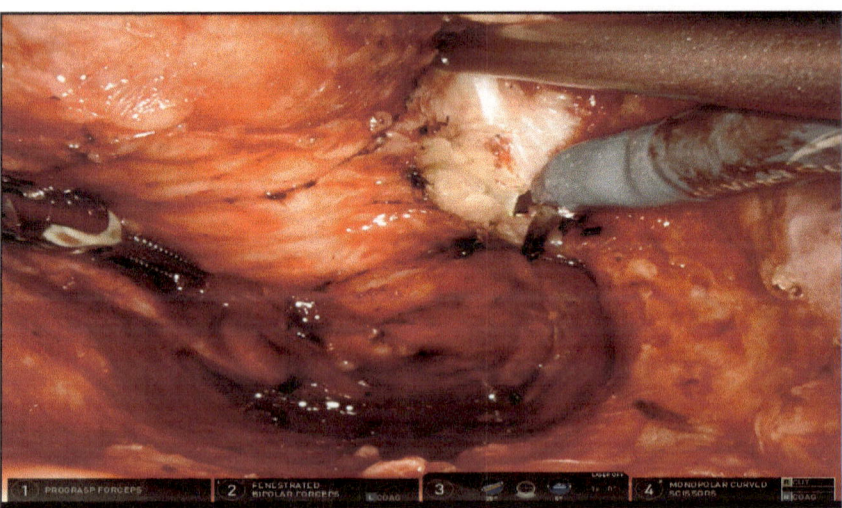

Fig. 8.11 Lateral Mesorectal dissection

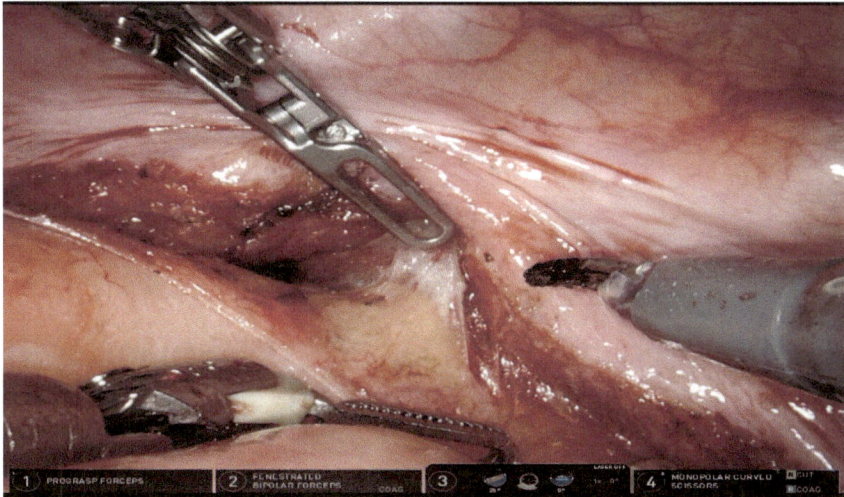

Fig. 8.12 Anterior Mesorectal dissection, Denonviliers fascia being grasped with robotic arm #4

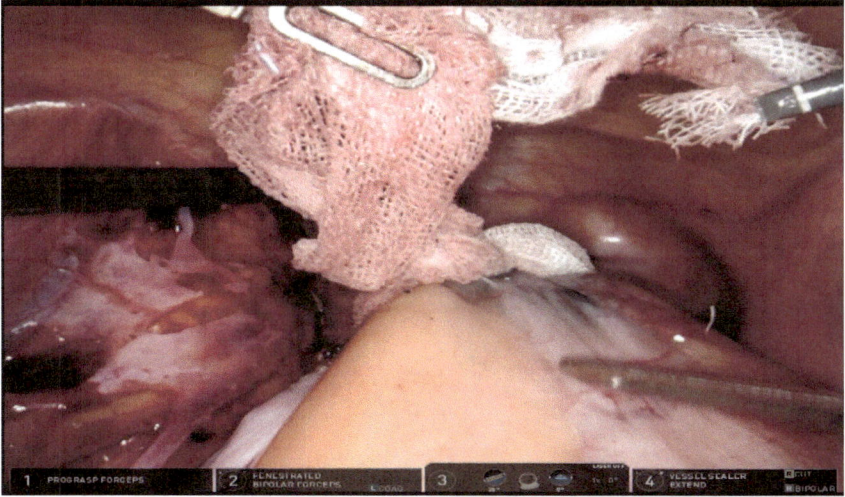

Fig. 8.13 Rectal "hanging maneuver" with vaginal tape to facilitate the low pelvic dissection

The Anvil of the circular stapler is secured to the descending colon with a 2–0 prolene purse-string suture; it is our preference to perform an end-to-end, coloanal-low colorectal anastomosis. The colon is reintroduced into the cavity, and the pneumoperitoneum re-insufflated.

The robot is re-docked, and an end-to-end stapled anastomosis is then performed under robotic assistance, checking that the descending colon is not twisted. Adequate blood flow to the descending colon is checked with indocyanine green using the

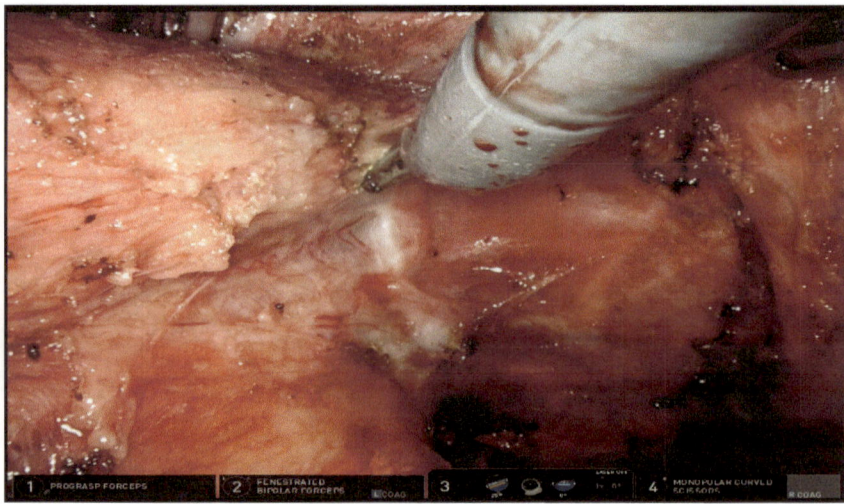

Fig. 8.14 Levator ani muscles exposed

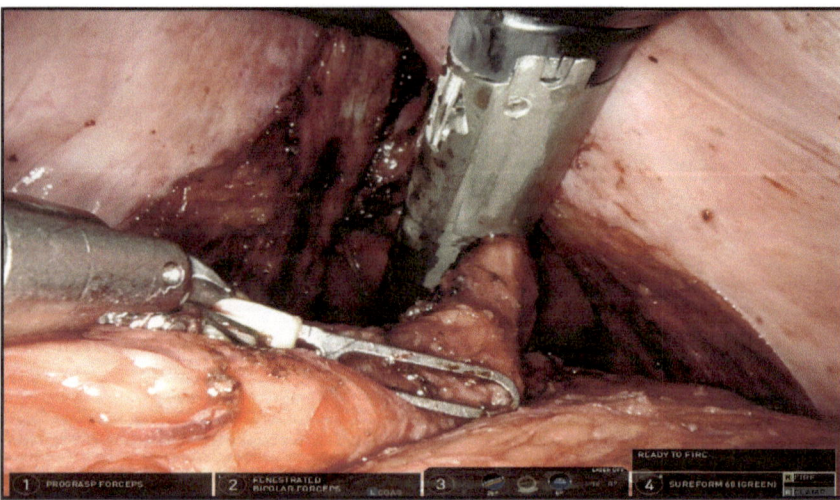

Fig. 8.15 Vertical rectal transaction from anterior to posterior

firefly mode (Fig. 8.16). Indemnity of the anastomosis is controlled with flexible sigmoidoscopy, performed with the pelvis filled with saline to check for air leaks.

A 19 Fr Blake drain is placed posteriorly to the anastomosis and extracted through a trocar in the left flank.

The 12 mm trocar site is closed under direct vision with a suture passer Thomason-Carter device.

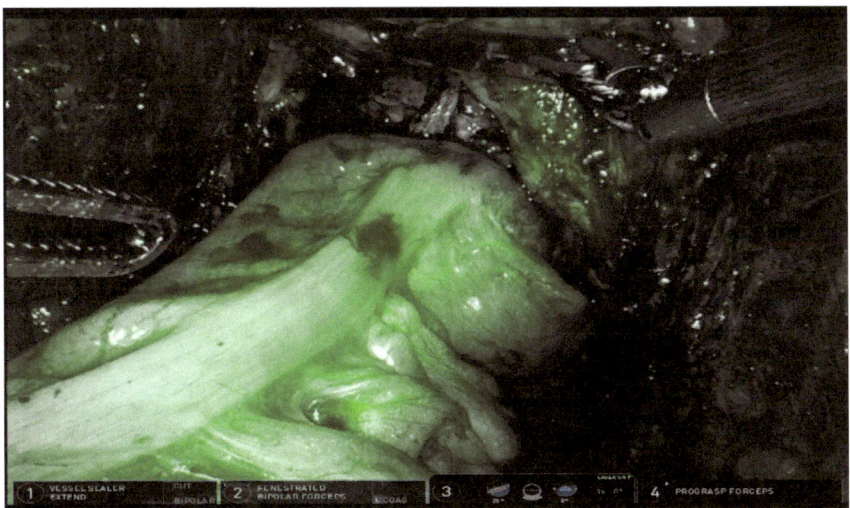

Fig. 8.16 Intraoperative evaluation of blood flow with indocyanine green

A diverting loop ileostomy is then constructed in the RLQ in a site previously marked by the stoma nurse; occasionally, the 12 mm trocar site can be used for this purpose.

The Pfannenstiel incision and the trocar sites are closed in the usual fashion.

Five Top Tips

- Positioning is Key. The patient should be appropriately secured to the table to avoid sliding, do not be shy with left tilt and Trendelenburg; consider gravity as an extra hand.
- Most of the dissection can be successfully achieved with the monopolar scissors on the right working arm. Become comfortable with it to minimize instrument exchange and be more efficient.
- We prefer the infra-mesocolic medial approach for splenic flexure mobilization. Access to the lesser sac is gained right on top of the inferior border of the pancreas without opening the transverse mesocolon.
- The "rectal hanging maneuver" facilitates the distal rectal dissection.
- Intraoperative flexible sigmoidoscopy is especially helpful to determine distal resection margin and check for anastomotic integrity and leaks.

Checklist

- Propper patient positioning.
- Exploratory laparoscopy and trocar placement.
- First docking targeting IMA/IVM.
- Pedicle Control, IMA/IVM high ligation.
- Medial to lateral Ascending/sigmoid Mesocolon dissection.
- Infra-mesocolic medial approach for splenic flexure mobilization.
- Total Mesorectal excision starting in the posterior aspect of the mesorectum.
- Lateral dissection following the plane obtained in the posterior dissection.
- Anterior dissection posterior to the Denonvillier's Fascia.
- Rectal Hanging Maneuver for distal rectal mobilization up to the levator ani muscles.
- Distal margin check with intraoperative endoscopy.
- Distal rectal transaction with a robotic linear stapler.
- Specimen extraction through Pfannenstiel incision.
- End-to-end stapled colorectal anastomosis.
- Indocyanine green test to check anastomosis perfusion.
- Intraoperative endoscopy to check for anastomosis integrity and leaks.
- Diverting loop ileostomy.

References

1. Rectal cancer. NCCN guidelines version 22021. 202;1–166.
2. Garcia-Granero A, Romaguera VP, Millan M, Pellino G, Fletcher-Sanfeliu D, Frasson M. A video guide of five access methods to the splenic flexure: the concept of the splenic flexure box. Surg Endosc. Springer US; 2020;34(6):2763–72.

Chapter 9
Robotic Low Anterior Resection Using Da Vinci Xi System

Seon Hahn Kim and Ju Yong Cheong

Abstract The Da Vinci Xi system™ (Intuitive Surgical, Sunnyvale) provides an excellent platform to perform low and ultralow anterior resection. In this chapter, we discuss ergonomic challenges in trying to operate on both the splenic flexure/rectum using the traditional port placement and we discuss the method to minimize robotic arm clashes. A step by step description of the ultralow anterior resection using the Xi system is presented.

Keywords Robotic rectal surgery · Low anterior resection · Ultralow anterior resection · Port placement · Ergonomics

Introduction

The robotic rectal surgery has been proposed as an improvement on the laparoscopic approach, with better three-dimensional visualization, seven degrees of motion (as opposed to 4°), the fluidity of motion allowing precise dissection, minimizing the tremor transmission, and ability to control four robotic arms [1]. In a comparison of the robotic versus laparoscopic approach, the ROLARR trial has shown no difference in conversion rate, circumferential resection margin (CRM) involvement, complication rate, and survival [2, 3]. However, in a large propensity-matched study, robotic surgery was found to be a good prognostic factor for overall survival and cancer-specific survival [4]. In this chapter, we discuss how to perform low anterior resection using the Da Vinci Xi System™ (Intuitive Surgical, Sunnyvale).

S. H. Kim (✉) · J. Y. Cheong
Division of Colon and Rectal Surgery, Department of Surgery, Korea University College of Medicine, Seoul, Republic of Korea (South Korea)
e-mail: drkimsh@korea.ac.kr

J. Y. Cheong
e-mail: Juyong.cheong@gmail.com

85

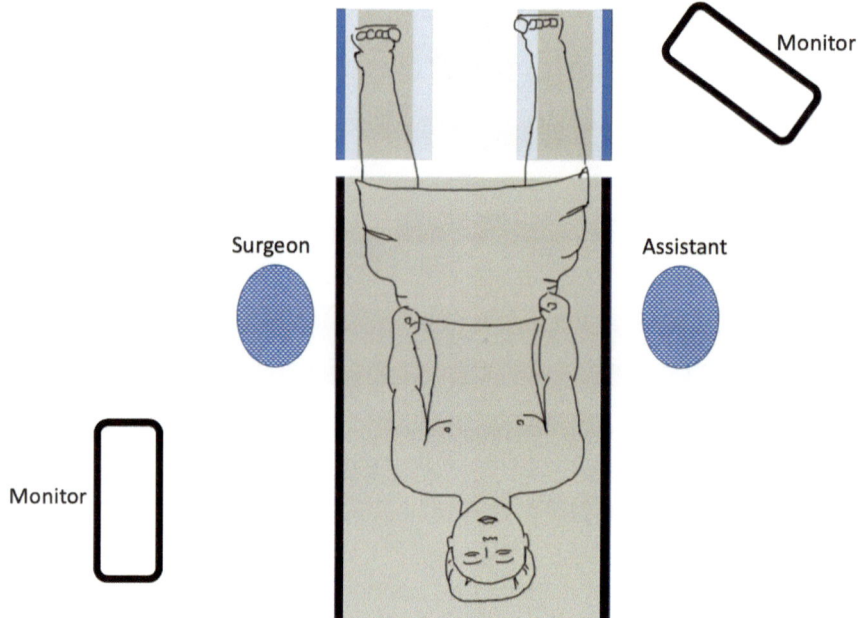

Fig. 9.1 Operating theatre setup

Positioning of the Patient and the Theatre Layout

The patient is placed in a lithotomy position with both arms by the side. The surgeon stands on the patient's left side and the assistant on the patient's right. There must be two separates monitors, with one on each side to allow both surgeon and assistant to see the insertion of ports (Fig. 9.1).

After all the ports are inserted, the robot approaches from the patient's left side (Fig. 9.2). The assistant stays on the patient's right side. The assistant must be able to see both monitors.

Placement of the Ports

The conventional principle of performing rectal cancer surgery using the Da Vinci Xi system™ (Intuitive Surgical, Sunnyvale) involves placing the four robotic ports in a linear line from the left upper quadrant to the right iliac fossa (Fig. 9.3a). The ports are placed at least 7–8 cm apart to prevent robotic arms from clashing. However, when the splenic flexure needs to be mobilized (for low rectal cancer), the ports are aligned more vertically (Fig. 9.3b). The dilemma with such port placement is that when pelvic dissection needs to be performed, the two left ports (arm1, arm2) are too

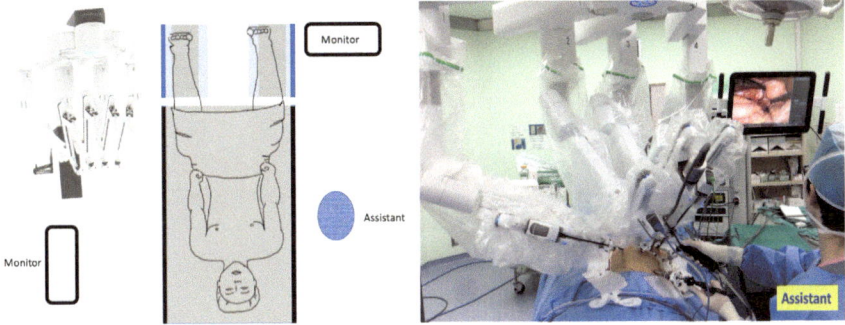

Fig. 9.2 The robot approaches from the patient's left, and the assistant stays on the patient's right side

close together cephalon-caudally, leading to clashing. Moreover, the right dissecting monopolar scissors arm (arm4) becomes too inferior and medial, hindering efficient pelvic TME dissection. Thus, colorectal surgeons are often left with the choice of aligning the robotic arms for splenic flexure or rectal dissection, with some surgeons opting for the first setup and taking down the splenic flexure laparoscopically.

At Korea University Anam Hospital, we have developed a novel six-port, double targeting, arm repositioning technique, which allows ergonomic access to both the

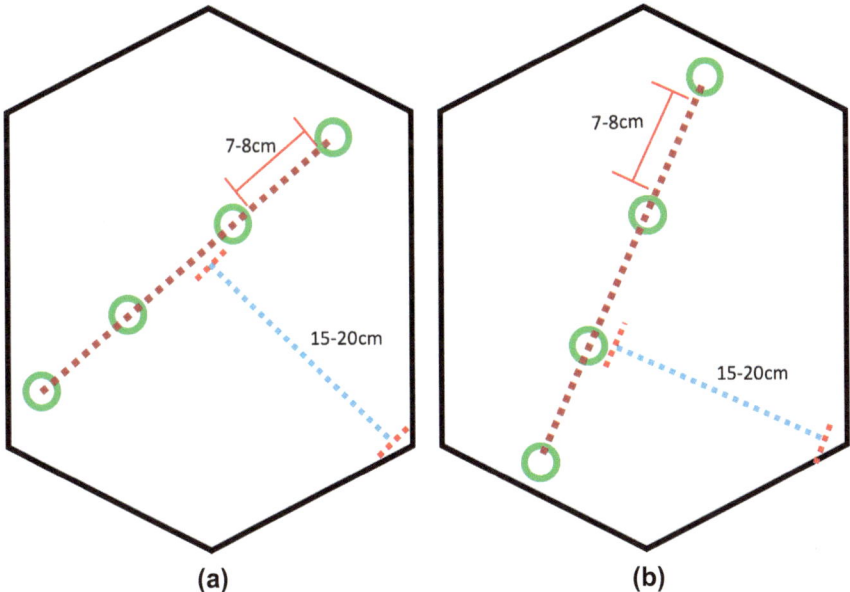

Fig. 9.3 a Traditional methods of port placement for robotic high/low anterior resection, **b** angulating the ports more vertically to allow for taking down the splenic flexure

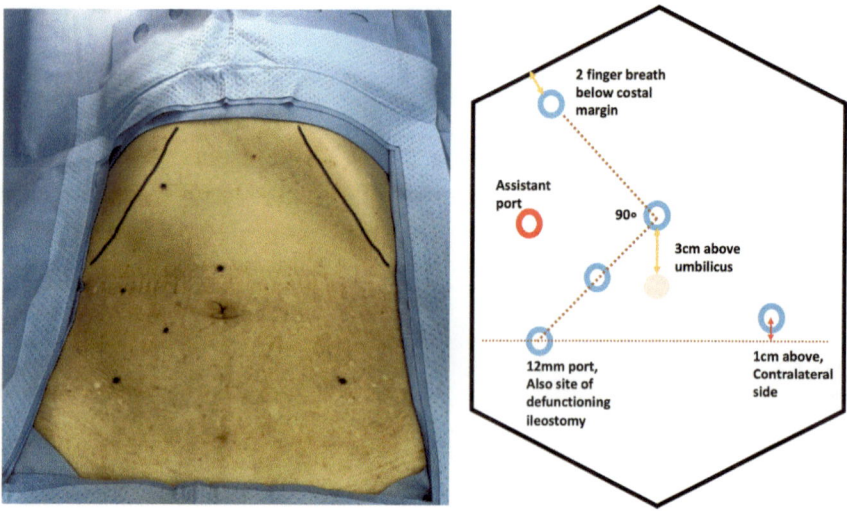

Fig. 9.4 Six port, double targeting technique for robotic low anterior resection

splenic flexure and the pelvis, allowing the entire operation to be performed robotically (Fig. 9.4). The first robotic port (8 mm) port is placed 3 cm cephalad from the
umbilicus. The second port (12 mm) is placed in the right iliac fossa, and through
this port, a defunctioning loop ileostomy can be created later. The third robotic port
(8 mm) is placed halfway in between. The fourth port (8 mm) is placed in the right
upper quadrant, two fingerbreadths below the costal margin, and is aligned at a right
angle to the two right quadrant ports. The fifth port (8 mm) is placed in the left iliac
fossa and is placed approximately 1 cm vertically above the right iliac fossa port. A
final 5 mm assistant port is placed on the right flank through which a grasper or a
suction device is inserted.

We recommend a 'two left-hand' approach with the camera placed into port 3
(Fig. 9.5). For colonic dissection, the camera is targeted to the mid-descending colon.
The right four robotic ports are utilized with Cadiere forceps (port 2) used to retract
the colon, the Maryland forceps (port 1), and monopolar scissors (port 4) used for
dissection. For pelvic dissection, the camera is retargeted to the mid pelvis. The
inferior four ports are used, with Cadiere forceps (port 1) used to retract the rectum,
Maryland forceps (port 2), and monopolar scissors (port 4) used for total mesocolic
dissection.

In our experience, with the current setup, the ports can be placed as close as 4 cm
without clashing. Depending on the body habitus (BMI), a slight variation in the six-
port technique can be made (Fig. 9.6). The right upper quadrant port can be placed
closer to the midline (especially in tall thin patients with narrow costal angles), with
the angle between the supraumbilical port and right iliac fossa port increased up to
110°. The supraumbilical port can be placed closer to the umbilicus (or sometimes
through the umbilicus). If this is the case, the right paraumbilical port (arm3) must
be placed more inferiorly also.

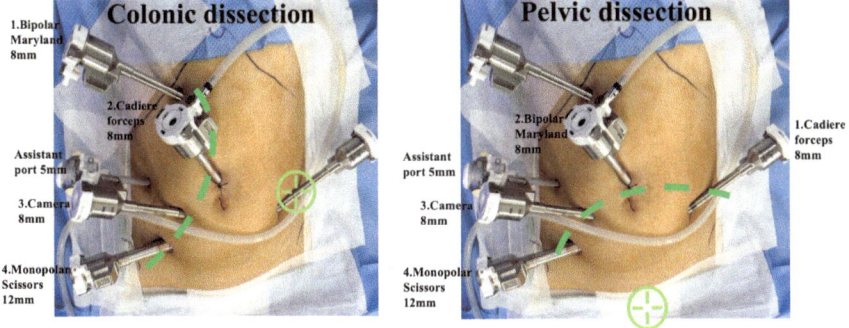

Fig. 9.5 Ports utilized for colonic and pelvic dissection. The green target indicates where the camera should be targeted

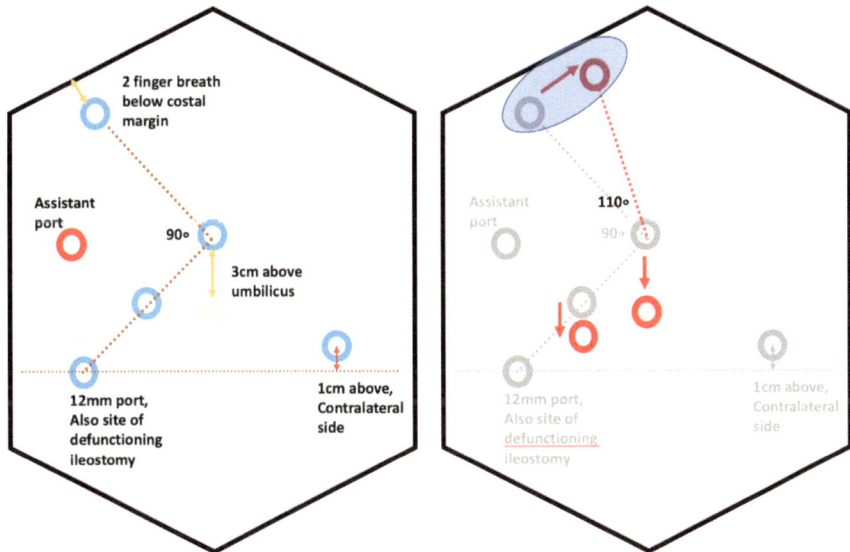

Fig. 9.6 Variation to the port placements

Moreover, using the inferior four ports has distinct advantage when an exenteration surgery needs to be performed. For the operation on the bladder, prostate, vagina, and the uterus, the four ports placed inferiorly is a familiar port layout for urologist and gynaecologist. This is also the case when lateral pelvic lymph node dissection needs to be performed.

As there are six ports in total, four are utilized by the robot, and the assistant can use the two remaining ports to aid the operation (Fig. 9.7).

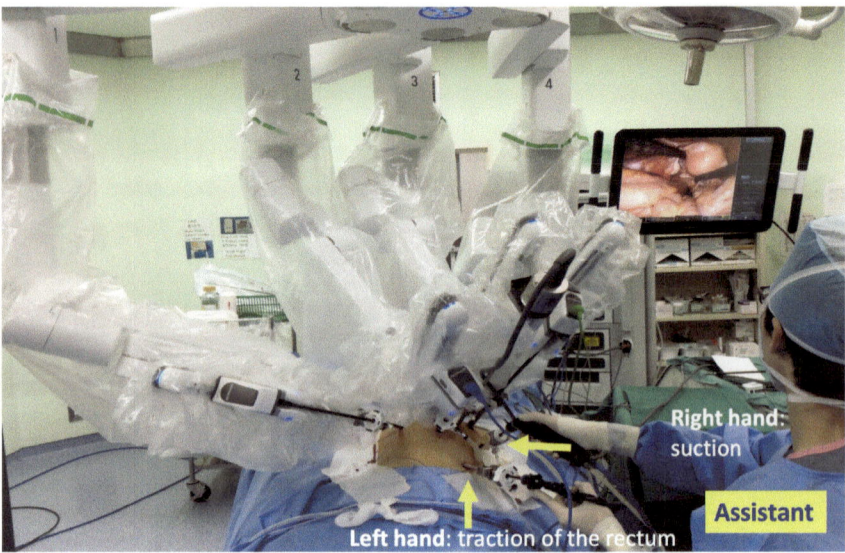

Fig. 9.7 Assistant utilizing two ports to assist with pelvic dissection

Equipment Needed

Da Vinci Xi system equipment:

1. Maryland forceps with bipolar diathermy
2. Cadiere forceps
3. Scissors with monopolar diathermy
4. Hem-o-lock™ (Weck Closure Systems, NC) using Da Vinci Xi system™ EndowristClip appliers (Intuitive Surgical, Sunnyvale)
5. Vessel sealer™ for Da Vinci Xi system™ (Intuitive Surgical, Sunnyvale)
6. Robotic stapler (Endowrist Stapler 45™, Intuitive Surgical Sunnyvale)

Wound protectors systems:

1. Alexis wound protector™ (Applied Medical, California) OR
2. Uni-port system™ (Daelim Medical, Korea).

Step by Step on Performing Robotic Low Anterior Resection

1. Time out is performed, and an indwelling catheter is placed. A dose of intravenous antibiotics is given.
2. The patient is placed in a lithotomy position. The patient is secured to avoid sliding during the operation. At our institution, we utilize a locally manufactured surgical bean bag suction positioner.

3. The patient is prepped and draped. The patient is prepped from xiphisternum to pubic symphysis. Costal margins are marked, and the port sites are marked (Fig. 9.8).
4. The right iliac fossa port is inserted first. A cut down is performed, and a 12 mm robotic port is inserted. This port will be utilized at a later stage for specimen extraction as well as forming a defunctioning ileostomy. Pneumoperitoneum is established, and other ports are inserted under vision. All the other robotic ports are 8 mm ports, and the assistant port is a 5 mm port.
5. The patient is placed head down at 30°, tilted with the right side down.
6. The robot is docked from the patient's left side (Fig. 9.9).
7. The camera port is connected to arm 3 of the robot. Targeting is performed with the camera pointing towards the left flank/mid descending colon (Fig. 9.10). The robot will adjust the other arms.
8. Other robot arms are docked to the ports (Fig. 9.11).
9. We utilize a '2 left hand' technique. For the robot's first arm, bipolar Maryland forceps are connected. For the robot's second arm, Cadiere forceps are connected. The robot's fourth arm is connected to monopolar scissors.
10. A medial to lateral approach is utilized. The Small bowel is medialised, and the duodenojejunal flexure is identified. The inferior mesenteric vein is identified (Fig. 9.12).
11. The inferior mesenteric vein is clipped with Hem-o-lock™ (Weck Closure Systems, NC) using Da Vinci Xi system™ EndowristClip appliers (Intuitive Surgical, Sunnyvale) and transected (Fig. 9.13).
12. The medial to lateral dissection is extended superiorly, over the anterior surface of the pancreas until the splenic flexure is visualized from Fig. 9.14.

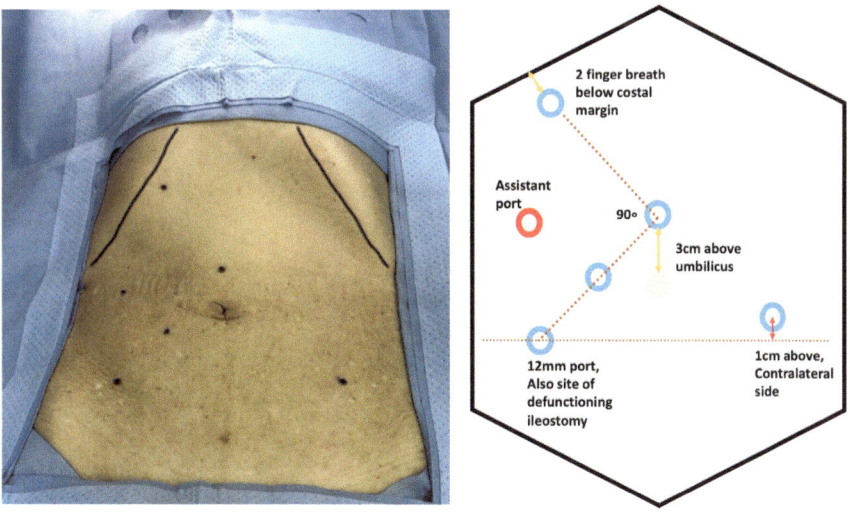

Fig. 9.8 Marking of port sites

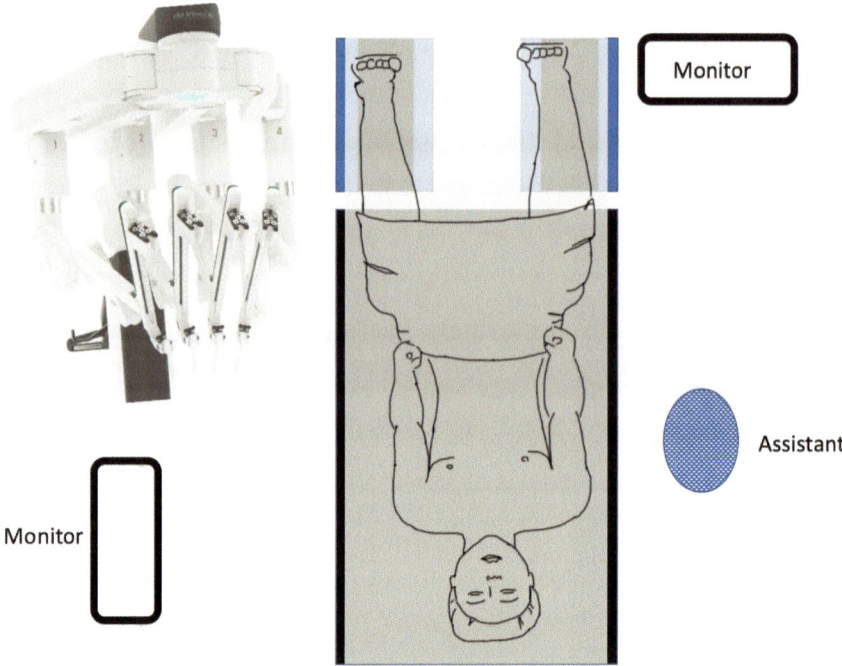

Fig. 9.9 Theatre setup

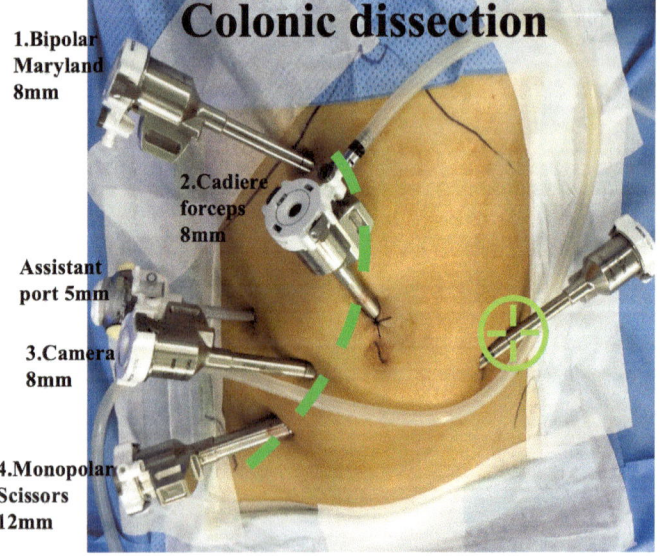

Fig. 9.10 Targeting the left flank

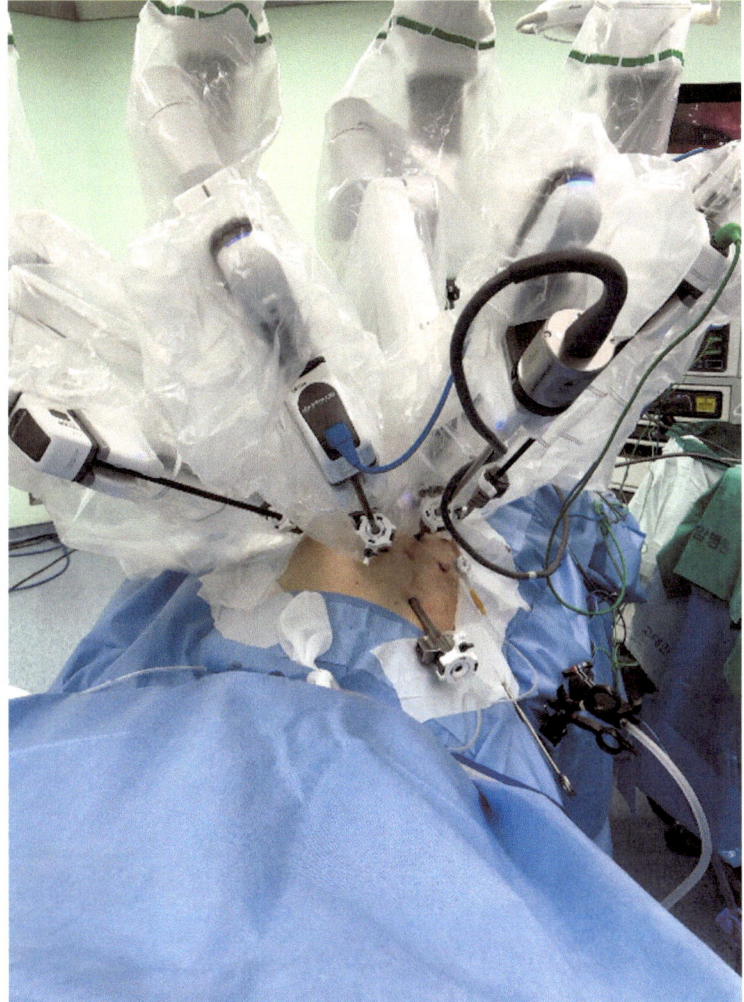

Fig. 9.11 Robotic arms docked

13. The medial to lateral dissection is extend inferiorly, and the inferior mesenteric artery is dissected (Fig. 9.15). Care is taken to avoid injury to the superior hypogastric plexus. The inferior mesenteric artery is clipped with Hem-o-lock™ (Weck Closure Systems, NC) using Da Vinci Xi system™ EndowristClip appliers (Intuitive Surgical, Sunnyvale) and transected.
14. The left gonadal artery and left ureter are identified (Fig. 9.16).
15. Medial dissection is extended laterally along descending colon and sigmoid colon (Fig. 9.17).
16. Laterally the sigmoid/descending colon is mobilized, and splenic flexure is brought down (Fig. 9.18).

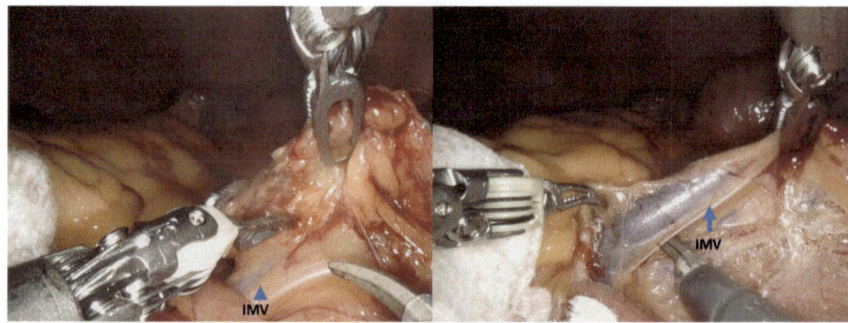

Fig. 9.12 IMV identified in paraduodenal fossa

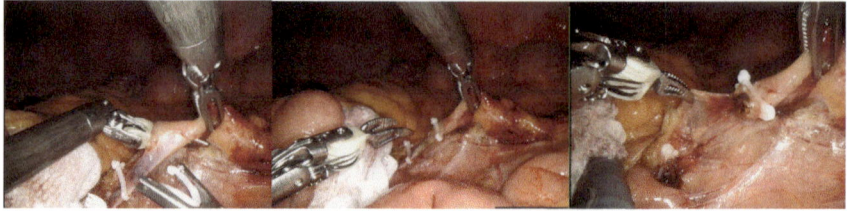

Fig. 9.13 IMV is transected

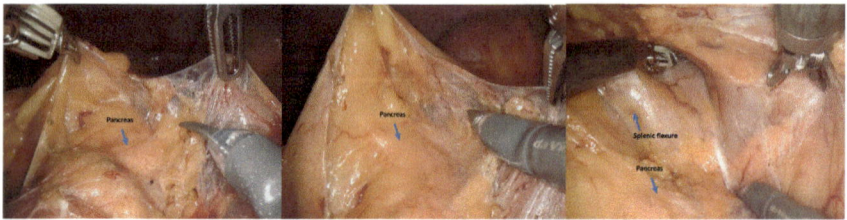

Fig. 9.14 Dissection over the pancreas

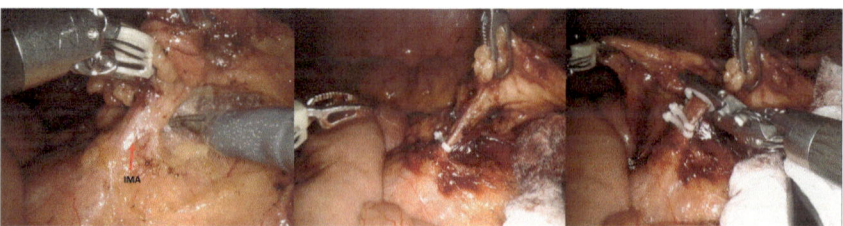

Fig. 9.15 IMA

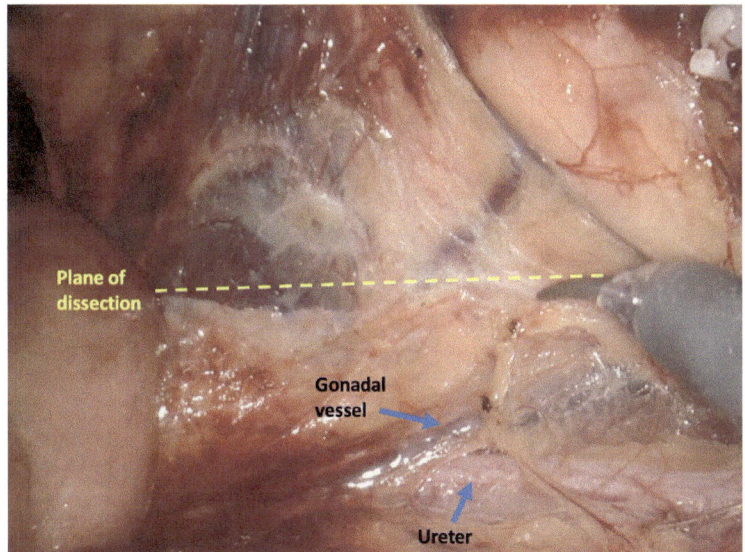

Fig. 9.16 Left gonadal artery, ureter

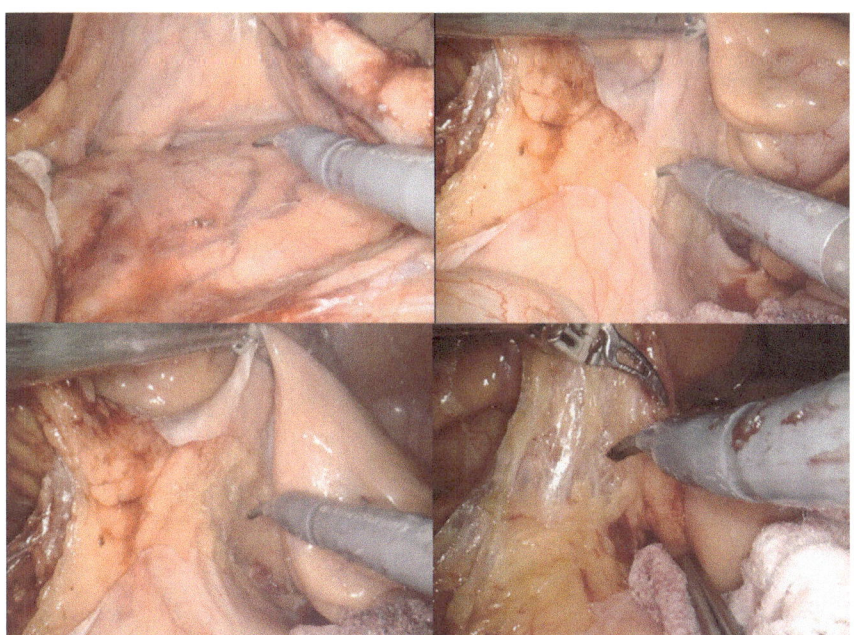

Fig. 9.17 Medial to lateral dissection

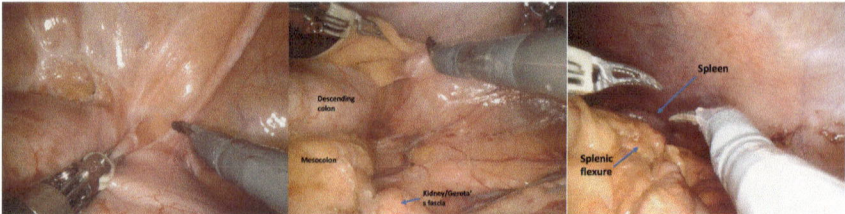

Fig. 9.18 Splenic flexure brought down

17. For the pelvic dissection, the camera is retargeted to the mid pelvis (Fig. 9.19). The inferior four ports are used, with Cadiere forceps (port 1) used to retract the rectum, Maryland forceps (port 2), and monopolar scissors (port 4) used for total mesocolic dissection. A nylon tape tied around the recto-sigmoid junction is often used to help pull the rectum out of the pelvis using the assistant's grasper.
18. The total mesocolic dissection is performed posteriorly (Fig. 9.20).
19. Then TME dissection is performed anteriorly, through the Denonvillier's fascia. The seminal vesicle is identified (Fig. 9.21).
20. TME dissection is finally performed laterally. The middle rectal artery is identified and divided (Fig. 9.22).

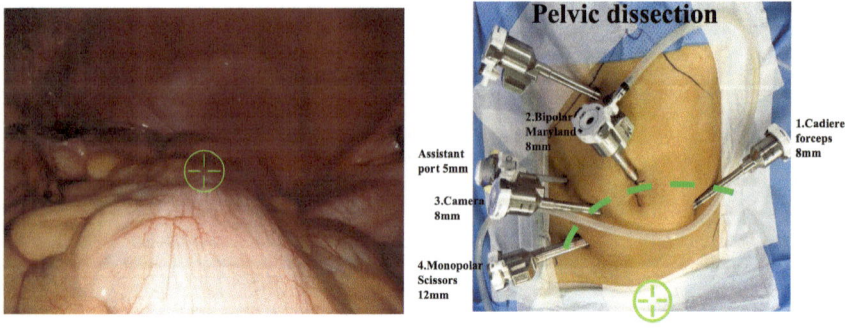

Fig. 9.19 Retargeting and redocking for pelvic dissection

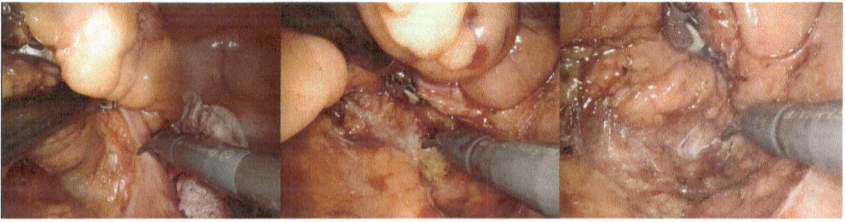

Fig. 9.20 Posterior TME dissection

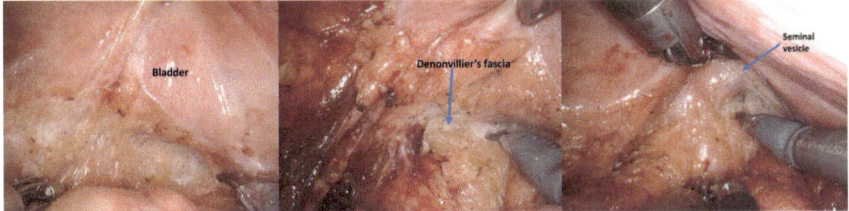

Fig. 9.21 Anterior dissection

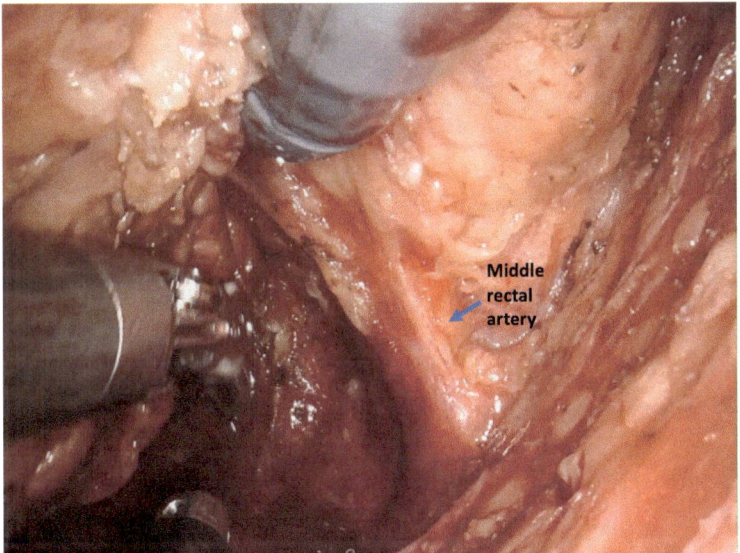

Fig. 9.22 Middle rectal artery

21. The dissection reaches down to the pelvic floor, and the puborectalis muscle is identified (Fig. 9.23).
22. The tumor is identified, and the point at which to divide the rectum below the tumor is identified. The mesorectum at this point is dissected, and the superior rectal artery is divided. We change the monopolar scissors to Vessel sealer™ for Da Vinci Xi system™ (Intuitive Surgical, Sunnyvale) for arm 4 (Fig. 9.24).
23. The 12 mm right iliac fossa port (arm 4) is used to insert a stapler (Endowrist Stapler 45™, Intuitive Surgical Sunnyvale) to transect the rectum below the tumor (Fig. 9.25).
24. The right iliac fossa 12 mm port is enlarged, and the specimen is delivered through a Uni-port system™ (Daelim Medical, Korea). The proximal end of the delivered colon is transected, the anvil of endocircular stapler inserted, and anastomosis is then formed.

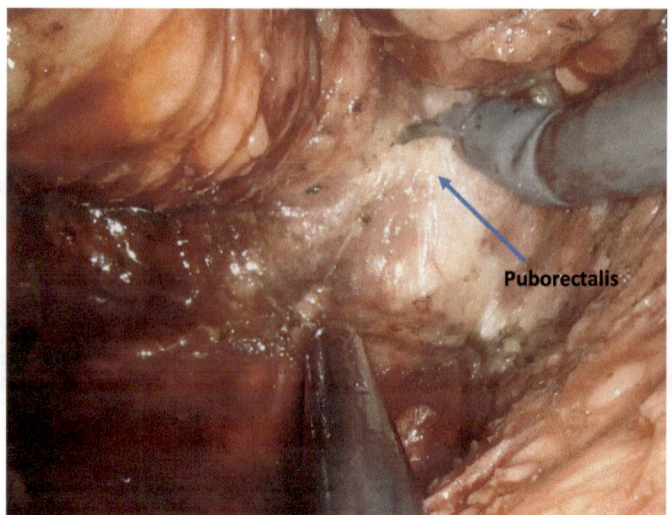

Fig. 9.23 Dissection down to the pelvic floor

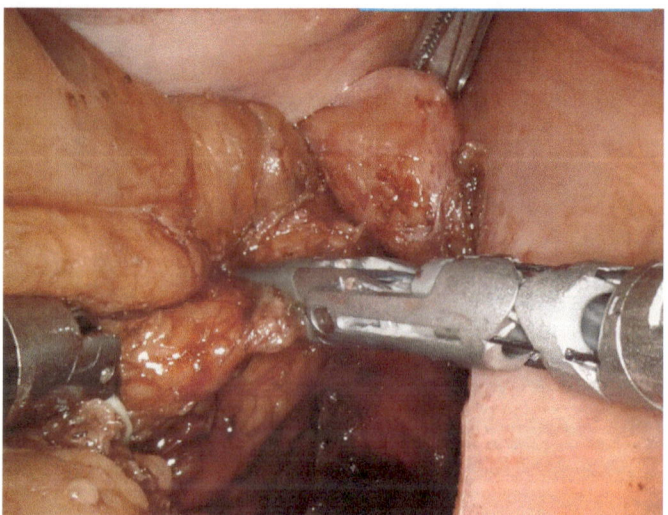

Fig. 9.24 Divide through the mesorectum

25. The lateral corners of the anastomosis are reinforced with interrupted sutures. A leak test is performed.
26. A defunctioning loop ileostomy is formed through the right iliac fossa port site.

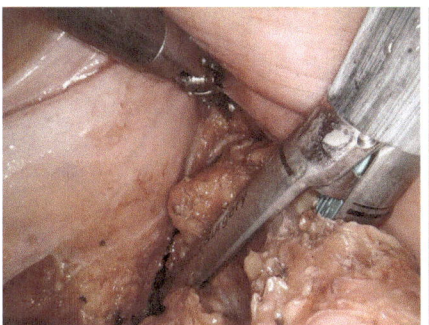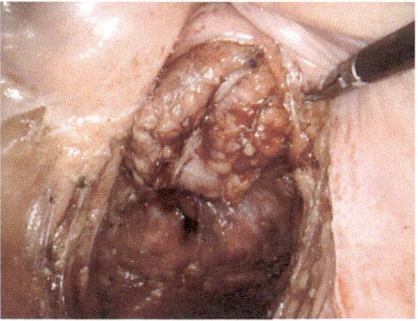

Fig. 9.25 Transecting the rectum

References

1. Baik S. Robotic colorectal surgery. Yonsei Med J. 2008;49(6):891–6.
2. Jayne D, Pigazzi A, Marshall H, Croft J, Corrigan N. Effect of robotic-assisted vs conventional laparoscopic surgery on risk of conversion to open laparotomy among patients undergoing resection for rectal cancer: the ROLARR randomized clinical trial. JAMA. 2017;318(16):1569–80.
3. Jayne D, Pigazzi A, Marshall H, Croft J, Corrigan N. Robotic-assisted surgery compared with laparoscopic resection surgery for rectal cancer: the ROLARR RCT. NIHR J Libr. 2019.
4. Kim J, Baek S, Kang D, Roh Y, Lee J, Kwak H, Kwak J, Kim S. Robotic resection is a good prognostic factor in rectal cancer compared with laparoscopic resection: long-term survival analysis using propensity score matching. Diseaes Colon Rectum. 2017;60(3):266–73.

Chapter 10
Robotic Abdomino-Perineal Excision of Rectum (APER)

Slawomir Marecik, Kunal Kochar, and John J. Park

Abstract Abdominoperineal resection (or excision; APR/APE) has always been considered a challenging procedure. The surgical robotic platform allows executing the previously difficult task in a much easier way. This chapter will explain how to perform a traditional mesorectal excision as part of APR and how to perform a novel technique of transabdominal levator transection. It will also discuss how the morbidity of the ELAPE technique can be minimized with robotic assistance and how some patients may benefit from selective (tailored) levator transection. In addition, a detail pelvic floor anatomy will be explained.

Keywords APR · APE · ELAPE · Abdominoperineal · Resection · Abdomino-perineal · Excision · Levator · Transection · Intraabdominal · Intra-abdominal · Rectal · Cancer · Pelvic · Floor · Anatomy · Adenocarcinoma · Carcinoma

Introduction

This chapter will discuss the technique of robotic abdominoperineal resection (APR, APER), also known as abdominoperineal excision (APE). Historically, APR has been considered a challenging procedure due to constraining anatomical conditions of the pelvis, unfamiliarity with deep pelvic anatomy, and frequently advanced tumor presentation. With its fatigue-less retraction ability, excellent visualization, stable exposure, and precise instrumentation, the robotic platform allows executing the previously difficult task in a much easier way.

S. Marecik (✉) · K. Kochar · J. J. Park
Advocate Lutheran General Hospital, Park Ridge, IL 60068, USA
e-mail: smarecik@uic.edu

J. J. Park
e-mail: jpark18@aol.com

The University of Illinois, Chicago, IL, USA

Several concepts will be presented in this chapter, including (1) robotic total mesorectal excision with conventional perineal resection, (2) the use of transabdominal levator transection to simplify the perineal dissection (including the extra levator concept), and (3) selective (tailored) levator transection for eccentrically located tumors.

Background

Historically, APR procedure has been associated with much worse oncological and functional outcomes when compared to sphincter-saving operations, regardless of the open or laparoscopic approach [1, 2]. Higher local recurrence rates and worse survival were closely related to higher perforation rates of the resected specimens and a higher rate of positive circumferential resection margins (CRM) [3].

In 2007, Holm and colleagues from Karolinska University, Sweden, published encouraging results on a new radical technique called extra levator abdominoperineal resection (ELAPR, ELAPE) [4]. This procedure expanded pelvic floor resection to involve the coccyx, coccygeus muscle, and lateral portion of the iliococcygeus muscles. Unfortunately, improved oncological results were later paralleled by worsened functional outcomes related to genito-urinary dysfunction and perineal wound healing [5–7]. One must remember that the ELAPE technique was born as a method of choice to remove the most advanced pathology, as Karolinska University is Sweden's quaternary institution, frequently addressing the recurrent and neglected disease. The degree of ELAPE technique application for less advanced tumors is still under question [8]. Its universal application is probably unnecessary if the surgeon understands the true extent of the disease, has deep knowledge of pelvic floor anatomy, and possesses good technical skills. In any case of APR, as in any case of rectal cancer resection, the surgeon's good pelvic MRI reading skills are crucial.

Robotic APR has been performed since the early years of the 2000s [9]. For many years, the extent of robotic dissection has not differed much from what was performed during ultra-low anterior resections (total mesorectal excision, TME). The subsequent improvements of the robotic platform (Xi version being the latest one) allowed for easier access to the deep pelvis with less collision of the instruments and arms. An important step forward in the progress of robotic APR was the technique of intraabdominal (transabdominal) levator transection (IALT) described by Marecik et al. [10]. This technique, which was made easier by the robotic assistance, was meant to simplify the perineal dissection, thus decreasing the rates of specimen perforation and positive CRM. In addition, the utilization of transabdominal levator transection frequently reduced the size of pelvic floor defects compared to the formal ELAPE technique (Fig. 10.1). Preservation of the coccyx and bilateral coccygeal muscles is almost universal in the IALT technique.

In contrast, the ELAPE technique frequently relies on their resection to gain complete and unobstructed access to pathology while maximizing the amount of CRM. Resection of the coccyx and coccygeal muscles, routinely performed in prone

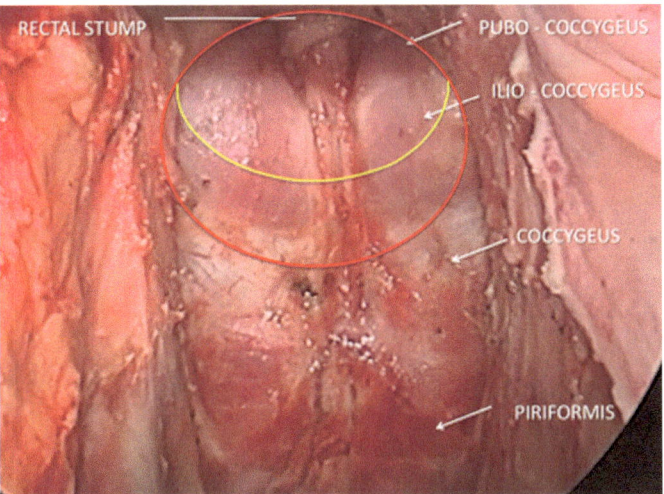

Fig. 10.1 Comparison of necessary levator resection during the formal ELAPE technique (red) and the robotic intra-abdominal levator transection (IALT) technique (yellow)

position during the ELAPE technique, increases not only the perineal defect but also endangers the structures of the lateral pelvic compartment (pelvic sidewall), especially in narrow pelvis. The injury of the pelvic plexus is of particular importance since it can lead to genito-urinary dysfunction [5–7] (Fig. 10.2). Avoiding radical pelvic floor resection associated with traditional ELAPE technique allowed us to evolve the IALT technique toward safe pelvic floor preservation in selected cases of eccentrically located tumors (tailored IALT APR) [11]. Apart from the levator defect, the skin and subcutaneous tissue defect in the IALT technique is frequently smaller when compared to the traditional ELAPE technique since deep and wide exposure during the perineal phase is unnecessary. In the authors' experience, smaller perineal defects associated with the robotic IALT technique can be frequently closed primarily without a need for mesh or flap reconstruction [10, 11]. Omental pedicle flaps remain a good option in selected patients.

Anatomy of the Deep Pelvis and Pelvic Floor

Surgeons performing APR procedures must understand how to safely navigate through the distal part of the pelvis while trying to preserve an appropriately wide circumferential resection margin around the tumor. The concept of total mesorectal excision must be modified during the APR procedure to prevent medial dissection toward the anorectal junction [8]. A certain amount of mesorectum near the tumor should not get detached from the levators, and the resected specimen should contain

Fig. 10.2 Pelvic plexus, right side, partially dissected mesorectum, visible sacral splanchnic nerves

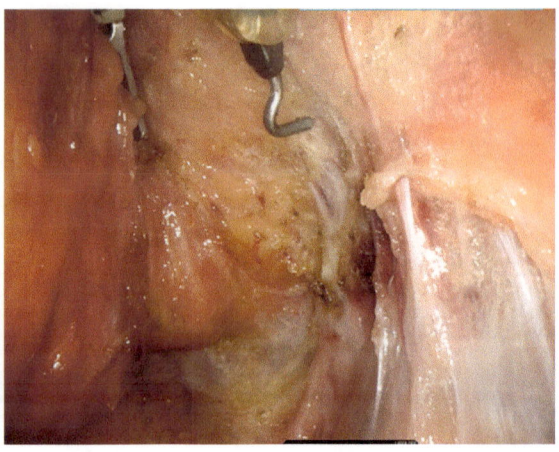

the corresponding levator segment [12] (Fig. 10.3). Levator resection can be accomplished during the perineal phase (traditional technique) or as presented in this chapter during the abdominal phase (robotic IALT technique).

During the distal part of the rectal dissection, while performing APR, the crucial question is when to stop the abdominal dissection and start the perineal phase? Or in the case of robotic IALT technique where exactly start the levator transection. Specific anatomical landmarks mentioned below will be helpful to guide the dissection.

1. During presacral dissection, a point of upward sacral deflection usually corresponds with the S-5 segment (Fig. 10.4). The deflection can be confirmed individually by an MRI analysis of the sagittal plane. The surgeon should also evaluate the length of the coccyx and the distance between the tip of the coccyx and the anus on MRI and digital exam.

Fig. 10.3 Levators still attached to the mesorectum (robotic IALT technique, coccyx was not removed)

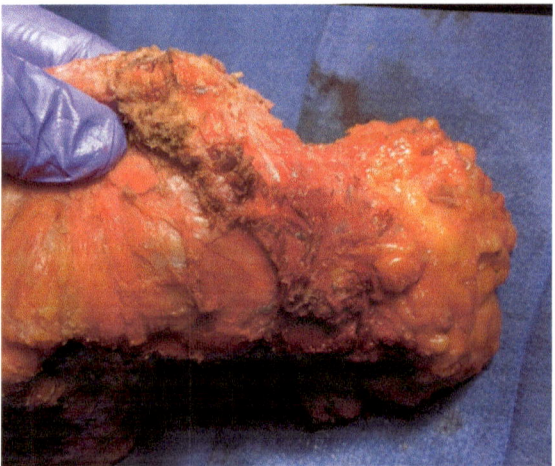

Fig. 10.4 Upward sacral deflection, usually at S-5 segment (cautery hook points to the sacro-coccygeal junction; visible domes of the ileo-coccygeal muscle anteriorly and flat coccygeus muscle posteriorly; both pelvic plexi preserved)

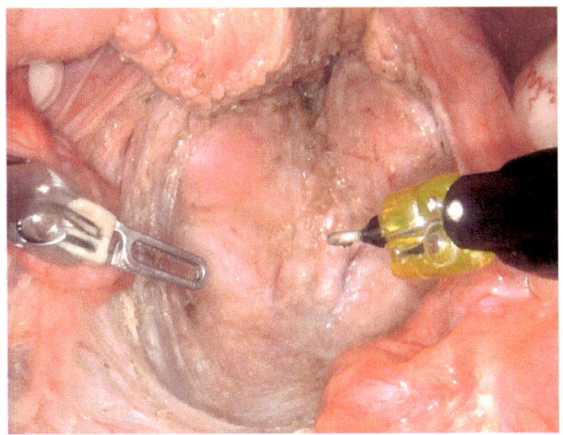

2. Piriformis muscles attach to the sacral segments S-2, S-3, and S-4 and exit the pelvis through the greater sciatic foramina. They don't belong to the pelvic floor; however, the floor begins just caudal to them. The sacrospinous ligament attaches to the lateral aspect of the sacrum, including the S-5 segment. The coccygeus muscle attaches to the S-5 and upper coccygeal segments and is situated ventrally to the sacrospinous ligament. When the distal sacrum and upper coccyx are removed, part of the coccygeal muscle is frequently removed, but the sacrospinous ligament should remain intact.

3. Distal and anterior to the coccygeus muscle, a convex part of the levators can be observed. This is the ileo-coccygeus muscle, which constitutes most of the levators supporting the mesorectal compartment (Fig. 10.4). A small portion of the levators supporting the anterior pelvic compartment (pubococcygeus muscle) also supports the mesorectum. Both the ileo-coccygeus muscle and the pubococcygeus muscle also support the lateral pelvic compartments. The convexity of the iliococcygeus muscles is caused by the push effect of the ischio-anal adipose tissue.

4. The levators attach laterally to the internal obturator muscle via the fascial attachment (*arcus tendineus*) (Fig. 10.5). The lateral attachment is located under the lateral compartment and is not under the mesorectal compartment.

5. Both the piriformis and internal obturator muscles can be bulky, contributing to the narrowing of the pelvic space.

6. Sacral splanchnic nerves can be observed at the periphery of the mesorectal compartment if the pre-hypogastric nerve fascia (the inner part of the presacral fascia) is lifted (Fig. 10.6). Together with the hypogastric nerves, the sacral splanchnic nerves converge laterally to form the pelvic plexus. The pelvic plexus is located between the lateral and the mesorectal compartment, just above (cephalad from) the ileo-coccygeus and coccygeus muscle (Fig. 10.2). The anterior portion of the pelvic plexus is covered by the lateral edge of Denonvilliers' fascia (Fig. 10.7).

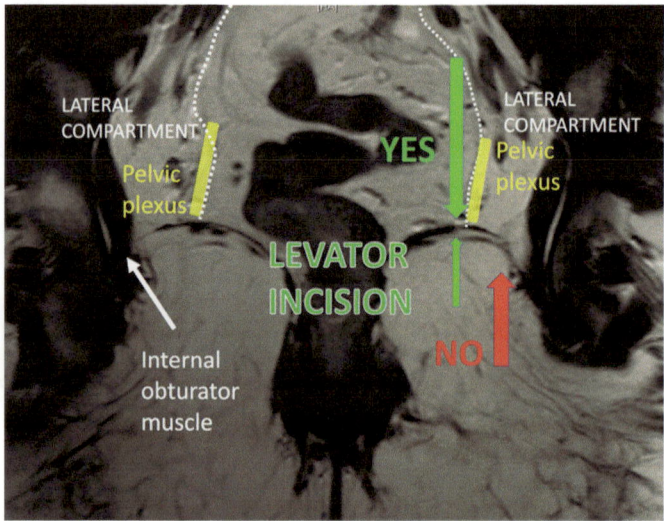

Fig. 10.5 Internal obturator muscle, levators, their origin, pelvic plexi and proper point of wide levator transection

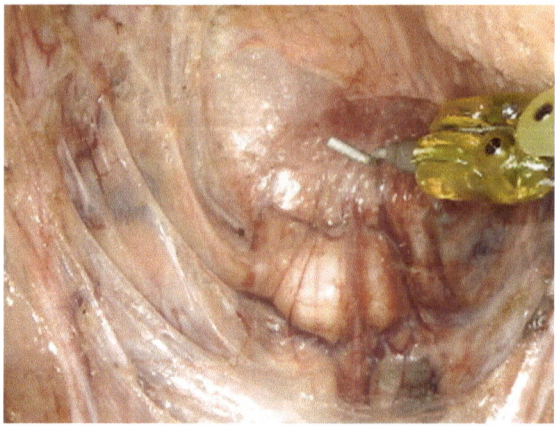

Fig. 10.6 Sacral splanchnic nerves converging in the pelvic plexus (all nerve structures well visible after the pre-hypogastric nerve fascia was removed with the mesorectal specimen)

7. Denonvilliers' fascia separates the mesorectal and anterior compartments in a curvilinear fashion, and its bottom edge rests on the pubococcygeus muscles. It protects the neurovascular bundles to the prostate and vagina (Fig. 10.7).
8. Two legs of the puborectalis muscle must be cut below Denonvilliers' fascia during APR procedures (Fig. 10.8).
9. The membranous segment of the male urethra may become exposed between the cut legs of the puborectalis muscle.

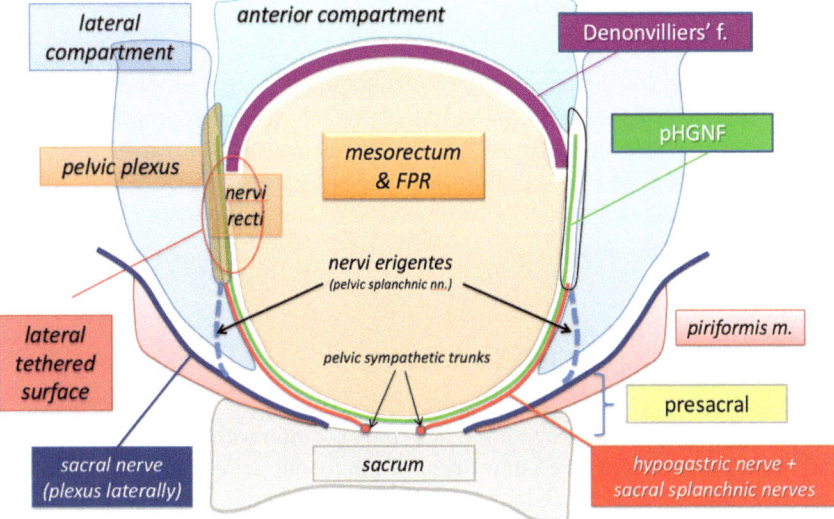

Fig. 10.7 Pelvic fasciae, compartments, and nerves

Fig. 10.8 The left
puborectalis leg seen under
the left levators, after
conservative (tailored)
levator transection

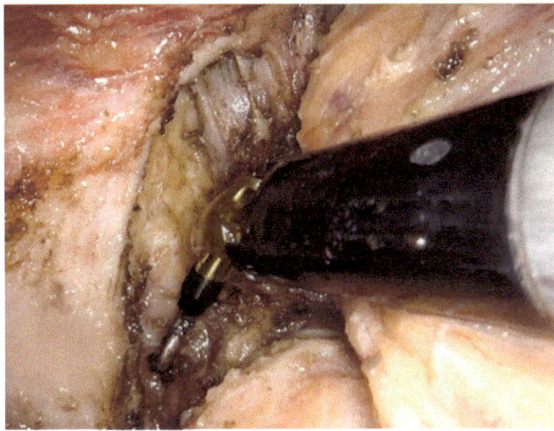

10. The mesorectal compartment is round and symmetrical (Fig. 10.7). This is an important feature to help guide the dissection when all other landmarks are distorted. The uninvolved part of the mesorectal excision can be used as a template to address the involved part.

Preoperative Preparation

The optimal site for the colostomy should be properly marked, preferably by the ostomy therapist. The surgeon should decide on the surgical approach after review of the preoperative imaging. Consideration should be given to intraabdominal levator transection, coccyx and coccygeal muscle resection (ELAPE), tailored approach (for eccentric pathology), beyond TME resection, and finally lithotomy versus prone perineal dissection.

Room Setup and Patient Positioning

The patient is placed in the modified lithotomy position with minimal flexion at the hips to allow for unrestricted movement of the robotic arms. The thighs should be relatively leveled with the abdominal wall. Trendelenburg position is used for most of the dissection, with a necessary right tilt of the table to keep the small bowel out of the dissection field. Frequently, no lateral tilt is needed for deep pelvic dissection. The robotic cart location should allow the assistant to be situated on patient's right side.

Port Placement

Ports are placed in a way that allows for free access to the inferior mesenteric artery (IMA), lateral attachments of the sigmoid, every aspect of the mesorectal compartment as well as the levators. Central camera placement (at umbilicus) is helpful in keeping the symmetry of the dissection and properly seeing each pelvic sidewall. Too cephalad port placement may result in arms hitting the pelvic brim and limiting the movements during the posterior part of TME. Four robotic arms are used, and the assistant can use two additional laparoscopic ports to maximize the exposure and control of the operating field (Fig. 10.9).

For the Xi system, the camera is placed through the umbilicus (R3). The right lower quadrant port (R4) is placed on the line from the umbilicus to the superior anterior iliac spine, about two-thirds the distance from the umbilicus. More medial port placement may be required for the narrow pelvis to allow unrestricted right-hand work along the right pelvic sidewall. This port will also be used for bowel stapling and thus can be upsized at the beginning of the case. The R1 port (left lateral) is placed as far to the left as possible, slightly above the lateral colon attachments, and just cephalad from the horizontal umbilical line. The remaining R2 port is placed at an equal distance between R1 and R3. One (or two) assistant ports are placed in the right mid-upper abdomen, between and cephalad from R3 and R4. Alternatively, one assistant port can be placed in the suprapubic region.

Fig. 10.9 Port placement for the Xi da Vinci platform; R—robotic, L—laparoscopic assistant ports

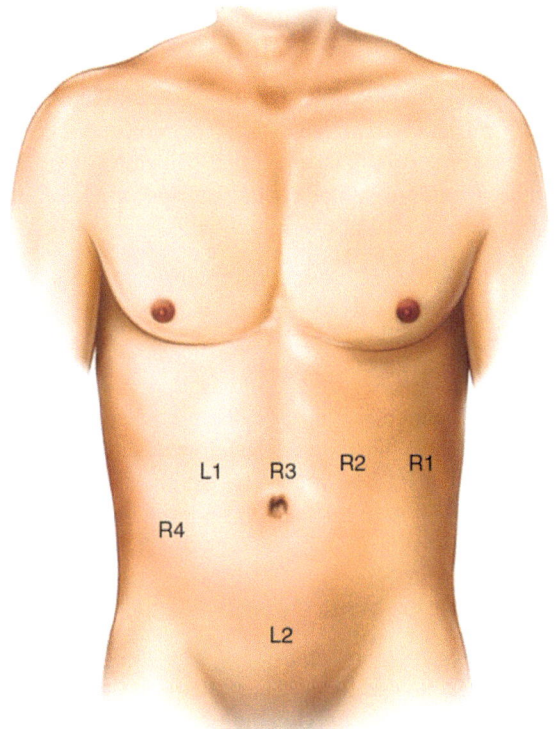

Instruments

The R4 port accommodates the dissecting energy instrument (hot sheers or monopolar hook), R2 uses a double-fenestrated bipolar grasper for micro-retraction. At the same time, R1 is supplied with a grasper (e.g., Cadière) to secure macro-retraction.

We don't try to accommodate the port placement to match precisely with the stoma site. Instead, we prefer a non-compromised robotic arm configuration that would translate into unrestricted dissection and no arm collisions throughout the case. The stoma site is usually located below and between R2 and R3.

The assistant is situated on the right side of the patient. The suprapubic port is usually a preferred site for the Airseal® system for more effective evacuation of pelvic fumes. In this case, the assistant can use the left hand to help with retraction, while the right hand can control the suction-irrigator.

Exploration

Exploratory laparoscopy is performed with the robotic endoscope. Most of the time, a 0° lens is used, although a 30° up scope can occasionally be used for very distal dissection (levators level). Splenic flexure is almost never taken down. However, if chosen, an omental pedicle flap can also use a 30° down scope. Liver evaluation can benefit from a 30° down lens as well.

Abdominal Phase

From the authors' experience, the "secret sauce" for successful robotic pelvic surgery involves three ingredients: (1) knowledge of pelvic anatomy and pathology location (2) efficient R1 arm macro-retraction, and (3) hemostatic dissection. The part of IMA-based lymphadenectomy, sigmoid mobilization, upper and mid rectal mobilization doesn't differ from a dissection discussed already in the low anterior resection chapter(s).

Only the most critical points will be mentioned here:

- Macro-retraction is usually provided by the left lateral (R1) arm. At the start of dissection, when identifying the plane between the pre-hypogastric nerve fascia/retroperitoneum and the mesorectal/mesocolic fascia, the grasping instrument pinches the rectosigmoid peritoneum, thus tensing it up at its base
- R1 arm provides the macro-retraction to the base of the sigmoid mesentery (along the superior hemorrhoidal vessels), while the medial-to-lateral dissection continues cephalad toward the IMA.
- Pre-hypogastric nerve fascia is kept intact during IMA and superior hemorrhoidal lymphadenectomy, thus protecting the preaortic nerve plexus.
- Retroperitoneal (Toldt's) fascia is kept intact during the entire dissection, thus protecting the left ureter and the gonadal vessels (Fig. 10.10). No attempt to find the ureter is often necessary if this fascia is kept intact and thorough hemostasis is maintained.
- Clips can be used for the IMA control. However, the mesenteric transection often requires a vessel sealer. The current ultra-fast robotic vessel sealer is one of the best sealing devices on the market. A laparoscopic vessel sealer may sometimes be cheaper.
- If the medial-to-lateral approach is or becomes difficult (lymphadenopathy, poor plane identification, obesity, small bowel in the field, aneurysm), the lateral-to-medial approach can be used instead. Contrary to standard laparoscopy, the robotic platform easily allows the surgeon to switch back to the medial approach after the lateral dissection is performed.
- Once the bifurcation of both hypogastric nerves is identified and the nerves are released toward the pelvic sidewalls, the pre-hypogastric nerve fascia can be incised, and the dissection plane switched into a deeper layer closer to the sacrum.

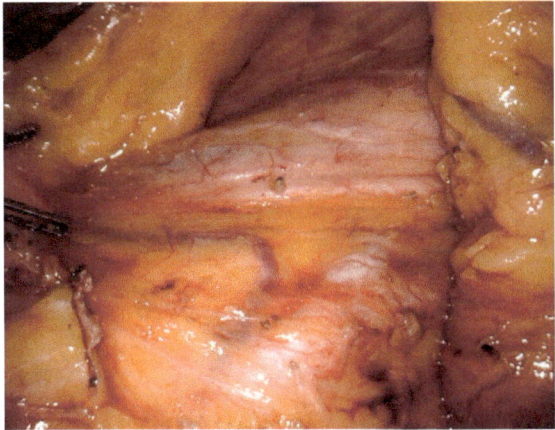

Fig. 10.10   An intact Toldt's fascia covering the left ureter just above the pelvic brim

If this occurs, the sacral splanchnic nerves become more visible (Fig. 10.6). These nerves provide additional sympathetic signal transmission to the pelvic plexus and are an excellent anatomical landmark for save pelvic dissection. Lifting the pre-hypogastric fascia together with the specimen also brings the dissection closer to the presacral vasculature (mainly venous).

- Macro-retraction with R1 during posterior mobilization of the rectum is provided by resting the mobilized specimen on the retracting instrument. Continuous macro-retraction adjustment takes place as dissection advances deeper into the pelvis.
- Macro-retraction with R1 during anterior mobilization is provided to the anterior pelvic structures. Almost never is there a need for suture retraction of the uterus.
- Macro-retraction with R1 for the left TME is applied to the left pelvic sidewall, while the micro-retraction is applied to the specimen with R2 or by the assistant.
- Macro-retraction with R1 for the right TME is applied to the specimen similarly as during posterior dissection.
- As for the lateral rectal attachments (this area is referred to as "tethered lateral surface"), they are taken down by cautery (Fig. 10.7). When most of the lateral mobilization is completed as a continuum of the posterior dissection around the rectum, this part of the dissection is relatively easy, especially if a line of anterior dissection has been marked. Care should be taken, however, not to injure the lateral pelvic plexi, which are a place of convergence of the sympathetic hypogastric nerves and sacral splanchnic nerves, as well as the parasympathetic sacral pelvic nerves (nervi erigentes located in the posterior aspect of the lateral compartment) (Figs. 10.2, 10.6 and 10.7).
- Occasionally, the posterior-lateral mobilization can bring the surgeon next to the lateral edge of Denonvilliers' fascia ad then in front of it, putting the neurovascular structures in danger (Fig. 10.7).

Fig. 10.11 Optional bilateral transection of the uterine round ligament can help retrovert the uterus to fill in the post-resection deep pelvic space

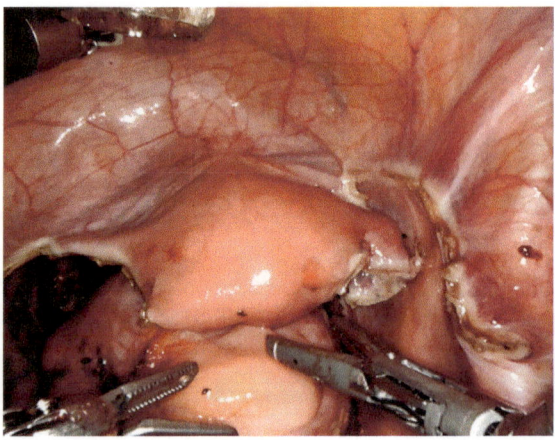

- The best point to first identify the levators before their intra-abdominal transection is laterally just medial to the pelvic plexus (Figs. 10.1 and 10.4). A decision on how much of the levators can be spared is made after the pelvic plexus is completely released from the mesorectum.
- In female patients, the uterus can often successfully obliterate the pelvic outlet after the APR procedure, with no need for additional flap reconstruction of the perineal wound. Occasionally, bilateral transection of the uterine round ligament can help retrovert the uterus to fill in the pelvic space (Fig. 10.11). If possible, an omental pedicle flap or redundant sigmoid mesentery can also be used for that purpose.

Levator Transection

When approaching the pathology in the distal third of the rectum, the surgeon must decide how to handle this most crucial part of the dissection. Two options exist: (1) complete this part of dissection from the perineal side in a conventional way or (2) perform robotically-assisted intra-abdominal levator transection to facilitate the perineal phase (IALT).

Conventional Perineal Dissection

The traditional perineal dissection requires proper training and appropriate exposure [8]. Today the ELAPE technique frequently replaces the classic, "old-fashion" technique, which creates a clear "waist" of the specimen. The "waist" was the result of TME completion before the levators were incised.

Coccygectomy (or very distal sacrectomy) is a helpful maneuver in the ELAPE technique because it widely opens the operative field, allowing for excellent exposure (Fig. 10.1). A frequent recommendation to divide the levators "close to the pelvic bone" is ill-advised because the levators originate from the internal obturator muscle along the arcus tendinous (Fig. 10.5). It must also be repeated that the lateral portion of the levators constitutes the floor of the lateral compartment and should remain intact during standard, not extended resections. The benefit of excellent exposure provided by the ELAPE technique, frequently associated with coccygectomy and wide levator resection, must be weighed against the morbidity of a large perineal defect. The ELAPE technique is an inherently maximally invasive approach to the perineum. It can be associated with large post-resection tissue defects frequently necessitating flap closure, complicated wound healing, chronic postoperative pain partly related to coccyx resection, perineal hernias, and GU dysfunction [5].

When one aims to use the robot only for TME during APR and complete the procedure using the traditional perineal ELAPE technique, the robotic dissection should be stopped posteriorly at the level of the sacrococcygeal junction, and laterally, where the levators, precisely flat coccygeus muscle, are visualized and when the pelvic sidewall is separated from the mesorectum (Fig. 10.1). Anteriorly the dissection should be carried as distal as it is possible and safe.

Robotic-Assisted Intra-Abdominal (Trans-Abdominal) Levator Transection

Intra-abdominal transection of the levators was introduced into clinical practice by Marecik et al. for multiple reasons, including (1) to perform the most challenging phase of the abdominoperineal resection under a direct vision, with complete control of the operating field, (2) to simplify the perineal part, and (3) to maintain the minimally invasive approach of the whole procedure with its postoperative benefits (preserving all tissue that can safely be preserved) [10]. The concept of minimally invasive (robotic) intra-abdominal levator transection has further evolved into a more conservative approach in appropriate cases with eccentrically situated tumors [11]. The evolution mentioned above aims not only to improve control over the operating field but also to take advantage of the minimally invasive benefits that the robotic technique offers.

For the robotic intra-abdominal levator transection (RILT), the first goal is to identify and expose the posterolateral surface of the iliococcygeus muscle (with its characteristic dome-like shape) (Fig. 10.1). This part is routinely excised during a standard ELAPE technique. Only then can these muscles be obliquely incised, starting just off the midline while extending the incision laterally along the contour of the mesorectal compartment and ending with an incision of the pubococcygeus muscle in the anterolateral aspect of the mesorectal compartment (Figs. 10.12, 10.13, 10.14, 10.15, 10.16, 10.17, 10.18 and 10.19). If the tumor is not threatening the anterior rectal aspect, the mesorectal dissection can be carried down to the perineal body posterior to Denonvilliers' fascia. The perineal body transection is usually done from the perineal side. If the cancer is threatening the anterior CRM, the mesorectal dissection should be carried out in front of Denonvilliers' fascia or it can be stopped, with a plan to complete the dissection from the perineal side.

Once the levators are transected, the fatty tissue of the ischioanal fossa can be visualized. The iliococcygeus and pubococcygeus muscles are not thick (usually 2–3 mm), and they may be significantly attenuated in older or asthenic individuals. Anterior part of the levators in individuals with narrow pelvis is frequently short and positioned more vertically than horizontally. In addition, during transection one can appreciate a thick levators fascia. For surgeons willing to try the intra-abdominal levator transection for the first time, the authors suggest ending the abdominal phase with posterolateral levator transection only [13]. The posterior midline part of the

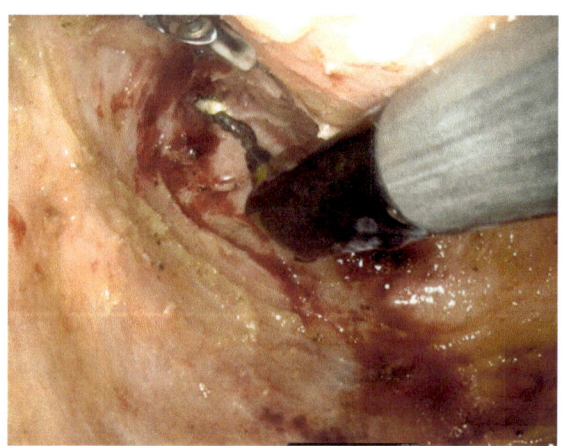

Fig. 10.12 Robotic intra-abdominal levator transection, starting in the left posterior aspect (female)

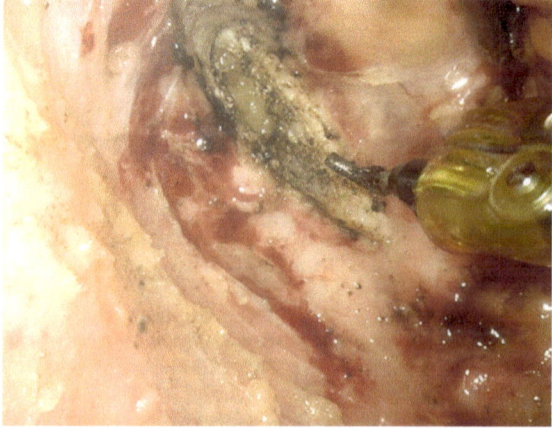

Fig. 10.13 Robotic intra-abdominal levator transection, medial extension of the levator incision

Fig. 10.14 Robotic
intra-abdominal levator
transection, incision in front
of the tip of the coccyx

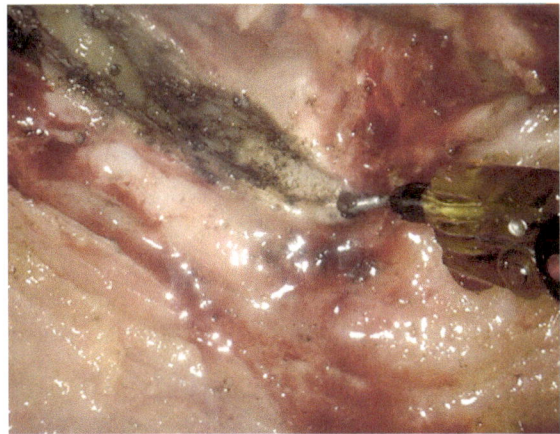

Fig. 10.15 Robotic
intra-abdominal levator
transection, incision
extended to the right side

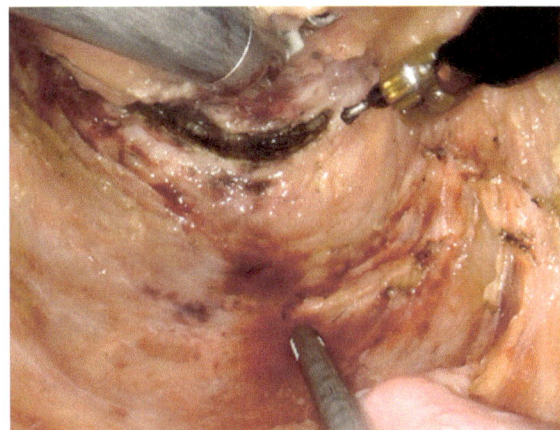

Fig. 10.16 Robotic
intra-abdominal levator
transection, incision into the
right ischio-anal fossa on the
right side (visible fatty
tissue)

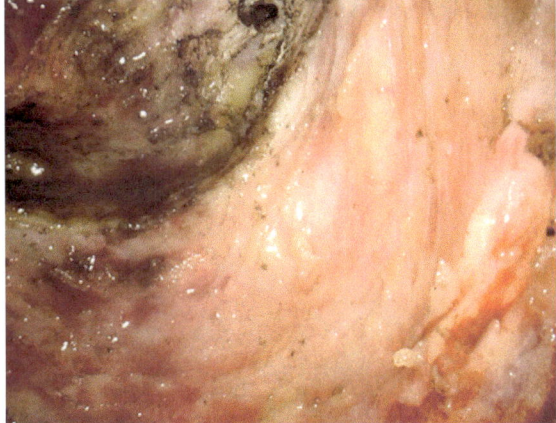

Fig. 10.17 Robotic intra-abdominal levator transection, completed posterior and postero-lateral incision

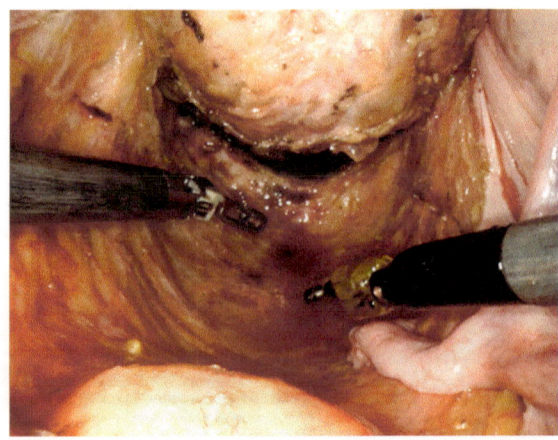

Fig. 10.18 Robotic intra-abdominal levator transection, transection of the left pubo-coccygeus muscle along the inferior border of Denonvilliers' fascia (a tight antero-lateral space in the obese male

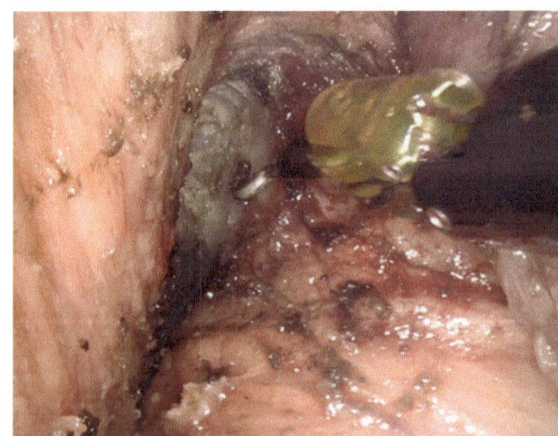

Fig. 10.19 Robotic intra-abdominal levator transection, a tight antero-lateral space in the obese male

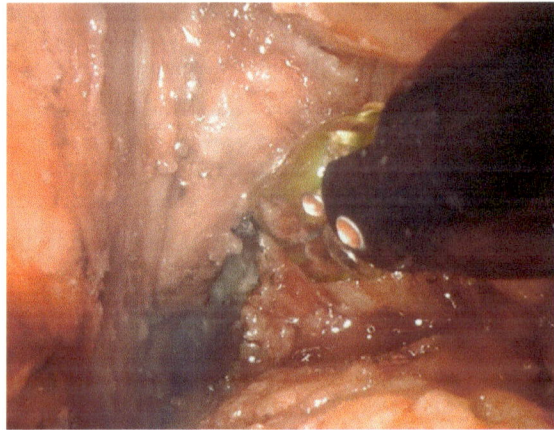

pelvic floor transection does not need to be completed. This leaves the levators raphe and the anococcygeal ligament intact to be divided during the perineal completion phase. Because the levators were properly incised posterolaterally, the surgeon should easily identify and access the dissected pelvic space, hook the raphe and the ligament with the index finger, and divide them during the perineal phase.

The second goal of IALT is to spare the coccyx (unless threatened by the tumor), thus sparing the coccygeus muscle, which part is frequently removed during a conventional ELAPE technique. We believe that saving the coccyx is important for patients who undergo the APR procedure (Figs. 10.20, 10.21 and 10.22). Coccyx preservation results in smaller postoperative defects, making it easier to close it primarily without flap reconstruction. In our experience, coccyx preservation leads to a less symptomatic perineal hernia rate. By standard calculations, a decrease of the wound diameter by half translates, on average, into a fourfold reduction in the area of the defect ($A = \pi r2$). No coccygectomy results in no exposed bone or cartilage at the site of disarticulation, which can be important since perineal wound infection can lead to osteomyelitis.

The third goal of IALT is to preserve all tissue that can be safely saved and is not close to the tumor. Because the pelvis can be very narrow, particularly in its distal part, this goal may not always be achievable, and oncological safety should dictate a more radical approach, which means complete ELAPE. The conservative (selective, tailored) approach should only be used for eccentrically located tumors by surgeons with a thorough understanding of tumor and patient anatomy, as well as experienced in intraabdominal levator transection [11].

There is a tendency among the surgeons who perform IALT for the first time to begin the intra-abdominal levator transection too proximal (cephalad), resulting in accidental exposure of the lower sacral or coccygeal segments. In addition, this could also result in bleeding from the lateral sacral arteries or even midline venous structures. If the surgeon identifies the mistake, by exposing the bone, the dissection should either start more caudal or continue along the bone's surface until the tip of the coccyx is reached.

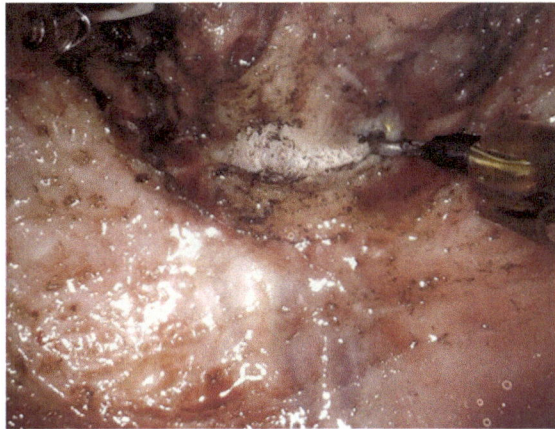

Fig. 10.20 Coccyx spared with the levator transection commenced at the level of the sacro-coccygeal junction. Subsequently, the dissection continues in front of the coccyx

Fig. 10.21 Bleeding control
in front of the coccyx

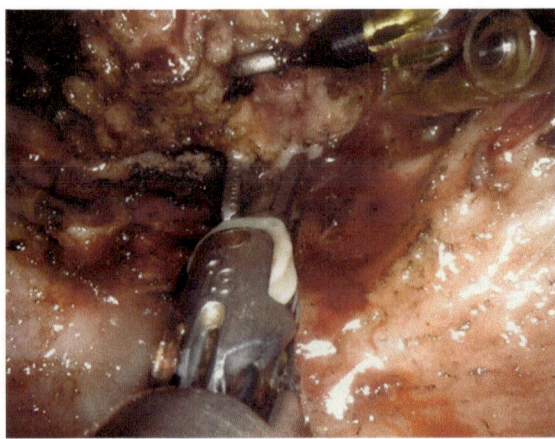

Fig. 10.22 Coccyx spared
during asymmetrical,
tailored robotic IALT; left
levators were also spared

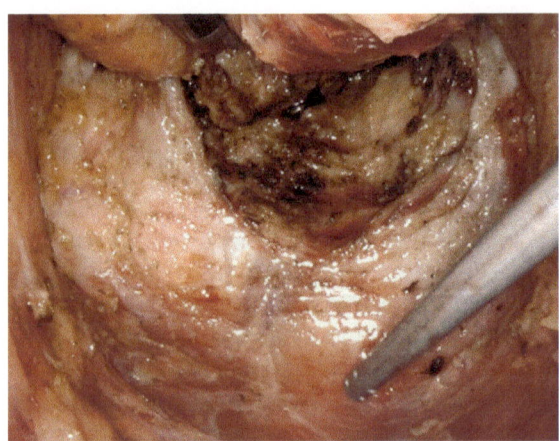

When the levators are transected too proximal, bleeding from the lateral sacral
arteries or levator feeders can be controlled using bipolar forceps (Fig. 10.21). Occasionally, simple vessel compression for 2–5 min with the robotic instrument may be
sufficient when cautery is not very effective.

The intra-abdominal levator transection along the periphery of the mesorectal
compartment allows for complete preservation of the autonomic nerve structures
(pelvic plexi and neurovascular bundles of the prostate and vagina), thus minimizing
the risk of GU dysfunction (Figs. 10.1, 10.7, 10.18 and 10.19). This transection is
done under direct vision. One critique of the formal ELAPE technique pertains to
the levator transection, which is done from the perineal site and is too close to their
origin from the internal obturator muscle (along *arcus tendinous*) (Fig. 10.5). It is
difficult to pinpoint from the perineal side where the nerve structures are located
precisely in such a situation. The incision may be performed underneath the lateral
compartment, resulting in injury to the pelvic plexus.

Completion Perineal Phase of IALT

After levators are incised, the surgeon can continue the dissection through the adipose tissue of the ischioanal fossa. Most of the ischioanal fatty tissue can be preserved if the tumor doesn't penetrate the levators, as evident on MRI and clinical exam. Wide local excision involving the perianal and ischioanal fat and skin is rare in rectal cancer and mainly reserved for squamous cell carcinoma cases.

The perineal dissection can be completed in the lithotomy or prone positions. The lithotomy position is often sufficient for uncomplicated cases with low patient body habitus, wide pelvis, and non-advanced pathology. The completion of perineal work is relatively quick in the cases when IALT has been completed. The dissection involves the skin, perianal fat, some degree of ischioanal fat, and finally, anterior transection through the perineal body and two legs of the puborectalis muscle. The lithotomy position is also chosen for the planned rectus abdominal flap.

Prone position in authors' practice is reserved mainly for advanced pathology threatening the anterior and lateral resection margins and posterior margin when coccygectomy or distal sacrectomy has to be utilized. In reality, the prone position for perineal dissection is the most comfortable position for the surgeon and offers the best view of the entire pelvic floor and deep pelvis. Many surgeons don't feel comfortable with the prone position, which is directly related to a lack of good training. Once mastered, the prone dissection technique will become very helpful to address the most complex cases with confidence. In general, dissection at the prostate, lower vagina, and the perineal body level can be completed with good control during the perineal phase if the rest of the circumferential levator transection has been completed either by the formal/modified ELAPE technique or by IALT. The delivery of a partially mobilized specimen out of the pelvis can be helpful before the anterior dissection commences. Still, one needs to remember that excessive traction on the delivered specimen may pull into the field pelvic sidewall structures, thus endangering them. Ureteral injury close to the bladder is possible in a woman due to the laxity of the pelvic structures. Enlarged prostate, on the other hand, can also distort the anterior dissection plane. Frequently, an enlarged prostate may lead to elongation of the membranous segment of the urethra, which can become easily exposed and injured when two legs of the puborectalis muscle are transected.

Surgeons often have trouble finding the right plane just in front of the sphincter complex, which continues into the rectovaginal or rectoprostatic plane. As a general rule, in most patients without large rectocele or large prostate, the plane in front of the sphincter complex is very horizontal (parallel to the floor) in both the prone and lithotomy positions.

When IALT has been performed, it should be pretty easy to find the previously dissected tissues during the perineal completion phase. Rendezvous is the easiest and the safest in the postero-lateral aspects, where the iliococcygeus muscles were once incised. The ability to quickly connect with the pelvic dissection plane is the main benefit of the IALT technique. Preservation of a large amount of skin, perianal and ischioanal fat is often possible during this phase. Anterior or posterior vertical skin incision can be added to a small elliptical skin incision around the anus instead of creating a large elliptical perianal used to provide broad access to the ischioanal fossa and the levators.

Conclusion

A robotic platform is an excellent tool, which can be effectively utilized in challenging operating field like APR. Modern surgeons should become familiar with the ELAPE concept and robotic intra-abdominal (transabdominal) levator transection (IALT). The IALT technique allows for precise tumor dissection according to strong oncologic principles and significant pelvic floor preservation.

References

1. Marr R, et al. The modern abdominoperineal excision: the next challenge after total mesorectal excision. Ann Surg. 2005;242(1):74–82.
2. Heald RJ, et al. Abdominoperineal excision of the rectum—an endangered operation. Norman Nigro Lectureship. Dis Colon Rectum. 1997;40(7):747–51.
3. Nagtegaal ID, et al. Low rectal cancer: a call for a change of approach in abdominoperineal resection. J Clin Oncol. 2005;23(36):9257–64.
4. Holm T, et al. Extended abdominoperineal resection with gluteus maximus flap reconstruction of the pelvic floor for rectal cancer. Br J Surg. 2007;94(2):232–8.
5. Welsch T, et al. Results of extralevator abdominoperineal resection for low rectal cancer including quality of life and long-term wound complications. Int J Colorectal Dis. 2013;28(4):503–10.
6. Kamali D, et al. Oncological and quality of life outcomes following extralevator versus standard abdominoperineal excision for rectal cancer. Ann R Coll Surg Engl. 2017;99(5):402–9.
7. Han JG, et al. A prospective multicenter clinical study of extralevator abdominoperineal resection for locally advanced low rectal cancer. Dis Colon Rectum. 2014;57(12):1333–40.
8. Holm T. Abdominoperineal excision: technical challenges in optimal surgical and oncological outcomes after abdominoperineal excision for rectal cancer. Clin Colon Rectal Surg. 2017;30(5):357–67.
9. Giulianotti PC, et al. Robotics in general surgery: personal experience in a large community hospital. Arch Surg. 2003;138(7):777–84.
10. Marecik SJ, et al. Robotic cylindrical abdominoperineal resection with transabdominal levator transection. Dis Colon Rectum. 2011;54(10):1320–5.
11. Pai A, et al. Robotic site adjusted levator transection for carcinoma of the rectum: a modification of the existing cylindrical abdominoperineal resection for eccentrically located tumors. World J Surg. 2017;41(2):590–5.
12. Stelzner S, et al. Deep pelvic anatomy revisited for a description of crucial steps in extralevator abdominoperineal excision for rectal cancer. Dis Colon Rectum. 2011;54(8):947–57.
13. Chang G, Surgeon from MD Anderson Cancer Center. Houston: Personal Correspondence.

Chapter 11
Robotic Lateral Pelvic Lymph Node Dissection

Tsuyoshi Konishi

Abstract Neoadjuvant (chemo)radiotherapy followed by total mesorectal excision (TME) has been a standard practice for c-Stage II–III rectal cancer in the Western countries. With improved surgical management in the central pelvis, majority of pelvic local recurrence has now shifted to the lateral pelvic compartment (Fig. 11.1). Lateral pelvic lymph node dissection (LPLND) has been performed for decades by Japanese surgeons as a standard practice for mid-low rectal cancer extending below the peritoneal reflexion. A recent international observational studies by the Lateral Node Consortium demonstrated oncologic benefits of adding LPLND to TME after neoadjuvant (chemo)radiotherapy in patients with enlarged lateral lymph nodes. LPLND is a great armamentarium of colorectal surgeons in the setting of referral centers. Autonomic nerve-preserving technique is important for minimizing postoperative urinary and sexual dysfunction. Anatomical plane-oriented dissection of the obturator and internal iliac compartments is required to achieve safe and complete lymph node dissection. A robotic approach provides more advanced knowledge of pelvic anatomy particularly outside of the TME. Standardization of this procedure may facilitate the dissection and provide optimal early and oncological outcomes. In this chapter, step-by-step procedures and technical tips of robotic LPLND are presented.

Keywords Lateral pelvic lymph node · Neoadjuvant therapy · Robotic surgery · Minimally invasive surgery

T. Konishi (✉)
Department of Colon and Rectal Surgery, The University of Texas M.D. Anderson Cancer Center, 1400 Pressler Street, Unit 1484, Houston, TX 77030, USA
e-mail: tkonishi.tky@gmail.com

© The Author(s), under exclusive license to Springer Nature Switzerland AG 2022   121
P. Coyne and J. Khan (eds.), *Robotic Colorectal Surgery*,
https://doi.org/10.1007/978-3-031-15198-9_11

Indications for Selective Lateral Pelvic Lymph Node Dissection After Neoadjuvant Chemoradiotherapy

Oncological outcomes of surgical treatment for rectal cancer have been dramatically improved during the past decades with improved neoadjuvant therapy and total mesorectal excision (TME). With improved surgical management in the central pelvis, majority of pelvic local recurrence has now shifted to the lateral pelvic compartment. A recent study of 366 patients who were treated with neoadjuvant chemoradiotherapy and TME demonstrated that 83% of local recurrences developed in the lateral ompartment; and 27% of patients with enlarged lateral lymph nodes (>5 mm in diameter) before treatment developed local recurrence [1]. Another series from UK also indicated similarly high local recurrence after chemoradiotherapy and TME in patients with enlarged lateral pelvic lymph nodes [2]. These data clearly indicate that chemoradiotherapy alone without surgical dissection never eliminates lateral nodal disease. Importantly, lateral node metastasis is not systemic disease but reginal disease that can be cured by surgical dissection. Studies demonstrated that 42–48% of patients with lateral nodal recurrence did not have distant metastasis [1, 3, 4]. A retrospective study from Japan that combined neoadjuvant chemoradiotherapy and TME with selective lateral pelvic lymph node dissection (LPLND) reported 2.7% local recurrence and 84% 3-year-relapse free survival in patients with enlarged lateral nodes [5, 6]. An international multicenter observational study by Lateral Node Consortium showed neoadjuvant (chemo)radiotherapy and TME with selective LPLND resulted in a significantly lower 5-year-lateral pelvic local recurrence compared to those who received neoadjuvant (chemo)radiotherapy and TME alone without LPLND (5 year LLR, 5.7 vs. 19.5%; P = 0.042) [7]. These data suggest oncologic benefits of adding selective LPLND to TME after neoadjuvant therapy in patients with enlarged lateral pelvic lymph nodes. Given currently available data, indication criteria for LPLND typically include cT3-4 mid-low rectal cancer extending below the peritoneal reflection, with enlarged lateral pelvic lymph nodes in the obturator and/or internal iliac areas (Table 11.1). Although the exact size of lateral pelvic lymph nodes for indication of LPLND has been controversial, at primary staging, a threshold of ≥ 7 mm (short-axis diameter) may be used as a criterion to diagnose positive lateral pelvic lymph nodes as supported by the Lateral Node Consortium and a global multidisciplinary expert consensus [7, 8]. Patients with potentially suspicious lateral nodes post-chemoradiotherapy should always be discussed individually for indication of LPLND by a multidisciplinary team.

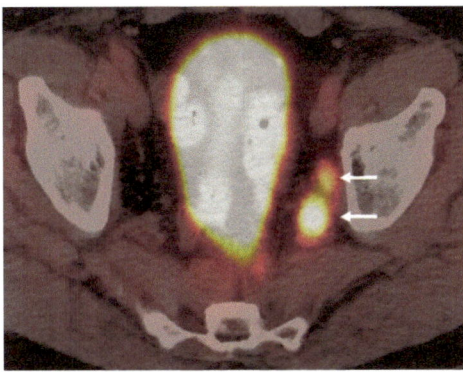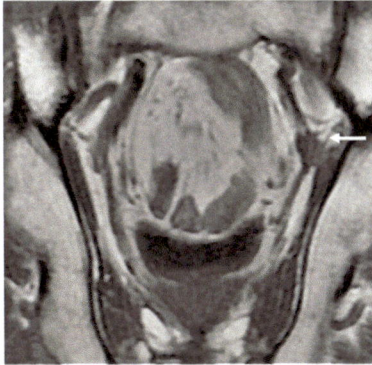

Fig. 11.1 MRI and PET images of a recurrent lateral pelvic lymph node after chemoradiotherapy and TME. Two enlarged metastatic lymph nodes with FDG uptake are observed in the left lateral compartment. The patient underwent salvage lateral pelvic lymph node dissection through a robotic approach, which revealed pathological metastasis in the lateral pelvic lymph nodes

Table 11.1 Indication for lateral pelvic lymph node dissection. Indication criteria typically include cT3-4 mid-low rectal cancer extending below the peritoneal reflection, with enlarged lateral pelvic lymph nodes in the obturator and/or internal iliac areas

Indication for lateral pelvic lymph node dissection
cT3-4 mid-low rectal cancer extending below the peritoneal reflexion
Enlarged lateral lymph node ($\geq$7 mm before neoadjuvant therapy)
Obturator and internal iliac areas

Anatomy of Lateral Pelvic Areas

Areas of Dissection and Anatomical Landmarks

Lateral nodal metastases from rectal cancer mainly occur in the obturator and internal iliac areas, and these areas are "regional" and can be cured by resection [9, 10]. In contrast, lateral nodes in the external and common iliac areas are rarely involved with disease and are more often associated with distant metastasis. As such, obturator and internal iliac areas are two major areas of dissection in LPLND for rectal cancer, while the other areas can be spared unless there are suspicious lymph nodes.

To simplify understanding of anatomic structures in the lateral pelvic compartment (Fig. 11.2), one should consider that obturator and internal iliac areas are surrounded by 3 planes: (1) lateral plane, psoas muscle and internal obturator muscle; internal plane, hypogastric nerve, pelvic plexus, ureter and urinary bladder; and posterior plane, internal iliac vessels and sciatic nerve (lumbosacral nerve trunk). Another plane divides the area into the obturator (lateral) and internal iliac (internal) areas: the vesicohypogastric fascia, which is an embryonic avascular plane of dissection composed by the internal iliac artery, vesical branches (umbilical artery, superior and inferior vesical arteries), and urinary bladder. The proximal (cranial) border of dissection is usually at the bifurcation of the internal and external iliac veins.

Dissection exposing these anatomic landmarks along with these planes results in complete dissection of the obturator and internal iliac lymph nodes in *en bloc* fashion. Importantly, metastatic nodes should be dissected in *en bloc* fashion without exposing or grasping the metastatic tissues. Piece-meal dissection of the nodes may lead to bleeding, spillage of cancer cells, and possibly recurrence [11].

Structures to Be Preserved

The ureter, hypogastric nerve, pelvic plexus, and obturator nerve are to be preserved in principle unless they are involved in cancer. A nerve preserving technique is important to preserve postoperative urinary and sexual function [12, 13]. Careful surgical manipulation is needed to avoid thermal and electric injury by electrocautery or energy devices.

Obturator artery and vein can be resected to facilitate obturator lymph node dissection as it does not cause dysfunction of any type after surgery. The umbilical artery and superior/inferior vesical vessels can also be resected if they are involved by metastasis. The inferior vesical vessels are often involved or abutted by metastatic nodes as this location is the most frequent site for metastasis [9]. For this condition, the obturator and internal iliac areas are dissected *en bloc* using the 3 planes and without using the vesicohypogastric fascia (Fig. 11.2). Preoperative radiologic images should be carefully evaluated for anatomic variation of the internal iliac vessels and their branches, particularly for the veins. It is important to evaluate whether the vessels are invaded or abutted by metastatic lymph nodes, particularly around the inferior vesical artery/vein. If invaded or abutted by metastatic nodes, combined resection is needed for vessel branches.

Step-by-Step Technical Details

Patient Positioning and Port Placement

LPLND is initiated after completion of TME. Patient positioning is the same as used in TME, typically placed in Trendelenburg position with right side tilt so that the small bowel and omentum are moved out from the pelvis by gravity. The degree of Trendelenburg position should be as minimal as possible, given the prolonged operating time expected for LPLND.

(i)

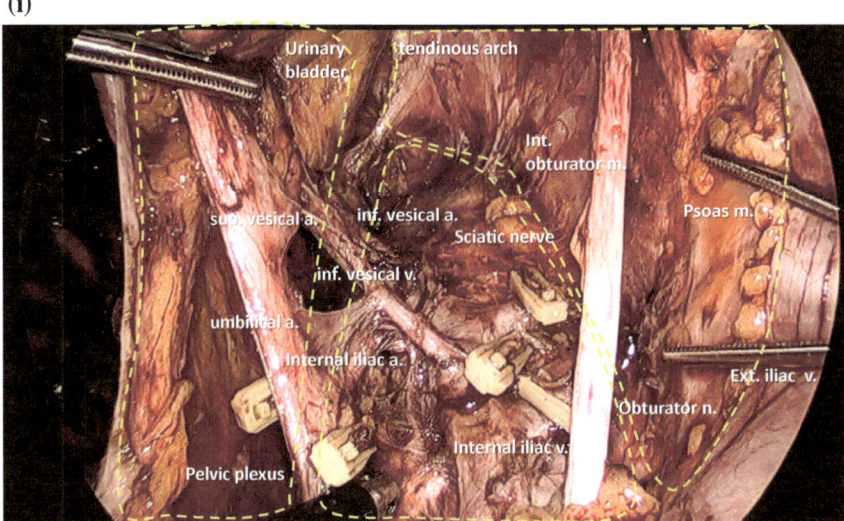

(ii)

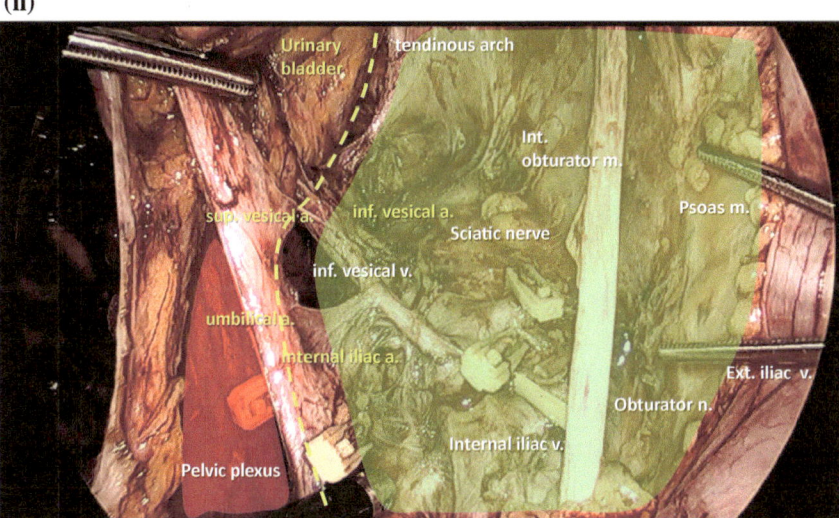

Fig. 11.2 Surgical view after right-sided LPLND preserving superior and inferior vesical vessels and autonomic nerves (2–1, distant view; 2–2, zoom-up view). Obturator and internal iliac areas are surrounded by 3 planes: (1) lateral plane, psoas muscle and internal obturator muscle; internal plane, hypogastric nerve, pelvic plexus, ureter and urinary bladder; and posterior plane, internal iliac vessels and sciatic nerve (lumbosacral nerve trunk). The obturator (green) and internal iliac (red) areas are separated by a plane called the vesicohypogastric fascia (yellow dotted line), which is composed by the internal iliac artery, vesical branches (umbilical artery, superior and inferior vesical arteries), and urinary bladder

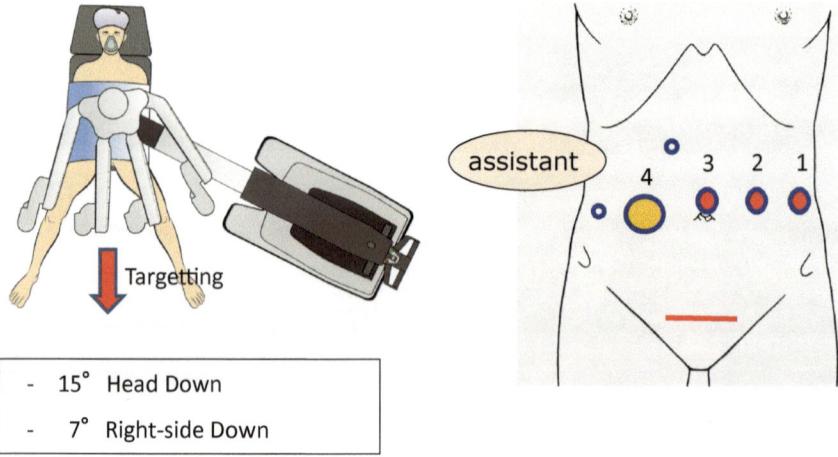

Fig. 11.3 Trocar positions (the same as regular TME). 1, 8 mm, Tip-up Fenestrated Grasper/Prograsp Forceps; 2, 8 mm, Fenestrated bipolar Grasper; 3, 8 mm, Camera; 4, 12 mm, Monopolar Curved Scissors/ Clip Applier/Vessel Sealer Extend/SynchroSeal/Stapler

Port placement can also be the same as used in TME with no need for additional ports. Typical port placement is described in Fig. 11.3. We typically place a 12 mm stapler port in the right lower ostomy site; three 8-mm ports at the umbilicus, left mid and left lateral quadrant in straight fashion; a 5 mm assistant ports at the right lateral abdomen and a 5 mm AirSeal port in the right upper abdomen. We also utilize at least one 12 mm port at the Pfannenstiel incision to be used so that gauze can be quickly inserted in case of bleeding.

Nerve and Vesical Vessel-Preserving LPLND

Isolation of Ureter and Pelvic Plexus

The ureter is identified, taped, and isolated distally. The hypogastric nerve and pelvic plexus are also mobilized together with the ureter in the same plane as a medial curtain, covered with the same connective tissue (i.e., prehypogastric-nerve fascia). Isolation of the pelvic plexus is stopped before the entry point to the neurovascular bundle to avoid injury. This first step ensures preservation of the ureter and autonomic nerves during the procedure.

Obturator Lymph Node Dissection

Identifying medial border of the external iliac vein

The external iliac vein is the first and easiest landmark to initiate dissection. The purpose of identifying the external iliac vein is to detect the psoas muscle just behind the vessel. Dissection of the external iliac lymph nodes on the vein surface is not necessary as this is an uncommon place for metastasis from rectal cancer and the dissection may cause postoperative edema in the lower extremities.

At the distal end of the external iliac vein, there is a lymphatic channel from the inguinal nodes to the obturator nodes. This lymphatic channel should be ligated with a clip to avoid postoperative lymphorrhea or lymphocele.

Dissection along psoas and internal obturator muscles

Once the psoas muscle is identified behind the external iliac vein, the dissection follows an avascular plane on the surface of the psoas muscle followed by the internal obturator muscle. Tiny perforating veins in this layer can be dissected with electrocautery.

Identification of the obturator nerve and vessels at the obturator foramen

Dissection is continued exposing the surface of the internal obturator muscle; and the obturator nerve, artery, and vein are easily identified anteriorly at the entry point to the obturator foramen. The obturator nerve is carefully preserved, and the obturator vessels are ligated at this entry point.

Dissection along the internal obturator muscle down to the tendinous arch of the levator ani muscle

Dissection is continued on the surface of the internal obturator muscle towards the pelvic floor down to the tendinous arch where the levator ani muscle attaches to the internal obturator muscle. Dissection is continued to expose the surface of the levator ani muscle, and the space is communicated with the TME space. Although communicating to the TME space is not needed, it ensures complete dissection of this area and avoids postoperative lymphocele as the discharge in lateral compartment is drained to the TME space through the communication. This is the end of the lateral border dissection of the obturator area.

Dissection along the umbilical artery and bladder (vesicohypogastric fascia)

Dissection now moves to the internal border of the obturator area. The first easiest landmark to identify is the umbilical artery. Just lateral to the umbilical artery, there is a clear entry point into an embryonic avascular layer that separates the bladder against obturator lymph nodes. Obturator lymph nodes are retracted laterally and this counter traction will expose the clear embryonic plane between the adipose tissue of the obturator lymph nodes and the adipose tissue of the bladder. This embryonic avascular layer is called the "vesicohypogastric fascia". Dissection continues following this layer, exposing the umbilical artery followed by lateral aspect of the superior and inferior vesical vessels and the surface of the bladder; and finally the dissection reaches to the levator ani muscle at the pelvic bottom which was previously exposed. This is the most distal medial end of the obturator area.

Preservation of the obturator nerve

Once the obturator nerve is identified at the obturator canal, the nerve is exposed and isolated from distal to proximal to the bifurcation of the internal and external iliac veins, detaching the obturator lymph nodes. At the iliac vein bifurcation, the nerve runs into behind the common iliac vein. Electrocautery or energy device should be used carefully around the obturator nerve as it might cause thermal or electric injury to the nerve with resultant postoperative obturator nerve palsy [14].

Ligation of proximal end of the obturator lymph nodes

After isolating and preserving the obturator nerve, the adipose tissue of the obturator lymph nodes is ligated at the bifurcation of the internal and external iliac veins. This lymphatic chain is to be ligated using a clip to avoid postoperative lymphorrhea or lymphocele. This is the proximal end of the obturator lymph node dissection.

Exposing internal iliac vessels and sciatic nerve (lumbosacral nerve trunk)

The dissection continues on the posterior plane by exposing the internal iliac artery and vein lateral to the vesicohypogastric fascia. It is critical at this point to keep the plane exactly on the surface of internal iliac artery and vein so that the branch vessels (e.g., obturator artery/vein, inferior vesical artery/vein) can be identified and ligated at the root. Laterally to the internal iliac vessels, dissection follows exposing the surface of sciatic nerve (lumbosacral nerve trunk). The surface of the sciatic nerve is covered with thin connective tissue, and dissection of obturator lymph nodes can be performed preserving this connective tissue. If this connective tissue is taken with the nodes, the surface of the nerve is exposed and patients may complain of lower extremity pain due to sciatic neuralgia.

Identification of inferior vesical vessels and infra-piriformis muscle foramen

Dissection of the posterior plane of the obturator area exposing the internal iliac vessels leads to identification of the inferior vesical vessels which are the last branches from main trunk of the internal iliac vessels, followed by the infra-piriformis muscle foramen at which the main trunk of the internal iliac vessels exit the pelvis behind the coccygeal muscle as the internal pudendal vessels. Dissection around the inferior vesical vessels and infra-piriformis muscle foramen is the most important as this area is the most frequent site for metastasis. If metastatic lymph nodes abut the inferior vesical vessels or internal pudendal vessels, then combined resection of the vessels is required. Down to the infra-piriformis muscle foramen, coccygeal muscle is exposed, and dissection reaches the distal obturator area which was previously dissected, and thus the dissection of the obturator area is finished.

Internal Iliac Lymph Node Dissection

Preservation of hypogastric nerve and pelvic plexus

As described at the beginning of the procedure, the hypogastric nerve and pelvic plexus are separated together with the ureter as a medial curtain from the piriformis muscle. The S4 pelvic splanchnic nerve sometimes runs adjacent to the inferior vesical vessels, which distally combine and form the neurovascular bundle at the entry point to the bladder. Isolation of the pelvic plexus can stop before the S4 pelvic splanchnic nerve to avoid injury to neurovascular bundle.

Dissection of internal iliac lymph nodes

Adipose tissue on the surface of the main trunk of the internal iliac vessels medial to the vesicohypogastric fascia is dissected, exposing the surface of these vessels. This area has relatively small volume of adipose tissue, but frequently carries metastatic nodes [15]. Complete removal of the lymphatic tissue in this area is important exposing the inferior vesical vessels.

Final Check and Drain Placement

The harvested lymph node tissues are removed from the abdomen with a plastic bag. It is important to inspect the specimen and ensure that targeted enlarged lymph nodes are harvested within the specimen before finishing the procedure, since metastatic nodes may adhere to the inferior vesical vessels or neurovascular bundle and are occasionally left in situ. If this is the case, combined resection of inferior vesical vessels or neurovascular bundle is needed. Finally, a drain is placed in the TME space.

Combined Resection of Vessels and Nerves in LPLND

Metastatic lateral nodes often involve or abut vesical branches of the internal iliac vessels. Particularly, the inferior vesical artery and vein are the most commonly involved as this is the most frequent metastatic site. Sometimes, the main trunk of the internal iliac artery/vein or pelvic nerve plexus are involved by large metastatic nodes. In either case, involved vessels and nerves must be resected. When the enlarged node involves the inferior vesical vessels, these vessels are resected preserving the main trunk of the internal iliac vessels and autonomic nerves. The vesical vessels are ligated at the root from the internal iliac vessels and distally at the entry point to the bladder. The umbilical artery can also be ligated to make the procedure easier. Dissection follows the lateral, medial, and dorsal planes, and *en bloc* combined dissection of the obturator and internal iliac lymph nodes is performed (Fig. 11.4).

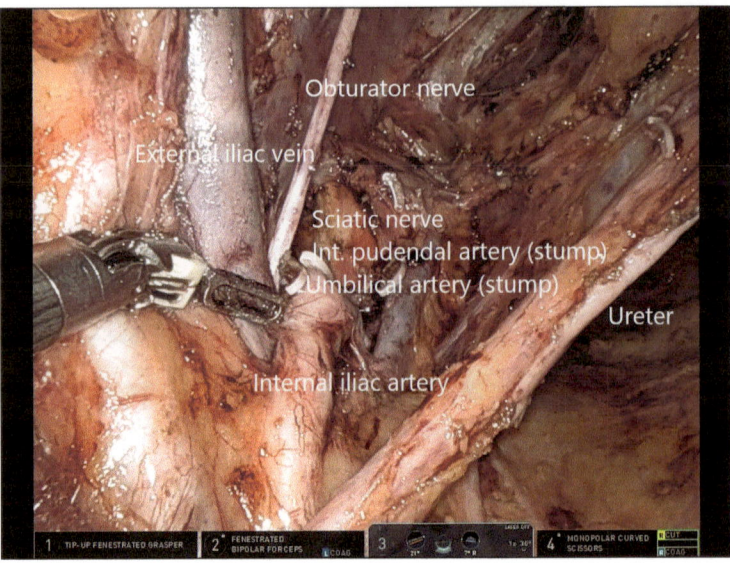

Fig. 11.4 Combined resection of the internal iliac artery including the main trunk and vesical arteries with preservation of the pelvic nerve plexus. Obturator and internal iliac areas were dissected in an *en bloc* fashion

When the metastatic nodes involve the main trunk of the internal iliac artery, it is ligated distal to the superior gluteal artery and distally at the entry point to the infra-piriformis muscle foramen. In this case, the dorsal dissection plane follows the surface of internal iliac vein and sciatic nerve. When the main trunk of the internal iliac vein is involved, dissection requires tremendous technical skill. Proximal ligation is similar with the artery, but the distal portion of the internal iliac vein often has multiple perforating branches to the pelvic wall. These must be carefully ligated to avoid bleeding. In this case, the dorsal dissection plane follows the sciatic nerve and piriformis muscle.

Postoperative genitourinary function after LPLND

Postoperative urinary or sexual dysfunction has been the biggest concern after LPLND. However, such genitourinary complications can be minimized by modern nerve-preserving techniques in LPLND. A secondary analysis after Japanese randomized controlled study reported no statistical differences in sexual and urinary dysfunction by adding LPLND to TME [12, 13]. For preservation of genitourinary function, careful preservation of the hypogastric nerve, pelvic nerve plexus and neurovascular bundle is important. Temporary urinary retention usually recovers in

1–2 weeks in unilateral LPLND as the counter side pelvic autonomic nerve and vesical vessels are preserved.

Conclusions

LPLND is a great armamentarium of colorectal surgeons in the setting of referral centers in combination with multidisciplinary management of rectal cancer. A robotic approach provides more precise dissection and improved visualization of pelvic anatomy particularly outside of the TME. Standardization of this procedure through a robotic approach may facilitate the dissection and provide optimal early and onco-logical outcomes. However, before such technique is implemented into clinical prac-tice, formal training with structured courses and most likely cadaveric dissections are to be considered to abbreviate learning curves and decrease the risk of intraoperative complications/injuries in early adoption phases. As refinement of precise indication for the procedure evolves, selection of ideal candidates will further achieve optimal outcomes.

References

1. Kim TH, Jeong SY, Choi DH, Kim DY, Jung KH, Moon SH, et al. Lateral lymph node metas-tasis is a major cause of locoregional recurrence in rectal cancer treated with preoperative chemoradiotherapy and curative resection. Ann Surg Oncol. 2008;15(3):729–37.
2. Kusters M, Slater A, Muirhead R, Hompes R, Guy RJ, Jones OM, et al. What to do with lateral nodal disease in low locally advanced rectal cancer? A call for further reflection and research. Dis Colon Rectum. 2017;60(6):577–85.
3. Kim MJ, Chan Park S, Kim TH, Kim DY, Kim SY, Baek JY, et al. Is lateral pelvic node dissec-tion necessary after preoperative chemoradiotherapy for rectal cancer patients with initially suspected lateral pelvic node? Surgery. 2016;160(2):366–76.
4. Kim MJ, Kim TH, Kim DY, Kim SY, Baek JY, Chang HJ, et al. Can chemoradiation allow for omission of lateral pelvic node dissection for locally advanced rectal cancer? J Surg Oncol. 2015;111(4):459–64.
5. Akiyoshi T, Toda S, Tominaga T, Oba K, Tomizawa K, Hanaoka Y, et al. Prognostic impact of residual lateral lymph node metastasis after neoadjuvant (chemo)radiotherapy in patients with advanced low rectal cancer. BJS Open. 2019;3(6):822–9.
6. Akiyoshi T, Ueno M, Matsueda K, Konishi T, Fujimoto Y, Nagayama S, et al. Selective lateral pelvic lymph node dissection in patients with advanced low rectal cancer treated with preoperative chemoradiotherapy based on pretreatment imaging. Ann Surg Oncol. 2014;21(1):189–96.
7. Ogura A, Konishi T, Cunningham C, Garcia-Aguilar J, Iversen H, Toda S, et al. Neoadjuvant (Chemo)radiotherapy with total mesorectal excision only is not sufficient to prevent lateral local recurrence in enlarged nodes: results of the multicenter lateral node study of patients with low cT3/4 rectal cancer. J Clin Oncol. 2019;37(1):33–43.
8. Lambregts DMJ, Bogveradze N, Blomqvist LK, Fokas E, Garcia-Aguilar J, Glimelius B, et al. Current controversies in TNM for the radiological staging of rectal cancer and how to deal with them: results of a global online survey and multidisciplinary expert consensus. Eur Radiol. 2022.

9. Kobayashi H, Mochizuki H, Kato T, Mori T, Kameoka S, Shirouzu K, et al. Outcomes of surgery alone for lower rectal cancer with and without pelvic sidewall dissection. Dis Colon Rectum. 2009;52(4):567–76.
10. Ueno H, Mochizuki H, Hashiguchi Y, Ishiguro M, Miyoshi M, Kajiwara Y, et al. Potential prognostic benefit of lateral pelvic node dissection for rectal cancer located below the peritoneal reflection. Ann Surg. 2007;245(1):80–7.
11. Liang JT. Technical feasibility of laparoscopic lateral pelvic lymph node dissection for patients with low rectal cancer after concurrent chemoradiation therapy. Ann Surg Oncol. 2011;18(1):153–9.
12. Ito M, Kobayashi A, Fujita S, Mizusawa J, Kanemitsu Y, Kinugasa Y, et al. Urinary dysfunction after rectal cancer surgery: results from a randomized trial comparing mesorectal excision with and without lateral lymph node dissection for clinical stage II or III lower rectal cancer (Japan Clinical Oncology Group Study, JCOG0212). Eur J Surg Oncol. 2018;44(4):463–8.
13. Saito S, Fujita S, Mizusawa J, Kanemitsu Y, Saito N, Kinugasa Y, et al. Male sexual dysfunction after rectal cancer surgery: results of a randomized trial comparing mesorectal excision with and without lateral lymph node dissection for patients with lower rectal cancer: Japan Clinical Oncology Group Study JCOG0212. Eur J Surg Oncol. 2016;42(12):1851–8.
14. Vailati BB, Juliao GPS, Mattacheo A, Habr-Gama A, Konishi T, Perez RO. Temporary lower-limb paresis due to excessive obturator nerve manipulation during lateral pelvic node dissection in rectal cancer surgery. Dis Colon Rectum. 2022;65(2): e71.
15. Schaap DP, Boogerd LSF, Konishi T, Cunningham C, Ogura A, Garcia-Aguilar J, et al. Rectal cancer lateral lymph nodes: multicentre study of the impact of obturator and internal iliac nodes on oncological outcomes. Br J Surg. 2021;108(2):205–13.

Chapter 12
Robotic Transanal Total Mesorectal Excision (taTME)

John Marks, Jane Yang, Rafael Perez, and Elizabeth Spitz

Abstract The treatment of low rectal cancers with the intention of sphincter preservation can be challenging given the anatomy of the pelvis and the ability to obtain adequate distal margins. Transanal total mesorectal excision (taTME) was developed to treat such cancers with good oncologic outcomes while preserving sphincter function after chemoradiation. Techniques for taTME have evolved significantly with the advent of new technology. This chapter illustrates the step-by-step procedure for performing taTME using the single port robot.

Keywords Robotic colorectal surgery · Transanal total mesorectal excision · Transanal abdominal transanal proctosigmoidectomy · Single-port robotics · Rectal cancer

Introduction

Operative treatment of low rectal cancers is difficult. Given the confines of the bony pelvis, it is difficult to achieve adequate distal and lateral margins without the need for a permanent colostomy. As the funnel of the pelvis narrows towards the anus, the space between the pelvic sidewall and the mesorectum becomes smaller, making the achievement of negative lateral margins challenging. The loss of a palpable mass when tumors respond to preoperative chemoradiation compounds the difficulty of obtaining negative margins at this time with respect to an adequate distal margin.

J. Marks (✉) · J. Yang · R. Perez · E. Spitz
Division of Colorectal Surgery, Lankenau Medical Center, Main Line Health, Wynnewood, PA, USA
e-mail: marksj@mlhs.org

J. Yang
e-mail: janeyangmd@gmail.com

R. Perez
e-mail: perezre@upmc.edu

E. Spitz
e-mail: spitzelizabeth96@gmail.com

By starting the dissection transanally, a known distal margin is assured by identifying residual scar and by relationship to fixed rectal landmarks identified pretreatment (rectal valves, anorectal ring/levators, and dentate line), and the most difficult portion of the operation is done first. Transanal total mesorectal excision (taTME) has expanded our capability of curing unfavorable low rectal cancers with sphincter preservation after high-dose chemoradiation [1]. A variety of approaches exist to perform TME surgery; open, laparoscopic, and robotic taTME can be performed. In our unit, our general approach is as follows: laparoscopic TME for tumors in the upper 1/3 of the rectum, Xi Robotic TME for tumors in the mid rectum, and taTME is ideally suited for cancers in the distal 3 cm, or lower 1/3 of the rectum.

Our approach has evolved over the last two decades, from laparoscopic TATA combining abdominal laparoscopy with an open transanal approach, to a flexible tip laparoscopic taTME approach, and now to robotic taTME using the single port robot (SP rTaTME) [2]. The 3D visualization, three-armed retraction and superior ergonomics provide tremendous advantage to the operative team. Here, we describe the setup and technique for taTME using a single port robot.

SP rTaTME Setup

Positioning

We prefer to position the patient prior to induction of anaesthesia. By engaging the patient, we ensure their maximum comfort and avoid pressure points. Patients' arms are tucked at their sides and padded. Their legs are placed in an extended lithotomy position. It is important to position the torso and legs so that the anus is overhangs the edge of the bed by four centimetres, providing the surgical team easy access to the anal canal. After induction of anaesthesia, a foley catheter is inserted and the patient is secured to the table with chest straps and tape. Shoulder bolsters are never used to position patients as they can lead to brachial plexus injury. It is important to ensure the patient is properly secured to the table, as the operation will require steep Trendelenberg and table tilting. The entire abdomen and perineum are prepped and draped in the standard sterile fashion (Fig. 12.1).

OR Layout

When docking the SP robot transanally, it is important to have a clear path for the robot to dock in between the patient's legs. Depending on the size of the OR, this may require turning the OR table at an angle to accommodate the path of the robot. We prefer that the robotic tower, laparoscopic tower and insufflation be positioned on the patient's left to maximize working space.

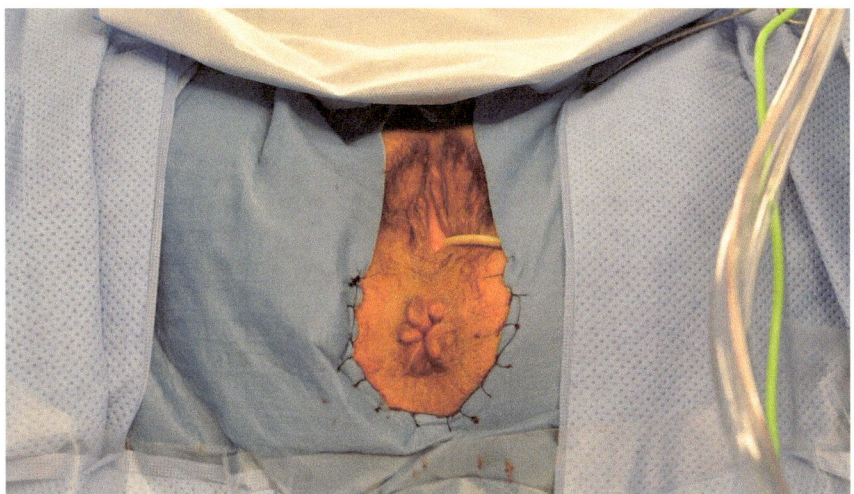

Fig. 12.1 Lithotomy position and draping of the perineum

Equipment Needed

Intersphincteric Dissection

1. Lighted bovie and suction/irrigator
2. Allis-Adair clamps
3. Richardson retractors
4. Deaver retractors

Robotic taTME

1. GelPOINT path transanal access platform
2. 25 mm SP robotic trocar
3. 5 mm AirSeal port for insufflation

Intraabdominal Portion

1. Standard laparoscopic instruments based on surgeon's preference
2. This could also be performed using a single port laparoscopic approach through the temporary ileostomy site or done robotically.

Steps of the Procedure

Open Transanal Intersphincteric Dissection

We begin by infiltrating the perianal skin and levator musculature with Xylocaine-epinephrine solution to minimize bleeding. The dissection is started by incising the mucosa circumferentially at the level of the dentate line using electrocautery. Completing this circumferentially and with care to avoid any mucosal bridges at the beginning helps to avoid radial tears at the distal margin during later dissection. To aid in this dissection, one can use Allis-Adair clamps at 12, 3, 6, and 9 o'clock to retract the perianal skin (Fig. 12.2), and a small Richardson retractor can be used to better visualize the dentate line. Some surgeons prefer to use a lone star retractor, but we find that the hooks often pierced our gloves or skin and therefore have avoided using the lone star.

Next, the Metzenbaum scissors are used to spread the tissue just off of the posterior midline to enter the full-thickness of the internal anal sphincter and into the intersphincteric plane. It is important to see the glistening white of the endopelvic fascia of the puborectalis (Fig. 12.3). This confirms identification of the correct plane of dissection between the levator ani complex and the mesorectum. It is critically important to be in the correct plane from both an oncologic and functional standpoint. If the dissection is carried out too superficially, the muscularis propria

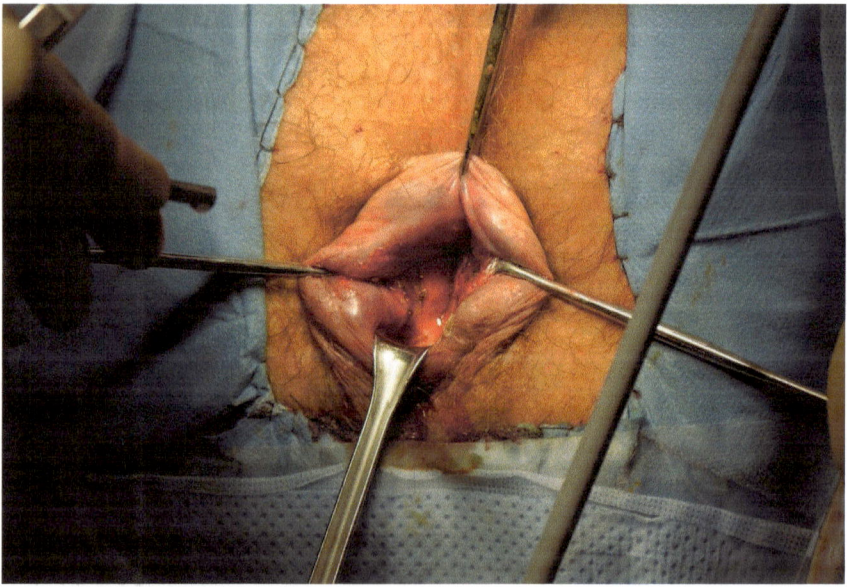

Fig. 12.2 Allis-Adair clamps at 12, 3, 6, and 9 o'clock

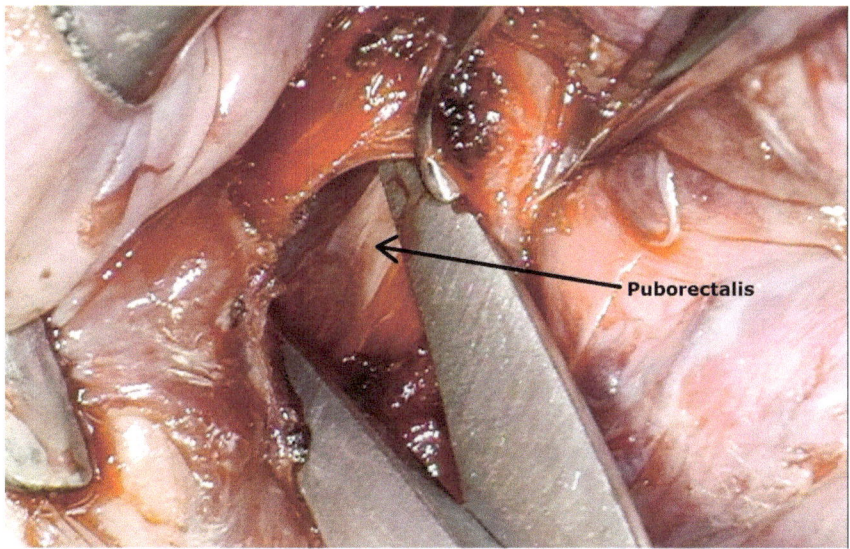

Puborectalis

Fig. 12.3 Intersphincteric dissection showing the puborectalis

or mesorectum is violated and oncologic outcomes are affected. Straying too deep can injure the puborectalis and cause significant bleeding intraoperatively and/or postoperative fecal incontinence.

After entering the correct plane, we place an Allis-Adair on the transected rectum and a baby Deaver retractor into the intersphincteric space to place the area of dissection on stretch. The dissection is carried circumferentially perpendicular to the axis of the anal canal and superiorly. Usually, we perform the lateral dissection on the left and right first, leaving the anterior dissection for last as this is typically the hardest part of the procedure. During the anterior dissection in men, the infraprostatic urethra and prostate must be identified and protected. In women, the anterior dissection can be facilitated by placing a finger into the vagina to better palpate the rectovaginal septum (Fig. 12.4). We prefer to carry the dissection as cephalad as possible during the open transanal portion; usually to the level of the cervix in women and the seminal vesicles in men.

The rectum is then sutured closed in a watertight fashion using an imbricating 0-Vicryl suture. The suture is placed in a seromuscular fashion on the mesorectum to invert the transected end of the anus (Fig. 12.5 a, b). The edges are turned inward using a horizontal-mattress suture; it is important to tighten after each stitch is placed to avoid contamination of the field with fecal matter or malignant cells. It is highly likely that problems achieving a watertight luminal closure played a large part in tumor spreading that lead to the Norwegian Moratorium of taTME. After completing the rectal stump closure, we proceed with the robotic SP rTaTME portion.

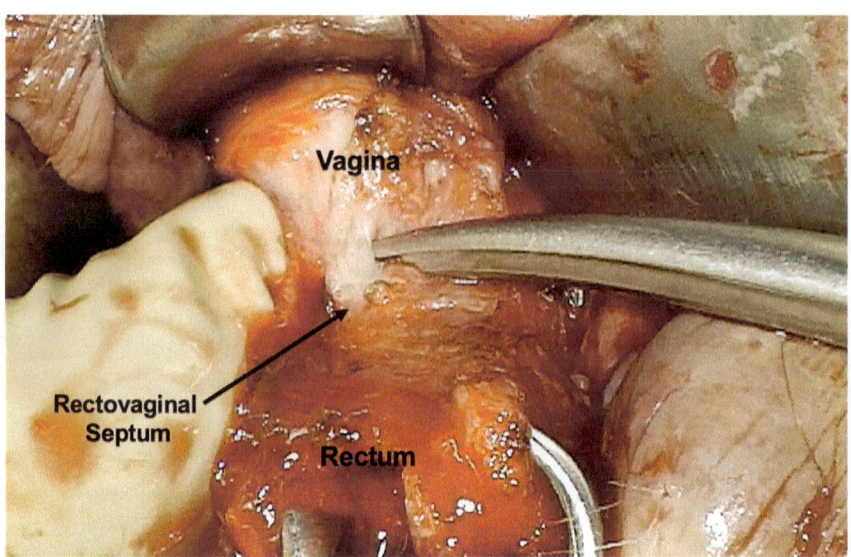

Fig. 12.4 Anterior intersphincteric dissection

SP Robotic Transanal TME (SP rTaTME)

A GelPOINT Path Transanal Access Channel is inserted transanally and secured to the perianal skin. A 25 mm DaVinci SP Trocar and a 5 mm AirSeal trocar are placed in a GelSeal Cap which is then secured to the access channel. The patient's legs are lowered so that the hips are slightly flexed to allow space for the robot arm. The DaVinci SP robot is brought in between the patient's legs and docked (Fig. 12.6). The robot is aligned so that the axis of the instrument cluster is along the axis of the rectum. This will allow movement of the instruments without friction. It is also important to ensure that the robotic boom is not fully extended prior to docking. This is how we ensure that there is sufficient space for the robot to extend as the dissection is carried cephalad and avoid the need to undock and redock multiple times. After docking, insufflation is started and the SP robotic camera is inserted (Fig. 12.7). We use Monopolar Scissors, Bipolar Fenestrated Forceps, and Cadiere forceps in arms 1, 2, and 3, respectively (Fig. 12.8) [3].

The taTME dissection is carried out in a circumferential fashion using sharp dissection with the monopolar scissors in arm 1 and bipolar fenestrated graspers in arm 2. By doing this, the avascular areolar tissue planes are encountered that define the proper plane of dissection (Fig. 12.9) and ensure a relatively bloodless plane. If small bleeders are encountered, monopolar energy can be used. It is important to note that if significant bleeding is encountered, the surgeon should re-evaluate the plane of dissection, but can use bipolar energy to obtain hemostasis. An additional benefit of sharp dissection is that it avoids creating smoke which, even in small quantities, can

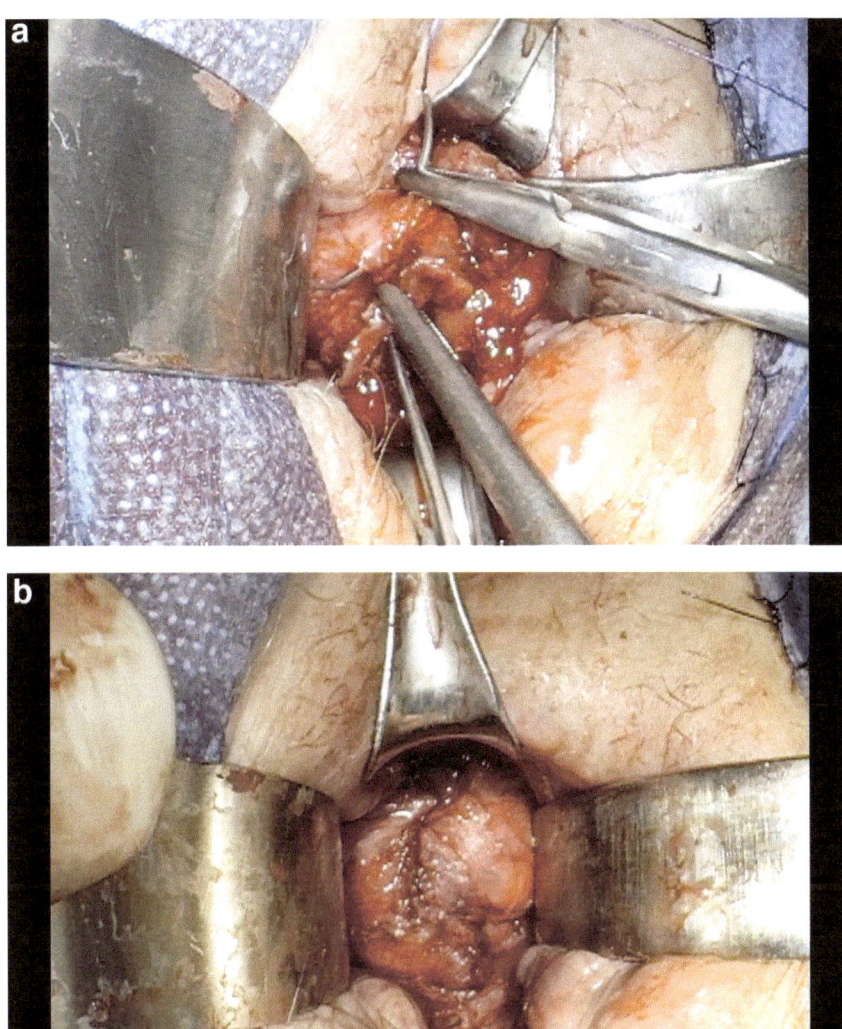

Fig. 12.5 **a** Closure of the rectum with seromuscular horizontal mattress sutures. **b** Final watertight closure of the rectum

severely limit visualization in the confines of the pelvis. We use Cadiere Forceps in the third arm of the robot to facilitate the dissection by providing constant retraction on the rectum readjusting as needed.

We start with the anterior dissection, taking care releasing the rectum from the vagina or prostate. This is particularly important for anteriorly based tumors, in which prior radiation treatment may obscure the proper planes. The dissection continues

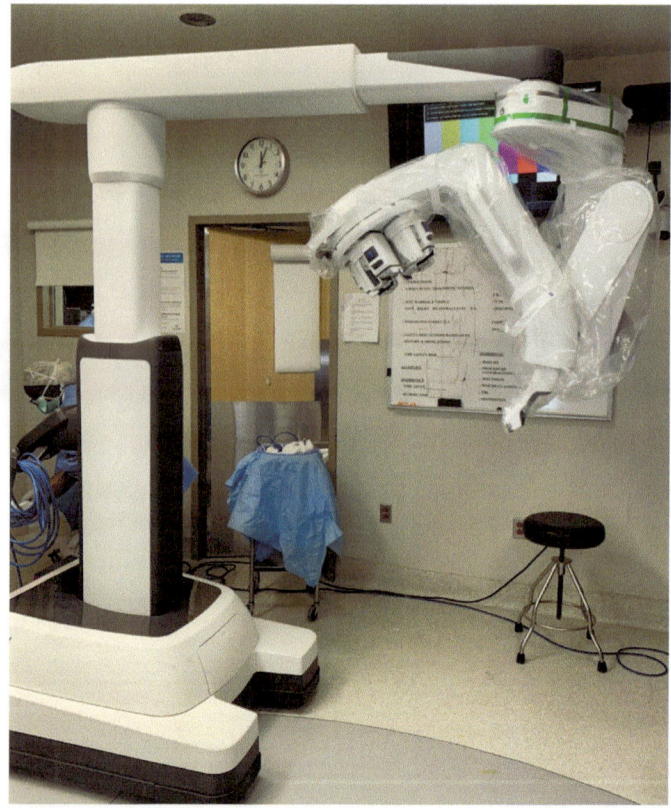

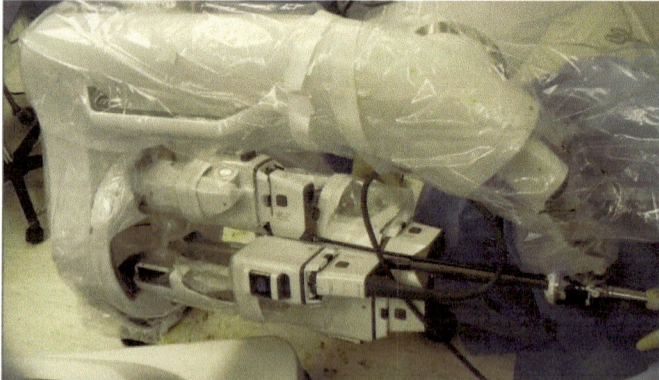

Fig. 12.6 Single port robot with the instrument channels turned for transanal surgery

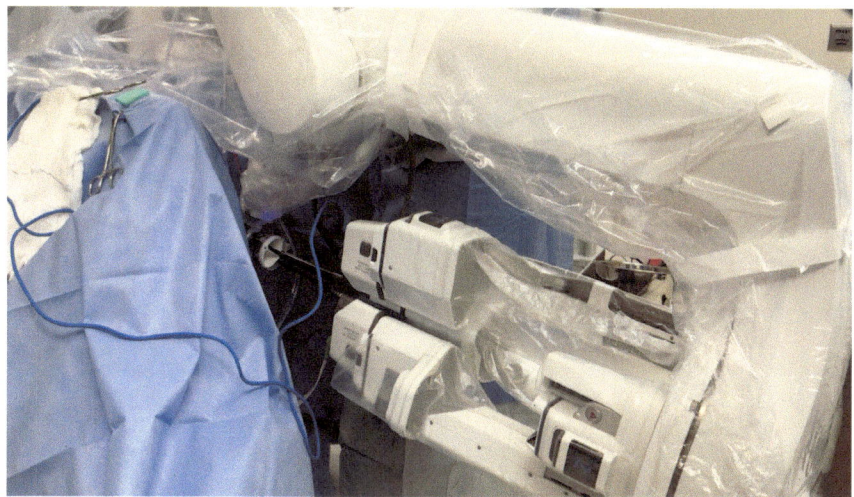

Fig. 12.7 Single port robot docked transanally

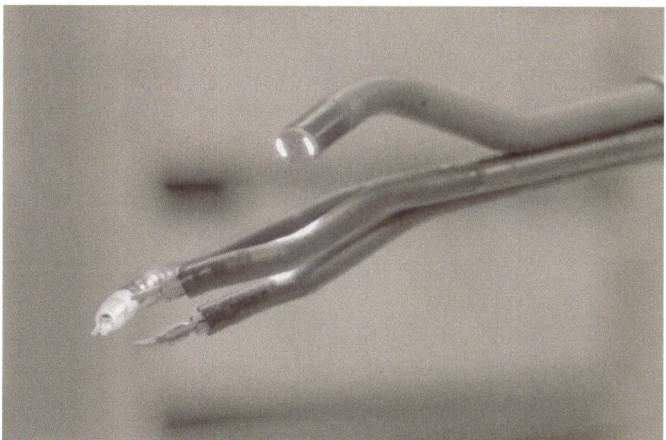

Fig. 12.8 Flexible three arms of the single port robot

in the posterior plane in a similar fashion. In the posterior midline, it is important to remember that the presacral hollow curves superiorly, and if dissection is taken straight back and fails to follow the curve of the sacrum, the presacral veins will be injured and significant bleeding is possible. Lastly, the lateral attachments are dissected. However, as the dissection is carried cephalad, the surgeon must continually reorient himself/herself and avoid straying laterally into the obturator fossa. The dissection continues in this circumferential fashion after entering through the peritoneum.

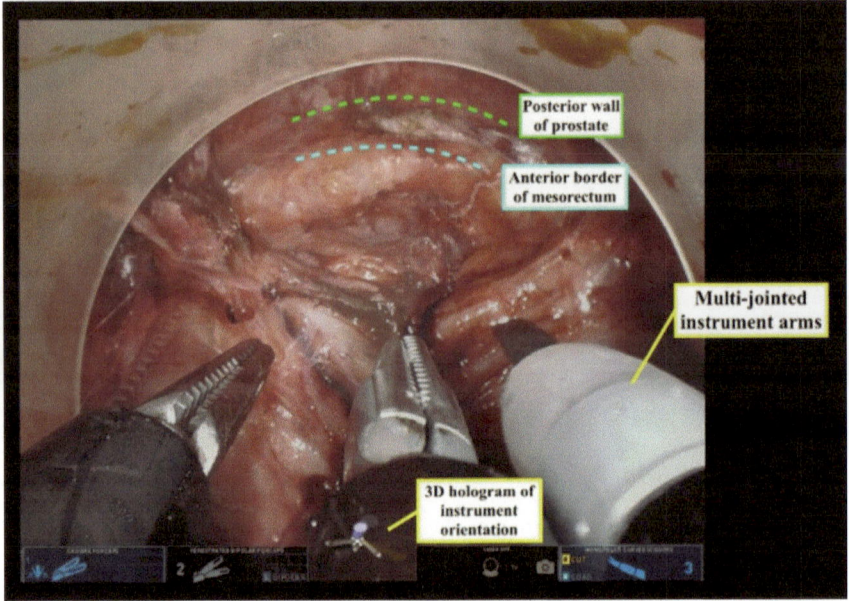

Fig. 12.9 SP robotic transanal view of the plane of dissection

The transanal portion of the procedure is complete after dissecting out the mesorectum completely up to the sacral promontory (Fig. 12.10). The SP robot is then undocked, gowns and gloves are changed, and we proceed with the transabdominal portion of the procedure. If an area of anatomy is unclear, that attachment is left to be approached transabdominally.

Transabdominal Portion

The transabdominal portion can be completed laparoscopically or robotically and can be performed simultaneously with the transanal dissection via a two-team approach. However, when using the SP robot transanally, we find that it is difficult to position the table to facilitate a two-team approach. Regardless of the approach selected, the transabdominal portion proceeds in a similar step-wise, reproducible fashion completing eight defined steps [4].

Step One: Splenic Flexure Takedown. We begin by mobilizing the splenic flexure in a supramesocolic fashion. The table is positioned with 5° of reverse Trendelenberg and 18° right tilt. The lesser sac is entered and dissection is carried medial to lateral. Following this, we mobilize the upper portion of the white line of Toldt, developing the fusion plane between the descending mesocolon and retroperitoneum to release the descending colon toward the midline. The splenic flexure mesenteric release is

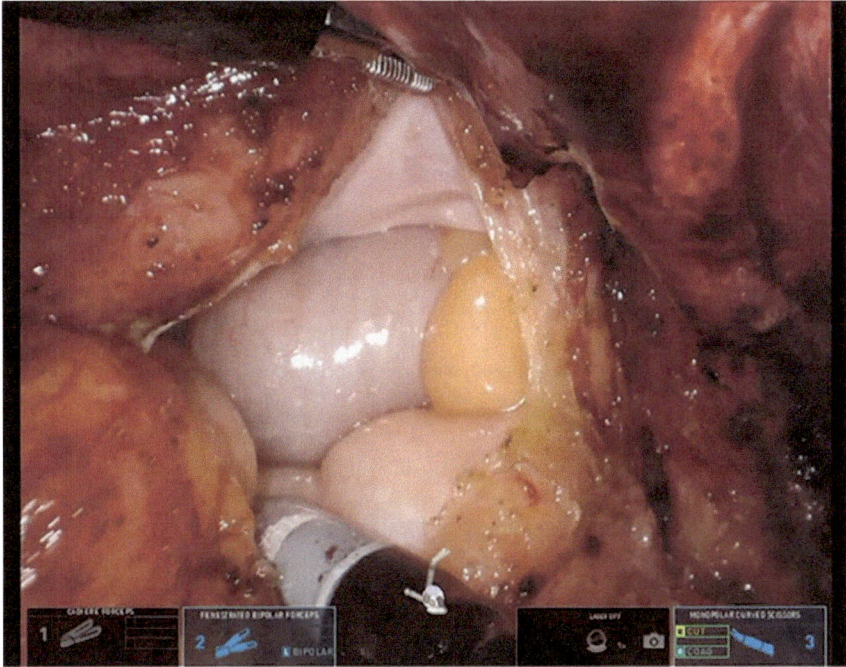

Fig. 12.10 Entering into the peritoneum transanally

facilitated by incising the peritoneal membrane 1 cm from the inferior border of the pancreas.

Step Two: Positioning of the Small Bowel. Next, the patient is positioned in 18° Trendelenberg and 18° right tilt to use gravity to help displace the small bowel and omentum from the pelvis. The greater omentum is retracted cephalad up and over the transverse colon which helps to "corral" it in the upper abdomen. The small bowel is retracted toward the right and superiorly to expose the IMA, IMV, and the pelvis.

Step Three: High Ligation of the Inferior Mesenteric Artery (IMA) and Vein (IMV). We then incise the peritoneum from the sacral promontory (at Gruber's ligament) to the duodenojejunal junction. By opening this superficially, it allows for pneumodissection to proceed in the embryologic fusion plane. The sigmoid colon mesentery is retracted anteriorly, and the hypogastric nerves are identified and swept posteriorly. This establishes a proper plane of orientation and will allow identification of the left ureter, followed by the gonadal vessels lateral to this. The key to the dissection is to identify the hypogastric nerves and sweep them posterior to protect the nerves and direct the dissection into the proper plane.

The IMA is dissected circumferentially and transected with a bipolar energy device, *proximal to the takeoff* of the left colic artery. It is important to visualize the back of the bipolar device to avoid inadvertent injury to the left ureter. We advocate placing an Endotie on the IMA stump in patients with a history of coronary or peripheral vascular disease or hypertension because of the higher incidence of vessel calcification and vessel sealer failure. The IMV is identified centrally, inferior to the lower border of the pancreas, dissected free, and transected in a similar manner.

Step Four: Mobilization of the Left Colon. Remaining attachments in the avascular plane between the colon mesentery and the retroperitoneum are divided working cephalad to meet with the mobilized splenic flexure. Much of this dissection has already been carried out in the medial to lateral dissection in the previous step. Finally, we complete the left colon mobilization by dividing the white line of Toldt and releasing the sigmoid colon attachments laterally.

Step Five: Complete the Pelvic TME. In many cases, this has already been completed from below. If not, the aim of this step is to join with the TME initiated transanally. The right and left pararectal sulci are incised. The hypogastric nerves direct the dissection as they are swept posteriorly as we dissect in the posterior midline until we meet the dissection from below. The mesorectum is retracted cephalad and to the left shoulder, and the hypogastric nerves and nervi erigentes are used as a landmark to carry the dissection down toward the pelvis and finish the dissection on the right side. This is completed in a similar fashion on the left, retracting the rectum up to the right shoulder to put this area on stretch. The mesorectum is fully mobilized circumferentially and is in continuity with the dissection from below. The rectum is brought out of the pelvis. The pelvis is inspected and hemostasis is achieved.

Step Six: Exteriorization of the Rectum and Sigmoid Colon. The mesentery of the descending colon is divided transversely from the level of the transected IMA to the sigmoid-descending colon junction. A suture or cautery mark is placed to identify the transection line at what will become the neorectum. An assistant inserts a Babcock clamp transanally to grasp the transected distal rectum (at the imbricating suture line), and under intraabdominal visualization and guidance, the rectum and sigmoid colon are delivered transanally, taking great care to assure the descending colon mesentery is not twisted or on tension.

Step Seven: Colon Transection, Coloanal Anastomosis (Specimen Delivery). The marked area of the colon is opened anteriorly as coloanal anastomotic sutures are first placed in the four cardinal positions at 12, 3, 6, and 9 o-clock. It is important to not completely transect the rectum before placing any sutures in order to prevent the neorectum from retracting back into the pelvis. A full thickness bite of the colon wall is taken with an 0-Vicryl stitch that is then passed through the previously transected anterior wall of the internal sphincter and anal mucosa. The remainder of the colon is transected, and a stitch is placed at the posterior midline. The four cardinal sutures are each secured with a hemostat to the drape and not tied. One to three additional sutures are placed between each of the cardinal position sutures being sure to take a full-thickness bite of the colon wall and of the internal sphincter and mucosa and are tied. Once these are complete, the cardinal stitches are tied. A visual inspection and a digital rectal examination are performed to confirm there are no defects in the anastomosis.

Step Eight: Loop Ileostomy Creation. After completing the coloanal anastomosis, gowns, gloves, and instruments are changed. We re-enter the abdomen, insufflate, and take one final look transabdominally. It is important to confirm again the neorectum is properly oriented, the mesentery is not on stretch, and there is no small bowl herniated under the mesentery of the left colon. Once this is done, the pelvis is irrigated and hemostasis is ascertained. A loop of distal ileum, approximately 20 cm proximal to the ileocecal valve, is brought out through the right lower quadrant with care taken to ensure proper orientation. It is then matured over a red rubber catheter in a standard Brooke fashion.

References

1. Marks JH, Salem JF. From TATA to NOTES, how taTME fits into the evolutionary surgical tree. Tech Coloproctol. 2016;20(8):513–5. https://doi.org/10.1007/s10151-016-1504-9.
2. Marks JH, Lopez-Acevedo N, Krishnan B, Johnson MN, Montenegro GA, Marks GJ. True NOTES TME resection with splenic flexure release, high ligation of IMA, and side-to-end hand-sewn coloanal anastomosis. Surg Endosc. 2016;30(10):4626–31. https://doi.org/10.1007/s00464-015-4731-7.
3. Marks JH, Salem JF, Adams P, et al. SP rTaTME: initial clinical experience with single-port robotic transanal total mesorectal excision (SP rTaTME). Tech Coloproctol. 2021;25(6):721–6. https://doi.org/10.1007/s10151-021-02449-0.
4. Marks JH, Perez RE, Salem JF. Robotic transanal surgery for rectal cancer. Clin Colon Rectal Surg. 2021;34(5):317–24. https://doi.org/10.1055/s-0041-1729864.
5. Knol J, Keller DS. Total mesorectal excision technique-past, present, and future. Clin Colon Rectal Surg. 2020;33(3):134–43. https://doi.org/10.1055/s-0039-3402776.

Chapter 13
Transanal Surgery and Single Port Robotic Platform

Tony W. C. Mak, Kaori Futaba, and Simon S. M. Ng

Abstract Colorectal cancer remains to be one of the commonest cancer in both developed and developing countries. The surgical management of rectal cancer has inherent technical challenges. To date, ingenious minimally invasive techniques such as TAMIS and taTME have been developed via conventional laparoscopic instruments or multiport platforms. These techniques have helped to solve some of the problems with difficult rectal surgeries but few remains. This chapter introduces the da Vinci single-port robotic platform with its indications, technical aspects, benefits and limitations for tran-sanal surgery.

Keywords TAMIS · taTME · Robotic surgery · Rectal cancer · Rectal neoplasm

Background/Introduction

Colorectal cancer has become the world's fourth most deadly cancer with almost 900,000 deaths annually [1]. In a study of anatomical distribution of colorectal cancers over a 10-year period, left sided colorectal cancers (defined as descending colon, sigmoid and rectum) represent 69%, with rectum being the most common site [2]. Operative treatments of rectal cancer have been proven to show better oncological results and survival benefits over other forms of therapy [3]. Surgery on rectal cancers can be difficult owing to the fact that most of the cases are narrow obese male pelvis, bulky tumour and which may have had neoadjuvant chemoradiotherapy. These difficulties in turn can translate to increased morbidity, positive resection margins and increased rate of local cancer recurrance, which may decrease survival. Recently Transanal Surgery has provided a surgical solution for both benign rectal polyps, early rectal cancers and advanced rectal cancers via a natural orifice. The Technique of Transanal total mesorectal excision (taTME) has provided a surgical alternative for unfavorable low rectal cancers with an aim for sphincter preserving surgery, decreased anastomotic leak rate with single staple anastomosis and more

T. W. C. Mak (✉) · K. Futaba · S. S. M. Ng
Division of Colorectal Surgery, The Department of Surgery, The Chinese University of Hong Kong, Hong Kong S.A.R., China
e-mail: tonymak@surgery.cuhk.edu.hk

© The Author(s), under exclusive license to Springer Nature Switzerland AG 2022   147
P. Coyne and J. Khan (eds.), *Robotic Colorectal Surgery*,
https://doi.org/10.1007/978-3-031-15198-9_13

accurate distal margin. Various techniques have been used which involved different platforms with conventional laparoscopic equipment such as transanal endoscopic microsurgery (TEMS), transanal endoscopic operation (TEO) and transanal minimally invasive surgery (TAMIS) or robotically with different generations of multi-port platforms. Commonly encountered difficulties amongst the laparoscopic systems are the loss of triangulation with the use of straight laparoscopic instruments, limited space for the operator and assistant and the loss of endo-wrists technology, external arm clashing, two-arm restrictions for the multi-port robotic systems.

We began our journey with training of the SP system at the da Vinci Sunnyvale Laboratory with porcine and cadaveric models [4]. Since then, the SP system has proven to be feasible and safe for SILS abdominal and Transanal surgery [5]. We would like to share our experience in this chapter.

Da Vinci SP

The da Vinci SP *("Single Port")* (Fig. 13.1) has been designed and purpose built to overcome the existing problems with single port minimally invasive surgery as well as incorporating the technological advantages of robotic surgery.

The Da Vinci SP Surgical System (Intuitive Surgical, Inc.) consist of three main components as per current multi-ports Da Vinci Surgical Systems (S, Si and Xi): surgeon console, patient-side cart and the vision cart. However, where it differs from the other Da Vinci systems is that the Da Vinci SP mounts three 6 mm flexible double-jointed instrument arms along with a flexible dual-channel 3-D laparoscope into an entry guide into a 25 mm single port cannula on the patient-side cart (Fig. 13.2**a**).

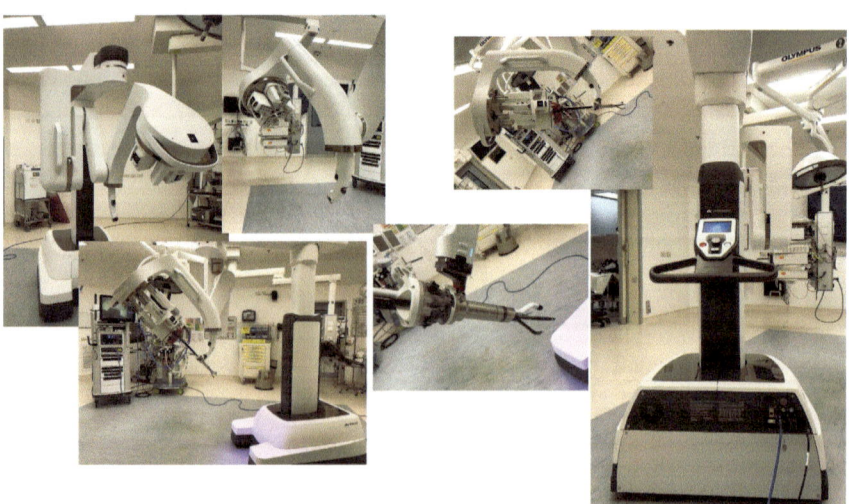

Fig. 13.1 Da Vinci SP system

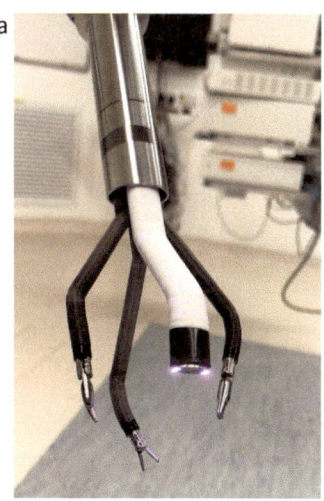 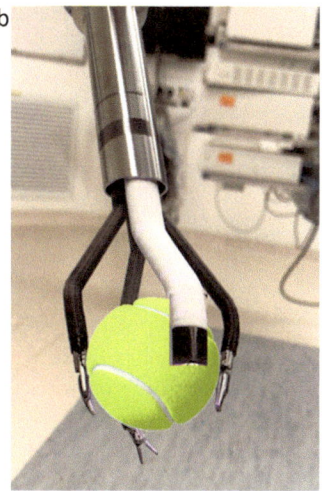

Fig. 13.2. a "Cobra-like" camera and three double-jointed instrument arms through the SP Cannula, which allow triangulation. **b** All instruments and arms work in the space of a tennis ball

On the surgeon console, there is an extra relocation pedal controls the movement of the instrument arm and at the central bottom of the screen there is a holographic navigator where the camera and arms are positioned which are colour-coded for optimal positioning.

There are seven 6 mm endowristed instruments available for the da vinci SP: monopolar curved scissors, monopolar cautery hook, Maryland bipolar forceps, fenestrated bipolar forceps, round tooth retractor, medium-large clip applier and needle driver.

One of the unique designs of the instrument arms is that they are double jointed (elbow/joggle and wrist joints) which creates triangulation of the instruments and camera which in turn improve handling, retraction and better view. However, one must note that both joints need to be inserted through the SP cannula before the surgery can benefit from this triangulation. Therefore, the end of the SP cannula cannot be too close to the surgical/target site for it to have the benefit of triangulation. During training of the SP, we were told to utilize the arms within a sphere of a tennis ball (Fig. 13.2b). This advice has helped us tremendously as it allows precision surgery to be done within a tight space.

Transanal Surgery

Transanal surgery with the da Vinci SP are mainly for: (1) Transanal surgery inside the rectum for benign rectal polyps or early rectal cancers in the form of TAMIS or (2) Transanal Total mesorectal excision. Some of the steps below are common to both techniques.

SP Transanal Surgery Setup

Patient Positioning

TAMIS: Patient is set-up supine in a modified lithotomy position. Both arms are secured by the patient and padded. We do not feel it is necessary to strap the patient as excessive Trendelenburg position is not required. A gel-pad is placed to lift the patient's sacrum in order for the anus to be accessible for the surgical team. Note that as for conventional TAMIS cases, it is not necessary to position the patient (left/right lateral or prone) according to the position of the rectal lesion. This is because the SP camera and instruments on the patient cart can rotate both clockwise and anticlockwise so that lesion is at its "sweet-spot" at 6 O'clock position.

TaTME: Patient can be set-up Trendelenburg with modified lithotomy position. Patient may also be tilted left-side up in order to facilitate abdominal colonic mobilisation by the abdominal team. In our practice, we did not feel the need for shoulder strap as it may cause brachial plexus injury and generally patients in Hong Kong do not have a high BMI. A gel-pad is placed to lift the patient's sacrum in order for the anus to be accessible for the surgical team.

Operating Theatre Layout

The Patient Cart of the SP is positioned at the patient's leg end. The path of the Patient Cart is approached and docked at right angle to the surgical table. This can be done both at right and left side of the patient. Once the Patient Cart is positioned, the boom is then lowered so the camera and instruments are at the level of the anal canal (Figs. 13.3, 13.4, 13.5 and 13.6).

Other Equipments

GelPOINT path transanal access platform (Applied Medical, USA).

AirSeal system with 5 mm port is used for a controlled insufflated view of the rectum or pelvis although this may be substituted with the Gelpoint path insufflation stablisation bag (ISB).

Lone star retractor system.

Laparoscopic suction/irrigation device.

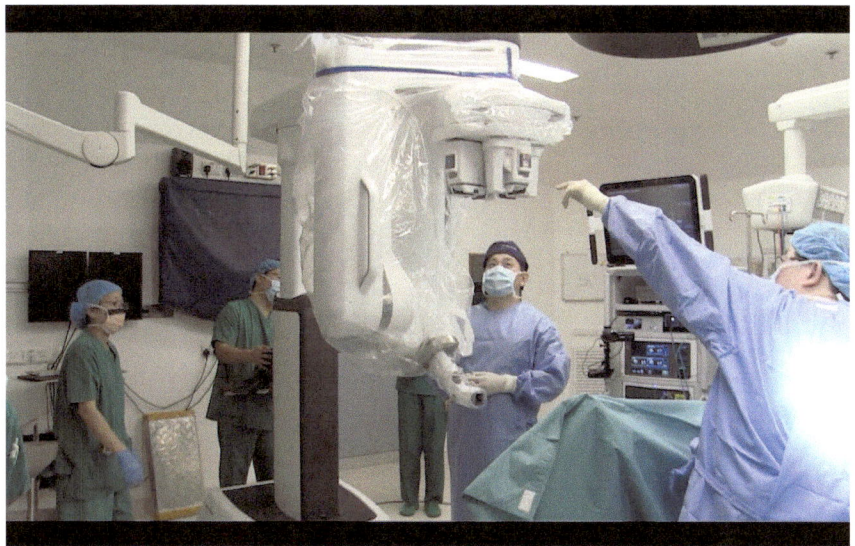

Fig. 13.3 Docking of the da Vinci SP with lowering of the boom for the alignment to the patient's rectum

Fig. 13.4 Insertion of the SP cannula, 5 mm AirSeal trocar and 5 mm port into the GelPoint cap

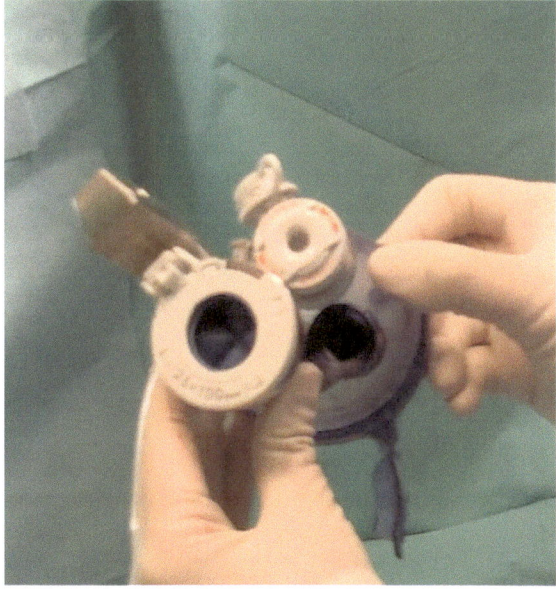

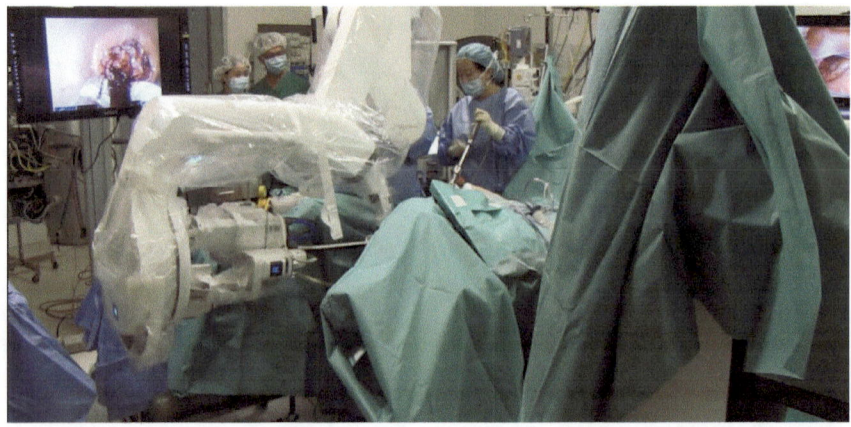

Fig. 13.5 da Vinci set up for Transanal surgery (TAMIS or TaTME)

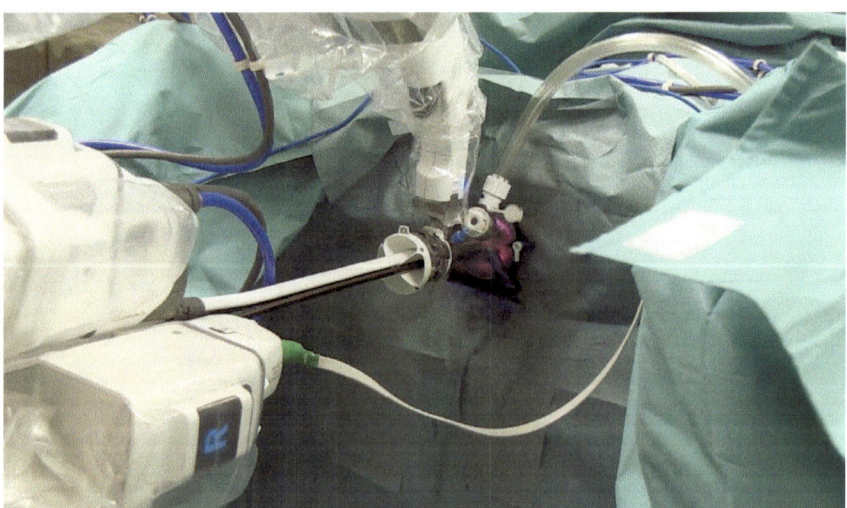

Fig. 13.6 Close up of Da Vinci SP performing transanal surgery (TAMIS or TaTME)

Additional energy device (e.g. ultrasonic energy or bipolar energy source).

Operative Steps

Transanal Minimally Invasive Surgery (TAMIS) (Fig. 13.7)

We begin by inserting the AirSeal 5 mm port, the 25 mm SP cannula port and × 1 5 mm port into silicon cap of the GelPOINT path. The GelPOINT path transanal access channel is inserted transanally and secured to the perianal skin. The da Vinci SP robot is then docked and aligned with the axis of the anorectum. Accurate alignment is important as it will optimize the positions of the flexible camera and 3 instrument arms inside the rectal cavity. 3 instruments used were: Arm 1-Monopolar scissors, Arm 2-Bipolar Fenestrated forceps and Arm 3-Cadiere forceps.

As the rectum is insufflated, the rectal lesion is then visualized. As mentioned above, rotating the SP so that the lesion is near the 6OC position will help with surgery. The dissection margin is marked with diathermy followed by excision of the lesion. The use of the three arms, with triangulation, provide better traction and easier for the surgeon to perform the operation. Diathermy from monopolar scissors or fenestrated bipolar forceps are used for haemostasis. Once the lesion is excised, the defect is then closed with barb sutures.

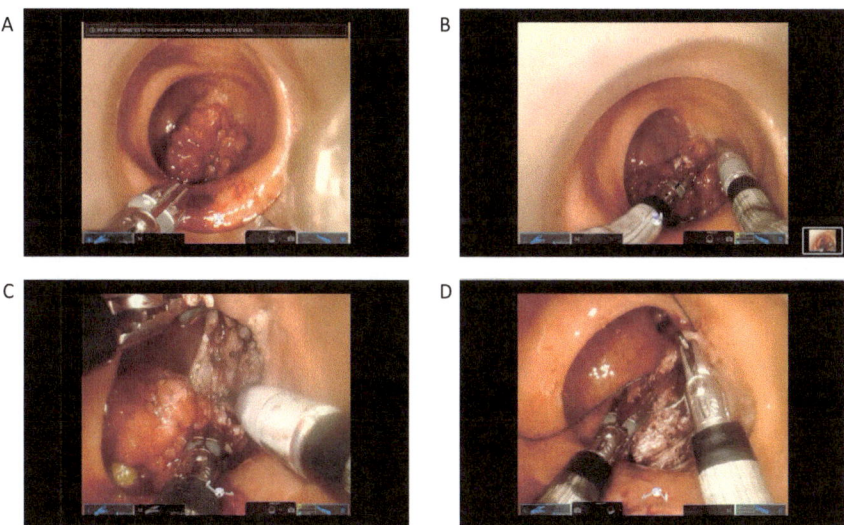

Fig. 13.7 Transanal Minimally Invasive Surgery (TAMIS): **a** Mid-rectal polyp **b** diathermy marking of dissection margin **c** partial thickness en-bloc dissection **d** defect closed with barb sutures

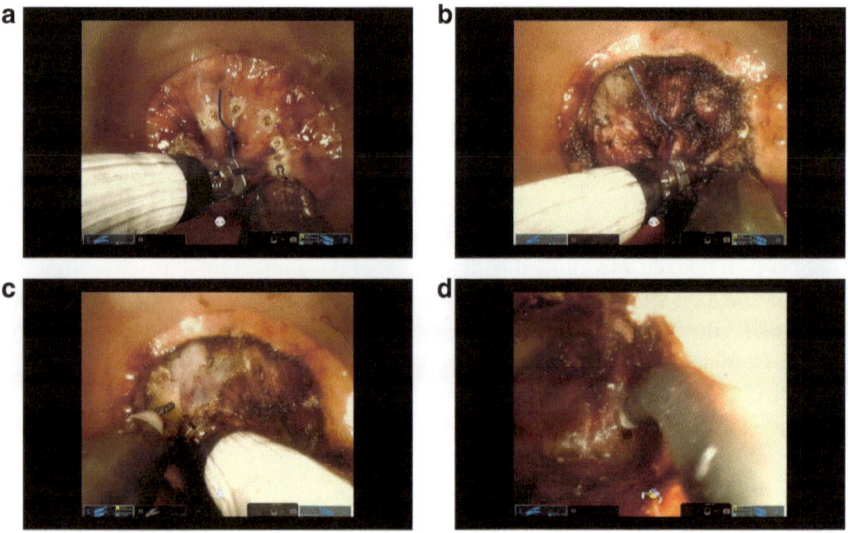

Fig. 13.8 Transanal Total Mesorectal Excision (TaTME): **a** Diathermy marking of the distal rectum for transection **b** Circumferential dissection **c** anterior dissection off the prostate **d** final dissection where "top meets bottom"

Transanal Total Mesorectal Excision (TaTME) (Fig. 13.8)

In TaTME, our unit practice the "two-team approach" with the abdominal part performed via conventional laparoscopic technique. For the "bottom approach", the insertion and setup are similar to TAMIS where the AirSeal 5 mm port, the 25 mm SP cannula port and × 1 5 mm port into silicon cap of the GelPOINT path. The GelPOINT path transanal access channel is inserted transanally and secured to the perianal skin. Prior to docking, distal margin of the tumour is identified and double tied with 2/0 PDS. The da Vinci SP docking and alignment needs to be on the same axis as the patient's anorectum (usually left tilt and head down). For the initial part of the dissection, two instrument arms are used instead of three in order to avoid instrument clashing as they are still inside the SP Cannula. As the dissection progress, the instruments and camera can that be advanced into the pelvic cavity thereby create better traction and handling with the aid of triangulation. We find that maintaining the surgical site within a sphere of an imaginary tennis ball will improve dissection and therefore the clutch on the surgeon console needs to be frequently used. Difficult areas at the 12 O'clock position can be overcome by rotating the SP Arm 180°. Identification of key landmarks for TaTME is the same as when performing with conventional laparoscopic instruments:

(1) Careful dissection of irradiated tissue for surgical plane

(2) Even circumferential dissection around the pelvis- don't be tempted to do the easy parts more than the difficult parts.
(3) Be aware of the sacral curve and not hesitate to optimize the position of the SP arm where necessary.
(4) Avoid straying into the obturator fossa.
(5) More active vascular pedicles (e.g. middle rectal artery) should be dealt with by ultrasonic or bipolar energy instruments.

We performed TaTME with a two-team approach. Once the two teams met, the tumour can then be delivered transanally or via the abdomen. Proximal end is then transected with anvil secured for anastomosis with a purse-stringed distal end.

Conclusion

Transanal robotic surgery with the da Vinci Single-port system is feasible and confers technological advantages over conventional laparoscopic and even multiport robots. Further evidence is required to confirm its advantages and it may pave the way to incision-less colorectal surgery in the future.

References

1. Bray F, Ferlay J, Soerjomataram I, Siegel RL, Torre LA, Jemal A. Global cancer statistics 2018: GLOBOCAN estimates of incidence and mortality worldwide for 36 cancers in 185 countries. CA Cancer J Clin. 2018;68:394–424.
2. Gomez D, Dalal Z, Raw E, Roberts C, Lyndon PJ. Anatomical distribution of colorectal cancer over a 10 year period in a district general hospital: is there a true "rightward shift"? Postgrad Med J. 2004;80:667–9. https://doi.org/10.1136/pgmj.2004.020198.
3. Wilkinson N. Management of rectal cancer. Surg Clin North Am. 2020;100(3):615–28. https://doi.org/10.1016/j.suc.2020.02.014.
4. Robotic transanal surgery (RTAS) with utilization of a next-generation single-port system: a cadaveric feasibility study. Tech Coloproctol. 2017;21(7):541–5. https://doi.org/10.1007/s10151-017-1655-3.
5. Da Vinci SP. Robotic approach to colorectal surgery: two specific indications and short-term results. Tech Coloproctol. 2022;26(6):461–70. https://doi.org/10.1007/s10151-022-02597.

Part III
Colon

Chapter 14
Robotic Standard Right Hemicolectomy with Intra-corporeal Anastomosis

Shinichiro Sakata, Jayson M. Moloney, and Andrew R. L. Stevenson

Abstract In this chapter, we offer a step-by-step description of the standard technique for robot-assisted right hemicolectomy with intra-corporeal anastomosis, which is our preferred approach for patients with right colon cancer. The benefits of the technique include optimising the quality of the pathologic specimen and lymph node harvest, while minimizing the extent of colonic dissection, mobilisation, and mesenteric traction placed on the ileo-colic anastomosis compared to an extra-corporeal anastomosis. This chapter is supplemented by a series of clinical images.

Keywords Colectomy · Right · Robotic · Da Vinci · Technique · Tips and Tricks

All authors have no financial support or conflicts of interest to disclose.

All authors provided intellectual contribution and have adhered to ICMJE authorship guidelines.

Authors agree with this submission.

There is no conflict of interest.

This article was not published previously.

This article is not under consideration elsewhere.

S. Sakata (✉)
Division of Colorectal Surgery, Department of Surgery, The Royal Brisbane and Women's Hospital, Brisbane, QLD, Australia
e-mail: shin.sakata@gmail.com

J. M. Moloney · A. R. L. Stevenson
School of Medicine, University of Queensland, Brisbane, QLD, Australia
e-mail: admin@ausces.com

Introduction

Robot-assisted surgical platforms were developed to overcome the ergonomic, technical, and visual limitations of laparoscopy, and have become ubiquitous throughout modern colorectal surgery. The latest iteration of the da Vinci® (Intuitive Surgical Inc.) multi-port robotic surgical system, the Xi robot, features simulated and magnified three-dimensional imaging, physiologic tremor filtering, motion scaling, Endowrist® technology and improved operating ergonomics [1–4].

Performing an intra-corporal anastomosis (ICA) reduces the extent of transverse colon dissection, small bowel handing, and mesenteric traction placed on the ileocolic anastomosis. An ICA may therefore result in a faster recovery of bowel function and allows for a safer off-midline, lower abdominal specimen extraction site rather than a vertical midline incision that is more prone to wound infection and incisional hernia [5–7]. Lower abdominal incisions for extraction are also associated with less pain, less consumption of post-operative analgesic drugs and reduced hospital stay [5]. For these reasons above, we believe that a robot-assisted right hemicolectomy with ICA is particularly valuable for patients who are obese. In our standard technique, described in more detail below, we place our 12 mm port in in the left lower abdomen for optimal ICA positioning and later extend this port incision for specimen extraction.

The aim of this chapter is to provide surgeons concise and practical information on our technique of standard robotic right hemicolectomy and intra-corporeal anastomosis, with reference to using the da Vinci® Xi surgical system. In addition, several emerging robotic platforms, such as the Versius® system (CMR Surgical, Cambridge, UK) and the Senhance™ (TransEnterix, Morrisville NC, USA) [8, 9], may become more accessible to colorectal surgeons in the future. Whilst port arrangement and patient cart positions may be different between these systems, the guiding principles of our technique remain the same.

Preoperative Considerations

Bowel Preparation

We recommend that all patients receive mechanical bowel preparation with polyethylene glycol or sodium phosphate, and oral antibiotic prophylaxis consisting of metronidazole (500 mg TDS) and erythromycin (400 mg TDS) is administered 24 hours before surgery, although neomycin or kanamycin can also be used, if available). This practice has been shown to reduce the incidence of surgical site infection, post-operative ileus and overall 30-day morbidity in patients undergoing elective colorectal surgery [10]. Mechanical bowel preparation also reduces the volume of bulky, bacteria-laden faeces. This allows for easier manipulation of the colon, more intra-operative space, minimizes faecal contamination during formation of an ICA, and a smaller incision required for extraction.

Patient Positioning

The patient is disrobed and positioned supine onto an anti-slip mat (The Pink Pad XL®; Xodus Medical Inc., New Kensington, PA). We consider anti-slip surfaces like the pink pad, crucial for minimizing hazardous displacement when the robotic-system is docked, and is especially important for obese patients in steep Trendelenburg. After general anaesthesia, the patient is repositioned in the low lithotomy position with both arms tucked-in at their sides. An indwelling urinary catheter is inserted, prophylactic parenteral broad-spectrum antibiotics is administered on induction, and both subcutaneous low molecular-weight heparin and sequential compression devices are utilised for deep vein thrombosis prophylaxis. An orogastric tube is inserted to deflate the stomach, increasing available operating space. The patient is then prepped and draped in the standard, sterile fashion.

Operative Technique

Abdominal Access and Port Configuration

Several port configurations for robotic right hemicolectomy have been described. We use a modified four-port suprapubic port technique utilizing a da Vinci Xi platform (Figs. 14.1 and 14.2; Intuitive Surgical, Sunnyvale, CA, USA) [3]. This arrangement provides excellent access to the entire abdominal colon, which is advantageous if extended right hemicolectomy is necessary). Further, this configuration lends itself to a low transverse extraction incision in either the suprapubic or left iliac fossa region, allowing for better cosmesis, and reducing the risk of port-site incisional hernias. However, the suprapubic port placement configuration limits access to the pelvis when the robot is docked. In cases where dissection in the pelvis is required, such as when the distal ileum is adherent to the pelvis, we suggest the traditional port placement [3].

We begin by a laparoscopic 5 mm optical entry in the left upper quadrant, 3 cm below the costal margin and lateral to the midclavicular line. We emphasise that placing this port too medial may result in instrument clasing during the operation. The peritoneal surfaces of the abdominal cavity and liver are routinely surveyed to exclude metastatic disease, and the abdomen inspected for pathology such as locally advanced cancers and adhesions that may influence port placement.

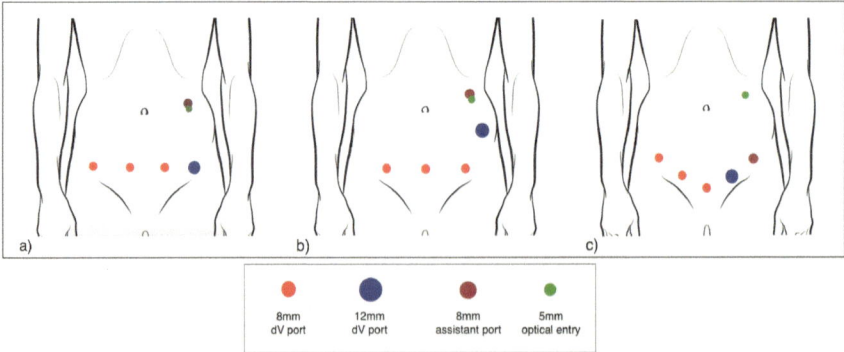

Fig. 14.1 Three variations of suprapubic port placements (SPPP) for robotic-assisted right hemi-colectomy. The patient cart approaches perpendicularly from the patient's right side, or alternatively from an (cephalo-caudally) oblique angle from the patients left

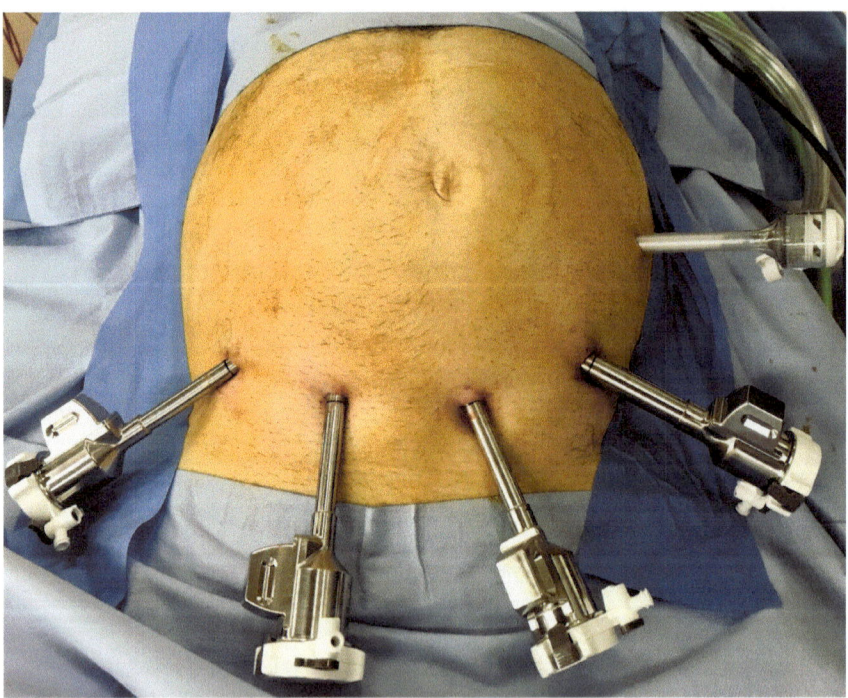

Fig. 14.2 The main variation of suprapubic port placement for robotic right hemicolectomy (Fig. 14.1: Variation A)

   Port positions are shown in Fig. 14.2. The optical entry port is exchanged for an 8 mm AirSeal® port (AirSeal® System, Conmed, CT, USA) and this is used as the assistant's working port and allows for suture exchange. For most patients, a relatively low pneumoperitoneum is maintained at 10-mmHg pressure. Three 8 mm robotic working ports are placed, and a 12 mm robotic working port (initially with an 8 mm reducer) is placed in the left iliac fossa. We tilt the operating table right-side up (10–15°) and laparoscopically manoeuvre the omentum over the stomach and small bowel away from the right iliac fossa prior to docking. A small amount of Trendelenburg tilt can also be used but this is not always required for adequate exposure.

   The robot is then docked, with the patient cart ideally positioned on the patient's right side. If the operating room configuration is otherwise limited, the patient cart may be positioned on the patient's left but on an angle from the left shoulder to provide access for the surgical assistant. We routinely use two left arms and one right arm. With this configuration the camera is placed in arm 3. Instrumentation includes a Small Graptor® (grasping retractor) utilized in the lateral-left arm (arm 1; the surgeon's "third arm"); either a SynchroSeal® advanced bipolar or Vessel Sealer® electrosurgical instrument utilized in the arm 2, while, and a scissor or hook is placed in the main operating/dissecting arm, arm 4.

Mobilization

The modified four-port suprapubic port technique lends well to a medial-to-lateral dissection. Mobilisation from lateral to medial is feasible, and we feel that it is important for colorectal surgeons to be facile with both approaches. With the medial-to-lateral approach, the fenestrated grasper is used to place the ileocolic pedicle on stretch, and the peritoneum along its undersurface is incised from medial-to-lateral. An inter-mesenteric dissection is carried through the loose fibers of Toldt's fascia, which is between the overlying mesothelial layer of the mesocolon and the underlying mesothelial layer of the retroperitoneum that covers the duodenum, right ureter, and gonadal vessels (Fig. 14.3A).

   Attention is returned to the ileocolic region where the ileocolic artery and vein are isolated, clipped with Hem-o-lok clips via the assistant port (Weck, Teleflex, Research Triangle Park, NC, USA) and individually divided using bipolar energy. Performing this manoeuvre facilitates further intermesenteric dissection towards the hepatic flexure, which can be performed at this stage. Then, mesenteric transection proceeds in a cephalad direction towards the origin of the right branch of the middle colic vein and artery. During dissection, the right colic vessels if present, are divided. Complete mesocolic excision for right colon cancer is based on high ligation of vascular pedicles and radical oncologic resection along the superior mesenteric vein. This technique is selectively used for right-hemicolectomy in our Institution and is covered by others in another chapter. The terminal ileum is then dissected from its peritoneal attachments along the pelvic brim. The dissection is continued laterally

Fig. 14.3 A–C Mobilisation of the right colon. Once the submesocolic plane is entered initially through a peritoneal incision along the undersurface of the tensioned ileocolic pedicle, the duodenum is dissected from the right colon mesentery (**A**)—the latter retracted anteriorly using the both the surgeon's 4th arm retractor and the bedside assistant. Active use of the assistant is helpful during all stags of mobilisation, including reflection of the greater omentum from the transverse mesocolon (**B**) and division of the colonic and ileal mesenteries (**C**)

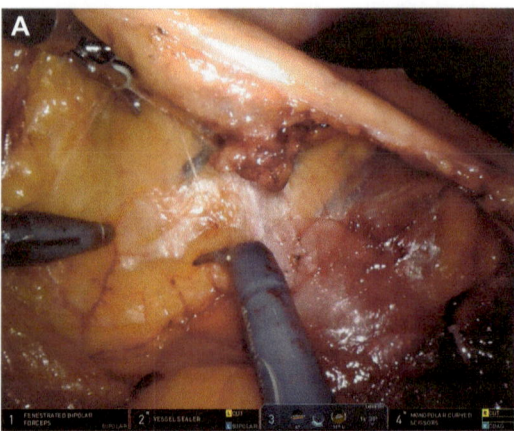

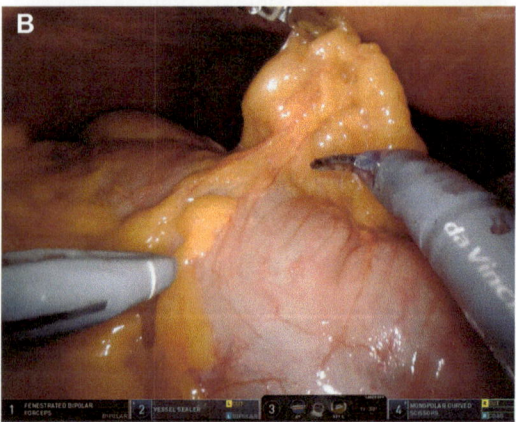

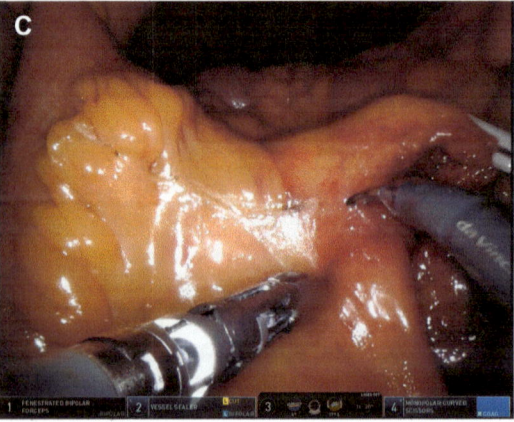

and the lateral peritoneal attachments of the cecum to the lateral abdominal wall are divided.

Intraoperative adjustment of table position is not usually needed during a standard robotic right hemicolectomy but occasionally, it can be useful to place the patient in a reverse Trendelenburg position for dissection of the hepatic flexure with the operating table tilted to the left side. Hepatic flexure dissection begins superiorly in the gastrocolic ligament to enter the omental bursa or greater sac (Fig. 14.3B). The dissection is then carried laterally so that the hepatic flexure and ascending colon are fully mobilized. The transverse mesocolon is completely mobilized off the pancreatic head and duodenum.

After the terminal ileum, right and proximal transverse colon are mobilized, the ileal mesentery (Fig. 14.3C) and transverse mesocolon are divided using the SynchroSeal® or Vessel Sealer®. To ensure adequate vascular perfusion at the resected margins before transecting and preforming an ICA, we routinely use indocyanine green fluorescence angiography (dose 0.2 mg/kg, administered intra-venously) viewed with the built-in Firefly™ vision mode (Intuitive Surgical, Sunny-vale, CA, USA). Bowel transection is performed using a robotic linear cutting stapler (Sureform 60, Intuitive Surgical Inc., Sunnyvale, CA, USA) introduced through the left iliac fossa 12 mm port (arm 4), with the 8 mm reducing sleeve removed.

Anastomosis and Specimen Extraction

An intracorporeal side-to-side isoperistaltic ileotransverse anastomosis is created (Fig. 14.4A–C). A small longitudinal colotomy is made 6–7 cm distal to the colonic staple line on the antimesenteric aspect to allow entry of the stapler's anvil (Fig. 14.4A). On the distal ileal remnant, a small enterotomy is made on the antime-senteric aspect 3 cm proximal to the stapled edge to allow entry of the stapler's cartridge. A gauze swab can be placed beneath the enterotomy and colotomy to control faecal spillage and minimize peritoneal contamination. An isoperistaltic, side to-side ileocolic anastomosis is made with firing of the stapler (Fig. 14.4B), and the resultant open-mouthed enteric end is sutured continuously with 15 cm 3′0 polydioxanone suture (Stratafix™, Ethicon Inc., Johnson & Johnson, Bridgewater, NJ, USA), beginning at the distal end of the enterotomy (Fig. 14.4C). This may be further reinforced with a second layer of continuous imbricating suture. The vascular integrity may be re-assessed after the anastomosis is completed with ICG and Firefly.

The specimen is then prepared for extraction by grasping the base of the appendix (if present) or the staple line. The pneumoperitoneum is then evacuated using a safe, closed system before the robot is undocked for specimen extraction. This may be performed via a muscle-splitting incision by extending the left iliac fossa 12 mm robotic port incision, or by unifying the median 2 in-line 8 mm working ports into single small Pfannenstiel incision. The specimen is then extracted via the incision using a medium Alexis wound retractor (Applied Medical, Rancho

166   S. Sakata et al.

Fig. 14.4 A–C An isoperistaltic, side to-side ileocolic anastomosis is performed by first creating enterotomies in the distal ileum and transverse colon (**A**), creating a lumen using a robotic stapler (**B**), and 2 layered suture closure of the common ileo-colotomy (**C**)

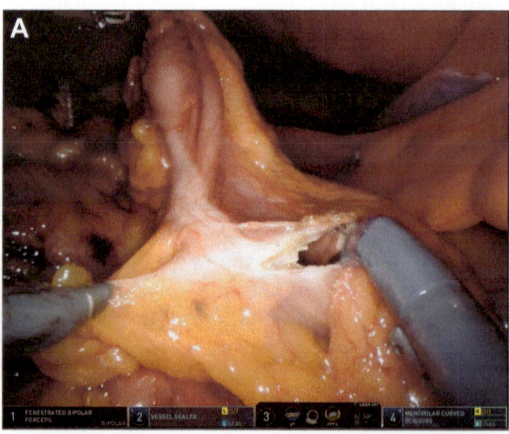

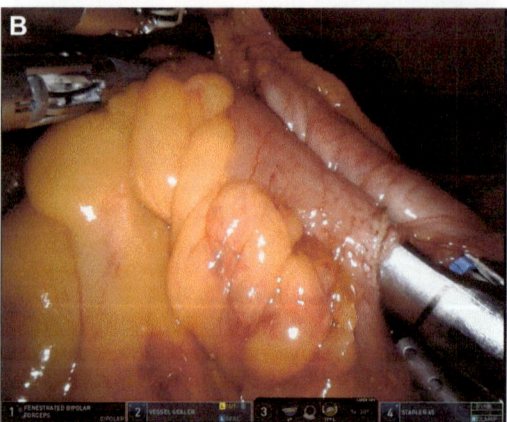

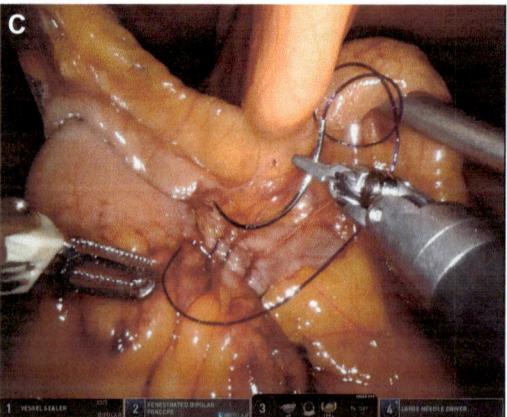

Santa Margarita, CA, USA). Closure is then performed in the usual manner using absorbable monofilament sutures.

Conclusion and Final Remarks

There is mounting evidence that robotic-assisted technology for right hemicolectomy delivers tangible clinical benefits over conventional laparoscopy. A recent systematic review has demonstrated that right hemicolectomy using modern robotic platforms significantly improves lymph node harvest and reduces anastomotic complications, as well as conversion to laparotomy, time to first flatus, incisional hernia rates, and length of stay [11]. However, it is important for readers to recognise that these conclusions were largely based on data from unmatched and potentially confounded, small, retrospective cohort studies [11]. Indeed, the call-to-arms for more robust data to guide clinical practice has become resounding over the past few years is currently being answered by a number of large-scale international randomised clinical trials (RCTs) including MIRCAST and RoLaCaRT, both currently in recruitment phase.

Robust data from these RCTs are needed to justify the rapid world-wide adoption of robot-assisted technology as routine practice for right hemicolectomy laparoscopy [12–14]. It is also important to conclusively identify any potential benefits of the robotic platform when performing an intra-corporal anastomosis and complete mesocolic excision, in the setting of a RCT.

Disclosure Statement

ARL Stevenson is a proctor and received educational financial support from Intuitive Surgical, Johnson and Johnson Ethicon Endosurgery, Medtronic, Olympus, Applied Medical and Cook Biotech. All other authors have no financial support or conflicts of interest to disclose.

All authors provided intellectual contribution and have adhered to ICMJE guidelines on authorship.

Authors are in agreement with this submission.

There is no conflict of interest.

This article was not published previously.

This article is not under consideration elsewhere.

References

1. Leal Ghezzi T, Campos CO. 30 years of robotic surgery. World J Surg. 2016;40(10):2550–7.
2. Liu H, Xu M, Liu R, Jia B, Zhao Z. The art of robotic colonic resection: a review of progress in the past 5 years. Updates Surg. 2021;73(3):1037–48.
3. Hamilton AER, Chatfield MD, Johnson CS, Stevenson ARL. Totally robotic right hemicolectomy: a multicentre case-matched technical and peri-operative comparison of port placements and da Vinci models. J Robot Surg. 2020;14(3):479–91.
4. Sakata S, Grove PM, Stevenson AR. Effect of 3-dimensional vision on surgeons using the da vinci robot for laparoscopy: more than meets the eye. JAMA Surg. 2016;151(9):793–4.
5. Vignali A, Elmore U, Lemma M, Guarnieri G, Radaelli G, Rosati R. Intracorporeal versus extracorporeal anastomoses following laparoscopic right colectomy in obese patients: a case-matched study. Dig Surg. 2018;35(3):236–42.
6. DeSouza A, Domajnko B, Park J, Marecik S, Prasad L, Abcarian H. Incisional hernia, midline versus low transverse incision: what is the ideal incision for specimen extraction and hand-assisted laparoscopy? Surg Endosc. 2011;25(4):1031–6.
7. Trastulli S, Coratti A, Guarino S, et al. Robotic right colectomy with intracorporeal anastomosis compared with laparoscopic right colectomy with extracorporeal and intracorporeal anastomosis: a retrospective multicentre study. Surg Endosc. 2015;29(6):1512–21.
8. Dixon F, O'Hara R, Ghuman N, Strachan J, Khanna A, Keeler BD. Major colorectal resection is feasible using a new robotic surgical platform: the first report of a case series. Tech Coloproctol. 2021;25(3):285–9.
9. Spinelli A, David G, Gidaro S, et al. First experience in colorectal surgery with a new robotic platform with haptic feedback. Colorectal Dis. 2018;20(3):228–35.
10. Rollins KE, Javanmard-Emamghissi H, Acheson AG, Lobo DN. The role of oral antibiotic preparation in elective colorectal surgery: a meta-analysis. Ann Surg. 2019;270(1).
11. Waters PS, Cheung FP, Peacock O, et al. Successful patient-oriented surgical outcomes in robotic vs laparoscopic right hemicolectomy for cancer-a systematic review. Colorectal Dis. 2020;22(5):488–99.
12. Larach JT, Flynn J, Kong J, et al. Robotic colorectal surgery in Australia: evolution over a decade. ANZ J Surg. 2021;91(11):2330–6.
13. Schootman M, Hendren S, Ratnapradipa K, Stringer L, Davidson NO. Adoption of robotic technology for treating colorectal cancer. Dis Colon Rectum. 2016;59(11):1011–8.
14. Halabi WJ, Kang CY, Jafari MD, et al. Robotic-assisted colorectal surgery in the United States: a nationwide analysis of trends and outcomes. World J Surg. 2013;37(12):2782–90.

Chapter 15
Robotic Right Hemicolectomy: Complete Mesocolic Excision and Intracorporeal Anastomosis

Marcos Gómez Ruiz, Carmen Cagigas Fernández, and Natatalia Suarez Pazos

Abstract Complete mesocolic excision (CME) as an oncologically optimal technique to treat right colon cancer has gained wide adoption in recent decades until it has become the Gold Standard today. Since 2008 and thanks to the work of the Erlangen group, the definition of CME has been clear. Its performance by a minimally invasive approach is one of the technical challenges faced by surgeons today. Although there are no RCTs that support its routine use, there are several meta-analyses that point to its better oncological outcomes. After oncological resection of the right colon, there are different technical options when constructing the ileocolic anastomosis. In this chapter, we present the completely intracorporeal mechanical isoperistaltic ileocolic anastomosis (ICA). There is some evidence in the literature that points to its potential benefit in the immediate postoperative period, although, like CME, its performance through minimally invasive approach is another technical challenge. Robotic surgery can help perform both CME and ICA through a minimally invasive approach. In this chapter we describe the robotic right colectomy technique with ESC and ICA step by step.

Keywords Robotic surgery · Right colectomy · Complete mesocolic excision · Intracorporeal anastomosis

M. Gómez Ruiz (✉) · C. Cagigas Fernández · N. Suarez Pazos
General Surgery Department, Colorectal Surgery Unit, Marqués de Valdecilla University
Hospital, 39008 Santander, Spain
e-mail: marcos.gomez@scsalud.es

C. Cagigas Fernández
e-mail: carmen.cagigas@scsalud.es

N. Suarez Pazos
e-mail: natalia.suarez@scsalud.es

Valdecilla Biomedical Research Institute (IDIVAL), 39011 Santander, Spain

M. Gómez Ruiz
Medical School, University of Cantabria, 39011 Santander, Spain

Introduction and Indications

Complete mesocolic excision (CME) with central vascular ligation (CVL) was first described by Hohemberger and Bokey. The concept of CME for treating right colon cancer has a similar philosophy to the total mesorectal excision (TME) for rectal cancer. Adequation of surgery with an optimal quality resection can contribute to improved outcomes over other treatment modalities. Precise terminology and quality surgery are vital factors [1].

Right colectomy with complete mesocolic excision has three main components [2]:

1. Dissection between the colonic mesenteric plane and the parietal fascia. Mesenteric excision with a complete envelope of the fascia and visceral peritoneum.
2. Central vascular ligation for complete excision of the central region lymph nodes.
3. Resection of the adequate length of the bowel to remove the affected pericolic nodes in a longitudinal direction.

Although there are no randomized studies, right colectomy with CME is associated with higher lymph-node retrieval and better oncologic outcome, especially for UICC stage II and III without increasing the morbidity and mortality [3].

Intracorporeal anastomoses (ICA) have been associated with several benefits in colorectal surgery, including accelerated recovery and decreased pain when compared to extracorporeal anastomosis after right colon resection [4].

Robotic surgery characteristics such as 3D improved vision, stable camera control, better ergonomics, physiologic tremor filters and precise dissection thanks to motion scaling and endowristed instruments may translate to a more precise and delicate dissection in a demanding and technically complex procedure. This could potentially overcome the technical limitations of conventional laparoscopy and shorten the learning curve of minimally-invasive right colectomy with CME and Intracorporeal Anastomosis while making it safe and effective [5].

Comparative studies between laparoscopic and robotic techniques (generally retrospective) have shown less blood loss, reduced postoperative complications, increased operative time and faster recovery of digestive function [6]. No large scale randomized clinical trials have compared laparoscopic and robotic right colectomy with CME and ICA.

When we refer to studies involving right hemicolectomy with CME comparing the three available techniques (open laparoscopic and robotic), we see that robotic surgery with CME improves the number of harvested lymph nodes and the specimen-node length ratio, which may reflect better quality of the specimen and mesocolic excision [7].

The team in Hospital Universitario Marques de Valdecilla has already performed more than 200 Robotic Right colectomies, with over 100 Robotic CME procedures performed so far. Our experience when comparing this cases with our laparoscopic cases is that thanks to Robotic instruments we have been able to safely introduce a technically demanding procedure such as minimally invasive CME with ICA, improving our postoperative and oncological outcomes in the last 10 years. This improvement is for sure due to multifactorial reasons, but robotic assistance has definitely helped us in this endeavor.

Procedural Cases

Position of the Patient

Patient is positioned supine on the table. The table is placed in a Trendelenburg position with a angle of 10°–15 and left tilt 5°–10°. To avoid collisions between patient legs and robotic arms during the procedure, legs should be in flex position to compensate the Trendelemburg (Fig. 15.1).

Theatre Layout

The anesthesia instruments and anesthesiologist are positioned at the patient's bedside over the left shoulder of the patient, the scrub nurse and assistant are positioned to the left side of the patient. At the same time, the robot cart enters from the right side of the patient either perpendicular, for Xi Robotic System, or 60° over the right shoulder of the patient, for X Robotic System (Figs. 15.2 and 15.3).

Care should be taken to avoid as far as possible the crossing of tubes and wires (pneumoperitoneum, monopolar/bipolar wires or sucker) on different sides of the patient as they may affect or be affected by the robot trolley or the arms if they are crossing in the right side of the patient.

- Port position for X and Xi system (Fig. 15.4):

1. Four robotic trocars are inserted along a transverse suprapubic line, about 6 cm above the pubis. Port number three (is placed 3–4 cm left from the mid

Fig. 15.1 Position of the patient

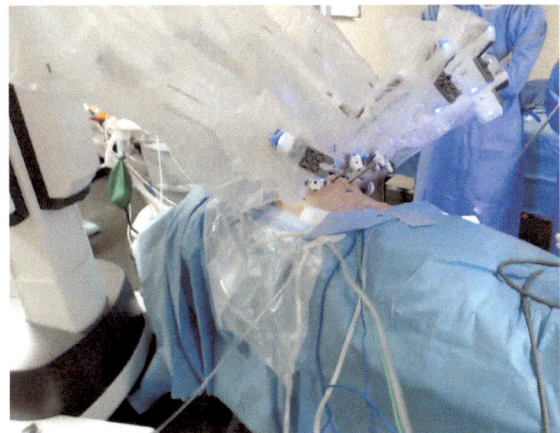

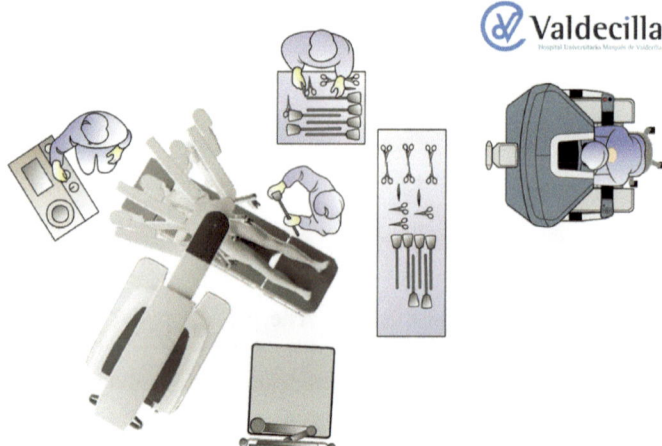

Fig. 15.2 Xi system theater setup

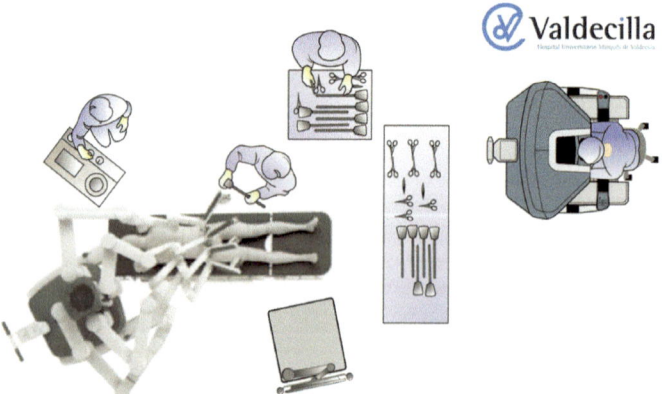

Fig. 15.3 X system theater setup

line (12 mm trocar), port number two (8 mm) is placed 3–4 cm right from the mid line. Ports one and four are positioned 6–8 cm lateral left and right from 2 and 3. Port configuration in Xi Robotic System is 1-2-3-4, whereas in X Robotic System is 4-1-2-3.

2. A 12 mm assistant port is placed lateral to the left mid clavicular line at the midpoint of the abdomen. When available, we recommend to use high flow insufflators, as they allow for more excellent stability of the pneumoperitoneum, which facilitates performing the procedure with lower pressure improving patient recovery.

Fig. 15.4 Port positioning (Suprapubic approach). Port numbers as per Xi robotic system

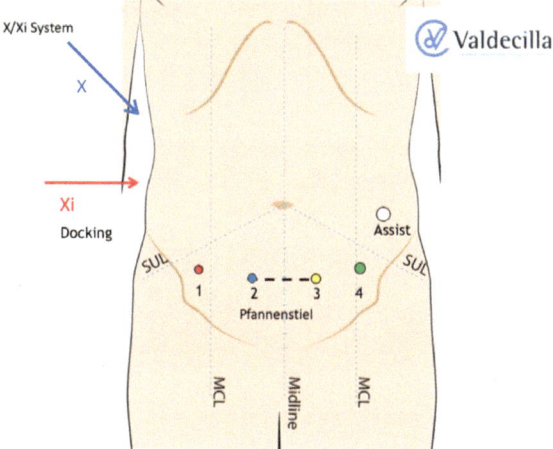

Safety/Adaptations Versus Lap or Open

Care should be taken to avoid any collision between the robotic arms and the patient. A 10–15° flex of patient legs is mandatory to avoid these during the procedure with suprapubic approach when Trendelenburg is used. Trendelenburg position often causes nerve injuries at the level of the shoulders. To avoid these, patients hands, arms and any support zones must be covered with a foam pad or a non-slip surface.

Equipment Needed [8]

Camera

A 30° scope is highly recommended during robotic right colectomy. Camera is placed in port/arm number X.

Dominant Hand Dissection Instruments

A monopolar energy instrument is often used during embryological or vascular dissection. Monopolar scissors or hook are both acceptable depending on surgeon preferences (Fig. 15.5).

Energy Devices, Traction and Counter Traction Instruments

A bipolar fenestrated instrument together with either Tip-Up fenestrated grasper or a Cadiere grasper are an optimal combination to achieve proper traction and countertraction during the dissection with the monopolar instrument. The bipolar fenestrated is specially helpful to perform hemostasis during vascular dissection. Some surgeons would alternatively use the Vessel Sealer as a grasping instrument (Fig. 15.6).

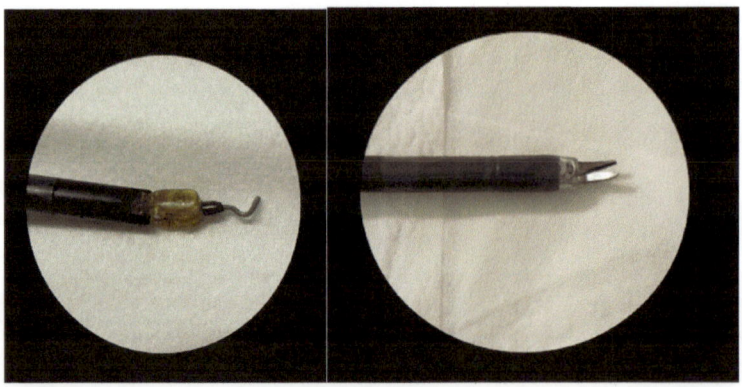

Fig. 15.5 Monopolar scissors and monopolar hook

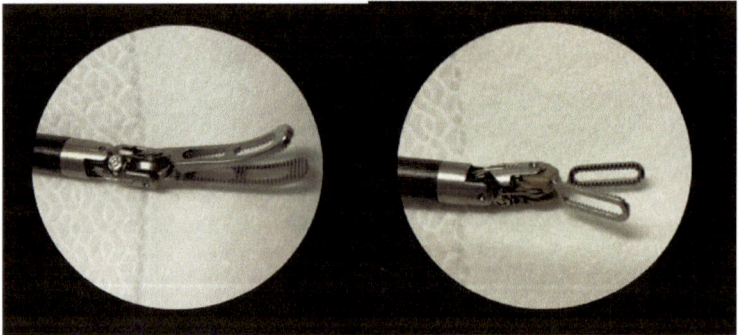

Fig. 15.6 Tip-up and bipolar fenestrated

Vascular Ligation/Division

Vascular ligation is usually performed with the endowristed Hem o Lock Clip applier mainly for the larger vessels (ileocolic, right colic or right branch of the middle colic vessels). Large clips are preferred for these vessels. Vessel sealer can also be used (Fig. 15.7).

Intracorporeal Anastomosis

During intracorporeal anastomosis, a large needle driver is used for suturing. Sure-form 60 mm robotic linear stapler with blue loads is recommended for bowel transection and side to side anastomosis (Fig. 15.8).

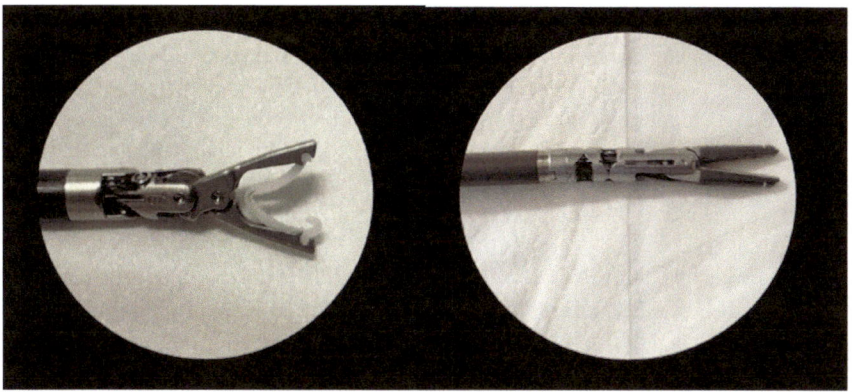

Fig. 15.7 Large Hem o Lock clip applier and vessel sealer

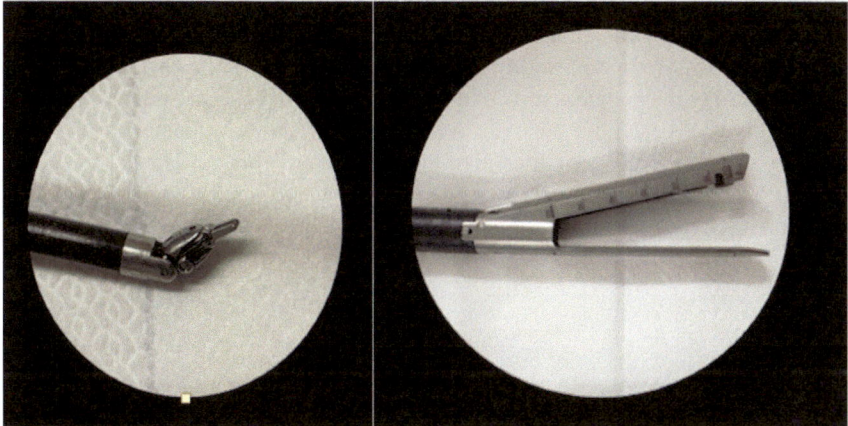

Fig. 15.8 Large needle driver and sureform 60 mm with blue loads

Steps of the Procedure

1. Sub-ileal dissection.
2. D3 Lymphadenectomy and Central Ligation of Ileocolic vessels (± right colic).
3. Central ligation of right branch of middle colic and colic branch of GCT.
4. Dissection of the Gastroepiploic arcade. Complete movilization of the hepatic flexure.
5. Transverse colon and ileal mesentery transection. Major omentum transection.
6. Intracorporeal anastomosis.
7. Specimen extraction (Transverse suprapubic incision).

After induction of pneumoperitoneum using a Veress needle in the left hypochondrium at the Palmer's point, four robotic trocars are inserted along a transverse suprapubic line, about 6–8 cm above the pubis; a 12-mm trocar for the assistant is inserted 2–3 cm lateral to the left mid clavicular line, at the level of the mid-point of the abdomen. Trocar layout is as shown in Fig. 15.1. The table is placed in a Trendelenburg position with a slight angle (5°–10°) and left tilt (5°–10°). Legs are flexed 10–15°. The robot is then docked from the patient's right side (60–90° depending on the System).

The procedure starts before docking the system with the adequate placement of the small bowel left upwards to allow us an optimal view of the terminal ileum posterior plane and fourth duodenal portion. The robotic platform is docked as shown in Figs. 15.2 and 15.3.

Sub Ileal Dissection

The dissection starts detaching the plane between the posterior aspect of the meso-ileum and the retroperitoneum (Fig. 15.9). Furthermore, it continues cranially, allowing us the identification of retroperitoneal structures as right ureter and gonadal vessels (SMV). We continue the dissection left lateral (patient) to reach the duodenum and the head of the pancreas on top of the Fredet fascia (anterior duodenopancreatic fascia) until we reach the posterior aspect of the superior mesenteric vessels and identify pancreatic and colic branch of the Gastrocolic Trunk of Henle (Fig. 15.10). At that level, we leave a small gauze protecting this area on top of the Fredet fascia and making it identifiable during the vascular dissection of the SMV.

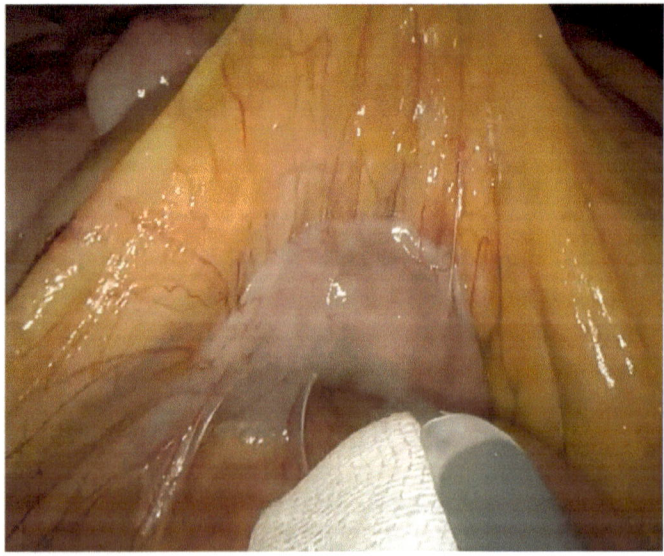

Fig. 15.9 Starting point for dissection during sub ileal dissection

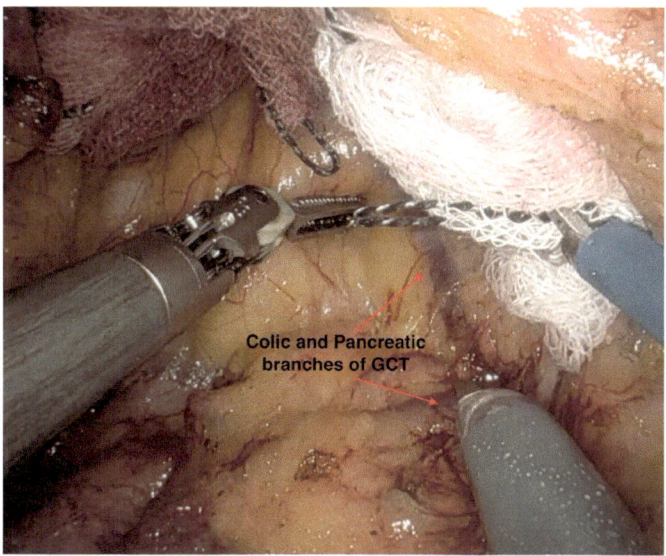

Fig. 15.10 Exposure and identification of coilc and pancreatic branches of GCT of Henle

Central Ligation of Ileocolic vessels (± right colic) and D3 Lymphadenectomy

The small bowel is placed back towards the pelvis with adequate exposure of the anterior aspect of the mesentery. The transverse colon is lifted cranially pulling at the midpoint (middle colic vessels) with the Tip-up forceps (instrument in Xi robotic system port number one); the assistant brings the terminal ileum towards the pelvis pulling from the ileal branch of the superior mesenteric vein (Fig. 15.11).

Vessel dissection starts at the level of ileal branch towards its confluence with the superior mesenteric vein (Fig. 15.12). The dissection is carried out cranially along the medial aspect of the vein (D3 Lymphadenectomy) identifying ileocolic vessels and right colic vessels (when present). These vessels are skeletonized, centrally ligated with hem-o-locks (veins and arteries) and divided.

Central Ligation of Right Branch of Middle Colic and Colic Branch of GCT

Once ileocolic and right colic vessels are divided, dissection along the middle colic artery is performed until the right branch of the middle colic artery and vein are identified. This branch is clipped centrally and divided between Hem o Locks. Proper traction and countertraction for ideal exposure of this vessel is achieved using the Tip-Up forceps at the level of the transverse colon for traction and countertraction with the Bipolar Fenestrated forceps. The mesocolic flap is lifted towards the right side of the patient with the Bipolar Fenestrated forceps and the colic branch of the Gastrocolic Trunk of Henle is identified. At this level it is key to distinguish between the colic and gastroepiploic branches. The colic branch is clipped with Hem o Locks and divided between them.

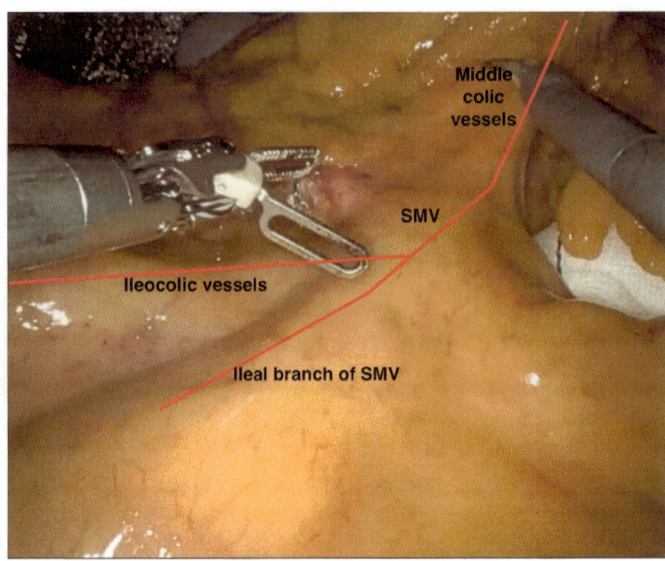

Fig. 15.11 Exposure of vascular axis

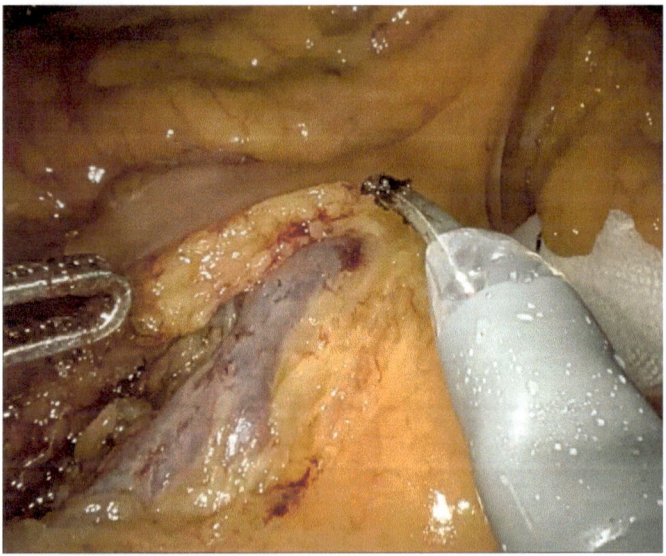

Fig. 15.12 Confluence between ileal branch, yeyunal branch and SMV

Dissection of the Gastroepiploic Arcade. Complete Mobilization of the Hepatic Flexure. Major Omentum Transection

Once all vessels have been clipped and divided, dissection follows on top of the transverse colon. First, the major omentum is divided either with the Vessel Sealer or with a combination of Bipolar Fenestrated and Monopolar Scissors. Then the gastroepiploic arcade is identified and followed towards the hepatic flexure. This can be either be done with the monopolar scissors or with the Vessel Sealer in obese patients. Right colon attachments to the parietal peritoneum are fully released.

Transverse Colon and Ileal Mesentery Transection

Transverse colon and ileal mesentery are completely divided using either the Vessel Sealer or with a combination of Bipolar Fenestrated and Monopolar Scissors.

Intracorporeal Anastomosis

Indocyanine green is administered intravenously (7.5 mg), and both ileum and transverse colon are evaluated for perfusion with the FireFly® fluorescence imaging system before dividing the bowel. The colon and ileum are then transected in a well perfused area with a 60 mm SureForm® stapler with blue loads. The specimen is placed in a bag over the liver to allow a comfortable performance of intracorporeal anastomosis.

A side-to-side isoperistaltic ileocolic anastomosis is performed with a a 60 mm SureForm® stapler with blue load; the enterotomy is closed with a hand-sewn running suture (using a 000 absorbable monofilament suture).

Specimen Extraction (Transverse Suprapubic Incision)

The specimen is finally extracted through a transverse suprapubic incision (Pfannenstiel incision) which usually includes the 12 mm trocar and is protected with a wound protector.

Top 5 Tips and Checklist

Top Tips

1. Patient in Trendelemburg position for optimal position of small bowel and subileal approach.
2. Inferior (subileal) approach first to perform the posterior dissection of the SMV until colic branch of the GCT of Henle is identified.
3. SMV exposure exposing middle colic vessels with the Tip-Up fenestrated.
4. Central lymphadenectomy and CVL with a combination of bipolar, monopolar energy and Hem o Locks.
5. Stapler in left lower quadrant for ileocolic isoperistaltic intracorporeal anastomosis.

Checklist

1. All instruments are available for the procedure.
2. Correct position and protection of the patient.
3. Table positioning (Tredelemburg and tilt left with legs down).
4. Step by step right colectomy with CME and ICA.

References

1. Hohenberger W, Weber K, Matzel K, Papadopoulos T, Merkel S. Standardized surgery for colonic cancer: complete mesocolic excision and central ligation-technical notes and outcome. Colorectal Dis. 2009;11(4):354–64; discussion 64–5.
2. Sondenaa K, Quirke P, Hohenberger W, Sugihara K, Kobayashi H, Kessler H, et al. The rationale behind complete mesocolic excision (CME) and a central vascular ligation for colon cancer in open and laparoscopic surgery: proceedings of a consensus conference. Int J Colorectal Dis. 2014;29(4):419–28.
3. Spinoglio G, Bianchi PP, Marano A, Priora F, Lenti LM, Ravazzoni F, et al. Robotic versus laparoscopic right colectomy with complete mesocolic excision for the treatment of colon cancer: perioperative outcomes and 5-year survival in a consecutive series of 202 patients. Ann Surg Oncol. 2018;25(12):3580–6.
4. Bollo J, Turrado V, Rabal A, Carrillo E, Gich I, Martinez MC, Hernandez P, Targarona E. Randomized clinical trial of intracorporeal versus extracorporeal anastomosis in laparoscopic right colectomy (IEA trial). Br J Surg. 2020;107(4):364–72. https://doi.org/10.1002/bjs.11389 Epub 2019 Dec 17 PMID: 31846067.
5. Bianchi PP, Salaj A, Giuliani G, Ferraro L, Formisano G. Feasibility of robotic right colectomy with complete mesocolic excision and intracorporeal anastomosis: short-term outcomes of 161 consecutive patients. Updates Surg. 2021;73(3):1065–72.
6. Xu H, Li J, Sun Y, Li Z, Zhen Y, Wang B, et al. Robotic versus laparoscopic right colectomy: a meta-analysis. World J Surg Oncol. 2014;12:274.
7. Widmar M, Keskin M, Strombom P, Beltran P, Chow OS, Smith JJ, et al. Lymph node yield in right colectomy for cancer: a comparison of open, laparoscopic and robotic approaches. Colorectal Dis. 2017;19(10):888–94.
8. Da Vinci X/Xi Instrument & Accessory Catalog. Intuitive Surgical SARL. 2020.

Chapter 16
Robotic Subtotal Colectomy

Sofoklis Panteleimonitis and Danilo Miskovic

Abstract In this chapter we describe the operative steps for subtotal colectomy. The preferred approach is a single dock from a suprapubic position with two right and one left hand, using 4th generation daVinci technology. The steps include subileal dissection, vascular pedicle transection of the right and transverse colon, supracolic and lateral dissection with transection of the terminal ileum, dissection of the splenic flexure, and transection of the IMA and IMV pedicle.

Keywords Colectomy · Robotic surgery · Colorectal cancer · 3D reconstruction · Indocyanine green

Introduction

Minimally invasive surgery has become an integral part of colorectal surgery over the last two decades. Laparoscopy has led to improved short-term outcomes [1] and as a result, laparoscopic colorectal surgery has become the standard of care for benign and malignant disease for much of the developed world [2].

Despite its accelerated adoption, laparoscopic colorectal surgery is limited by the inherit limitations of the laparoscopic instruments. The camera is assistant dependant and offers 2-D views (although 3-D platforms are available) and the instruments are straight with fixed endpoints. These limitations result in poor instrument ergonomics, an enhanced tremor effect and the tool endpoints moving to an opposite direction of the surgeon's hands, known as the fulcrum effect, making laparoscopy a non-intuitive motor skill that is hard to learn [3]. Currently, as shown in the 2020 National Bowel Cancer Audit, in the UK 72% of colorectal cancer surgery is performed laparoscopically, but the conversion rate remains relatively high at 11% [4].

S. Panteleimonitis · D. Miskovic (✉)
St Mark's Hospital, Watford Rd, HA1 3UJ London, UK
e-mail: danilo.miskovic@nhs.net

© The Author(s), under exclusive license to Springer Nature Switzerland AG 2022   181
P. Coyne and J. Khan (eds.), *Robotic Colorectal Surgery*,
https://doi.org/10.1007/978-3-031-15198-9_16

Robotic surgical systems were designed to overcome the technical limitations of laparoscopic instruments and since the first robotic colectomy by Weber in 2002 robotic colorectal surgery has increased in popularity [5]. Robotic instruments offer stable 3-D views and superior instrument ergonomics with 7 degrees of freedom enabling precise dissection.

While robotic rectal surgery has quickly gained acceptance among colorectal surgeons, its implementation for colonic surgery has been slower. This is because colonic procedures such as right hemicolectomy and sigmoid colectomy are confined within the abdominal cavity where there is relatively a lot of space. This makes colonic procedures reasonably straightforward when compared to pelvic procedures and they can therefore be more easily performed laparoscopically. As a result, the increased cost of the robotic platform has initially deterred surgeons from using it for colonic surgery. However, with competition for robotic platforms opening up and prices improving, robotic colonic surgery has become increasingly more common. Initially, its application in colonic surgery was mainly reserved for the complete mesocolic excision (CME) right colectomy, which requires a higher degree of dexterity in order to complete the vascular ligation. Robotic CME has been shown to be safe and feasible with an increasing number of studies reporting its short and long term outcomes [6–8]. However, extended colonic resections such as subtotal colectomy and proctocolectomy where multi-quadrant access is required, are more cumbersome to perform robotically due to the robotic platform's limitations in multi-quadrant access. With the 4th generation system, the da Vinci Xi®, addressing these limitations and providing better access to the abdomen without the need to reposition or undock and re-dock the robot, robotic extended colonic are becoming more common and increasingly reported in the literature [9, 10].

In our practice we routinely use the robotic system (da Vinci Xi®) for all colorectal cancer resections. This chapter describes a stepwise modular approach to robotic subtotal colectomy.

Procedure Preparation

Patient Preparation

Mechanical bowel prep with antibiotics is used for all patients. In addition to the hypothesised benefits of bowel prep with antibiotics in colonic resection surgery [11], it facilitates the formation of intracorporeal anastmoses. For subtotal colectomies, and when performing ileorectal or ileo-distal sigmoid anastomoses, we often choose to perform them in an open fashion through a Pfannenstiel incision (see below). For any anastomosis more proximally, an intracorporeal formation is preferred.

Position and Set Up

The patient is placed supine in a modified Lloyd Davies position with the arms wrapped besides the body. A vacuum bean mattress is used to prevent the patient

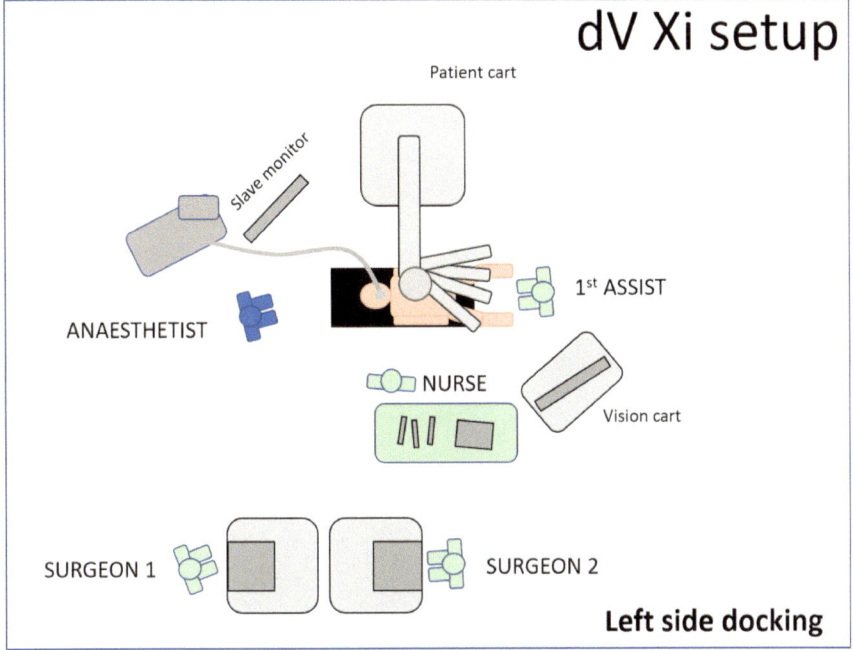

Fig. 16.1 Operating theatre setup with da Vinci Xi®

from sliding off the table and a protective cross bar is applied over the patients face to prevent it from being hit by the robotic arms. Sequential compression devices are applied on both legs and a prophylactic single-shot antibiotic is administered at the beginning of surgery. The assistant sits between the legs of the patient and the robotic cart is docked form the left side. The operating theatre layout is shown in Fig. 16.1.

Port Placement

First, we gain access into the abdomen via a Pfannenstiel incision. A small Alexis® wound retractor is inserted with a green cap and 12 mm port through it. Through the port pneumoperitoneum is created with an AirSeal® insufflator. Port positioning is drawn on the patient's abdomen and the ports are inserted under direct vision. Ports R1 to R3 are 8 mm in size, R4 is either 8 mm or 12 mm, when planning for a intracorporeal anastomosis. The ports are placed 8 cm (6–10 cm range) apart from each other in a straight line between the right and left anterior superior iliac spines. R1 and R4 are placed approximately 3 cm medial to the right and left anterior superior iliac spines respectively. Initially we used the AirSeal® port over the suprapubic incision for insufflation. More recently, we have been replacing the AirSeal® port with a 12 mm robotic port and maintaining pneumoperitoneum via an 8 mm robotic AirSeal® port, allowing us to use 8 mm ports for R1 to R4. Robotic port configuration is demonstrated in Figs. 16.2.

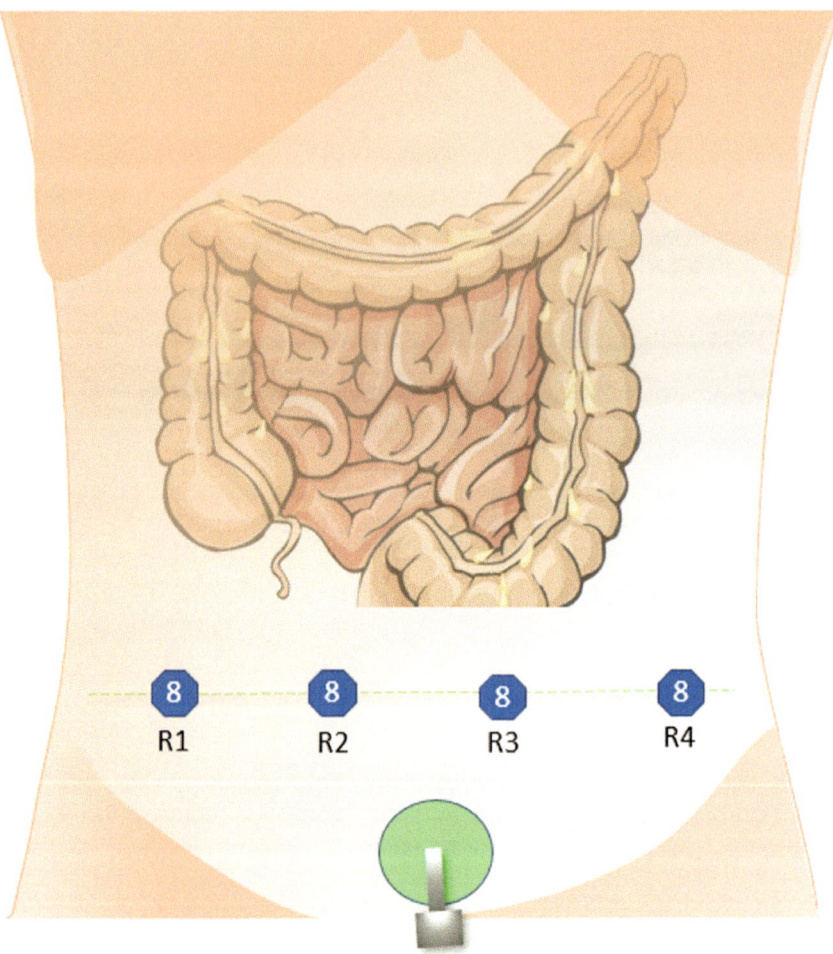

Fig. 16.2 Robotic port positioning. If we use a 12 mm AirSeal® port over the suprapubic extraction site, we have to replace the R4 with a 12 mm robotic port. Otherwise, we place the 12 mm robotic port through the suprapubic incision

Robot Docking

The robotic patient cart is set to the left upper abdomen anatomy setting and brought towards the patient from the patients left side. Thereafter, a laser guided system displaying a green target is projected from the cart's overhead boom, which is aligned to the camera port (R2). The camera is then inserted in R2, pointed towards the falciform ligament and selected as the target anatomy. The cart then automatically positions its boom in an optimised configuration for surgery. The remaining robotic arms are docked and the rest of the instruments inserted; fenestrated bipolar forceps are inserted in R1, scissors with monopolar diathermy in R3 and Cadiere forceps

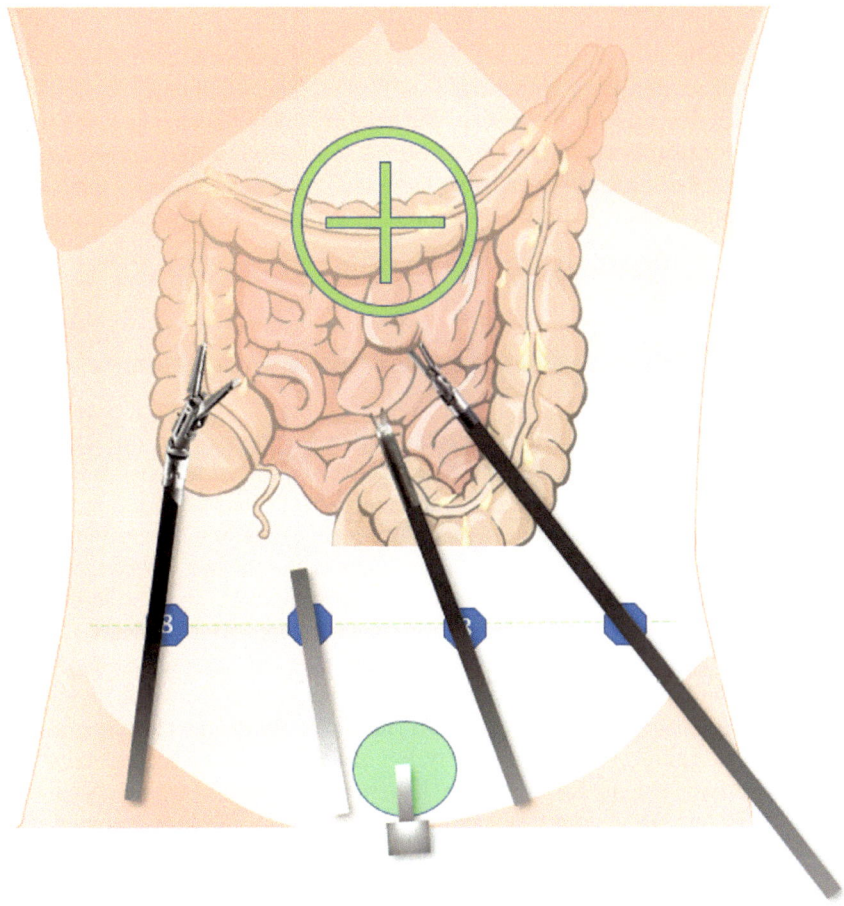

Fig. 16.3 Laser target position and instrument placement. R1: fenestrated bipolar forceps; R2: camera, R3: scissors with monopolar diathermy, R4: Cadiere forceps

in R4. The assistant uses the 12 mm robot port through the suprapubic incision for suction, retraction and the insertion and removal of tonsillar swabs as required. Figure 16.3 illustrates the laser target position and instrument placement. Before the instruments are fully inserted into the abdomen, we use the table motion feature to place the patient in the Trendelenburg-left tilt position (see procedure steps for details). The instruments are then fully inserted, the omentum and transverse colon is displaced cranially, with the small bowel being retracted towards the left side.

Equipment

The equipment we use includes a 30 degree camera, fenestrated bipolar forceps, scissors with monopolar diathermy, Cadiere forceps, robotic Hem-o-lok applicator and the SureForm® 60 robotic stapler. We favour using two right arms rather than two left arms. This means that we have two instruments on the right side of the camera. We believe this allows us to switch between using the scissors and fenestrated forceps for dissection and the fenestrated and Cadiere forceps for tissue manipulation and handling. The use of a Vesselsealer® can be very helpful, when performing the omento-colic separation. The robotic Hem-o-lok applicator is usually applied through R3 instead of the scissors. When using the robotic stapler, we undock the R3 arm from the 8 mm R3 port and dock it on the 12 mm robotic port over the suprapubic incision.

Step-by-Step Description of Robotic Subtotal Colectomy

The following description of the procedure relates to an oncological resection and applies all principles of complete mesocolic excision. This includes a sufficient longitudinal resection, preservation of the embryologic planes of the mesocolon and central ligation of the feeding vessels. The exact extent of the procedure (longitudinal) is obviously determined by the position of the tumour. These indications are rare, but surgeons may also choose to perform a subtotal colectomy for tumours in the splenic flexure or benign indications for inflammatory or functional bowel disease. The operative technique may change for such indications, as it may not be mandatory to follow a central vascular dissection throughout the whole mesocolon. Nevertheless, the advantage of central vascular dissection is the close spatial relationship of all central vessels. Robotically, this can be an advantage as operating on a small footprint is slightly easier. Despite this, robotic subtotal and total colectomies are probably one of the most challenging procedures, as it involves operating in all four quadrants of the abdomen. Port positioning (see above) is crucial, and some surgeons may to prefer to use a port position with a dual docking approach, as they are moving from the right to the left or vice versa. In our experience, the single-dock approach with a suprapubic port positioning works well for most indications and it allows to access the whole abdomen, bar the pelvis.

We prefer to start from the right side and move over to the left. The reason for this is to approach the main landmark on the right, the distal superior mesenteric vein (SMV), early and move along it towards proximally. The relevant vascular structures can be identified and taken up and including the middle colic artery (MCA). We then use the body of the pancreas as the guiding landmark and move to the left, by identifying the inferior mesenteric vein (IMV) and artery (IMA). This path describes a 'semicircle' and is often not bigger than within a field of 10×10 cm.

For some benign indications, some surgeons may prefer to tackle the MCA distally first and then move to the right and left. Our preference in those cases is still to start at the right side, mobilise laterally and then use a vessel sealing device (e.g. Vesselsealer advance® or Syncroseal®) to dissected through the mesocolon in relative vicinity to the colon.

The following steps describe the procedure using a daVInci® Xi system with integrated table motion. In theory, these steps can be translated to other robotic systems. The integrated table motion can be very useful for this procedure as it allows to reposition the patient without undocking.

Step 1. Subileal dissection

For the first step, the patient is in a steep head down position (around 25 degrees) and a slight right tiles (around 10 degrees). This allows for the small bowel to be positioned in the right upper quadrant and enables access to the base of the mesentery. The dissection is started below the terminal ileum, at the base of the mesoileum. The anatomical landmarks are the aorta and inferior cava vein posteriorly, and the mesoileum and the duodenal-jejunal junction superiorly. As soon as the peritoneum is incised, the intraperitoneal gas will travel outside of the posterior mesocolic envelope and posterior to the duodenum. In order not to Kocherise the duodenum too far, this layer needs to be incised at the duodenum (also referred to as fusion fascia of Fredet). Once incised, the duodenum can be dropped posteriorly and followed towards pars 2 and eventually pars 1 of the duodenum. During this manoeuvre, the uncinate process of the pancreas will become visible and the anterior surface of the pancreas can also be dissected, in order to drop the pancreas and the duodenum posteriorly. The posterior plane of the right mesocolon can be followed laterally and should be opened until the ascending and proximal transverse colon can be visualised from posterior. At the end of this step, the pancreas, duodenum and renal fascia (Gerota) should be completely exposed.

Step 2: Vascular dissection of the right and transverse colon

At this point, the patient is repositioned to a slight head down (5–10 degrees) and left tilt (15 degrees). The small bowel is now positioned towards the left side of the abdomen and allows exposure of the central vessels (SMA and SMV). The distal SMV can often be identified by 'tugging' on the ileocolic vessels with the left hand grasper and holding the middle colic vessels towards anterior and cranial with the right hand grasper. This manoeuvre demonstrates where the vessels come together and gives an indication of the position of the SMA/SMV. In thin patients the vessels are often directly visible, in obese patients it can be challenging and it may be safer to start the dissection below the ileocolic vessels and move centrally to find the SMV. The use of intraoperative ultrasound can be helpful but is not widely adopted. Once the SMV is identified, its anterior surface will be dissected completely. This is an avascular plane and allows for bloodless dissection on the vessel. The dissection follows the SMV towards proximal and the first branch is commonly the ileocolic artery and vein. The artery can cross over or underneath the SMV and preoperative assessment of the CT anatomy is recommended. After clipping of the ileocolic vessels, the SMV is followed further cranially. True right colic arteries and veins are rare and it is more common to get directly to the MCA and MCV. At the same level the gastropancreaticocolic trunk of Henle (GCT) can be found on the right side of the SMV. The Henle trunk is not always complete and can also be composed of only one or several elements (pancreatic, gastroepiploic and/or colic veins). In the video example it is a gastropancreatic trunk, without any colic vessels. MCA and MCV are clipped and transacted. We tend to preserve the GCT and only take colic vessels, unless there is an advanced tumour in the transverse colon, in which case the gastroepiploic vessels are removed from the greater curvature of the stomach.

Step 3: Supracolic and lateral dissection, transection of terminal ileum

The transverse colon is now moved causally and the gastroepiploic ligament is opened, usually just outside of the gastroepiploic arcade. The lesser sac is entered and the mobilisation of the hepatic flexure is completed. At this point, there should be only a thin layer left, as most of the dissection has been achieved from inferior. The right colon is released laterally, again, often only one thin layer is remaining. The distal mesoileum is transacted (a Vesselsealer® can be very helpful at this point). And followed to the terminal ileum. The terminal ileum can be transacted with a robotic or laparoscopic stapler.

Step 4: Left transverse colon and splenic flexure

The patient is now positioned in a neutral or slightly head up position (0–10 degrees) and tilt to the left (15 degrees). The dissection of the gastroepiploic ligament is followed to the left side and the splenic flexure released from adhesions towards the spleen. This complete mobilisation of the left transverse mesentery from cranially allows to lift the mesentery anteriorly and complete the mobilisation from below. In this position, the body of the pancreas is clearly visible and the mesentery can be dissected at its root.

Step 5: IMV and IMA

A consistent structure at the inferior border of the pancreas is the IMV. We prefer to dissect onto the Gerota fascia from medial before taking the IMV. This can be achieved easily by lifting up the IMV anterior and incising the peritoneum below. The pressure of the pneumoperitoneum allows the CO2 to enter the space of least resistance which is the plane anterior to the prerenal fascia. At this point the Gerota fascia should already have been defined from cranial and lateral and both medial and lateral approach can be joined up. The IMV is now taken with clips. Depending on the extent of the resection, the IMA will be taken at its root, or only the left colic artery is taken. The extent of the lymphadenectomy has to be adjusted to the positioning of the tumour.

Step 6: Lateral mobilisation of the sigmoid colon

The lateral adhesions to the sigmoid colon need to be fully released. The medial plane is completed from medial. Protection of gonadal vessels and left ureter have to be ensured. Access to the distal sigmoid is often limited when using a suprapubic approach. In some cases, temporary repositioning of the robotic arms may be considered, by undocking arm 4 (the port can be used by an assistant and redocking arm 3 in the suprapubic port (through the wound retractor). A robotic 12 mm port usually gives a better seal for this. This will allow to access the left lower quadrant with three robotic arms.

Step 7: Extraction and anastomosis

Once the sigmoid is fully mobilised, the colon is now completely positioned in the left abdomen, by pulling the transacted distal end of the terminal ileum in the left upper quadrant. This important manoeuvre will prevent strangulation of the small bowel mesentery when attempting extraction. The transacted terminal ileum is held with a laparoscopic instrument, the robotic is undocked and the specimen is extracted through the Pfannenstiel wound. The distal sigmoid/ rectosigmoid is lying directly underneath the Pfannenstiel incision and can be transacted with a linear stapler. We prefer a functional end-to-end anastomosis by swinging the terminal ileum anticlockwise in a parallel position to the distal sigmoid. We then perform a stapled side to side anastomosis ('Barcelona technique').

Top Tips

- Integrated table motion: subtotal colectomy with a single-docking approach are one of the procedures that benefit most from integrated table motion. If your system is not compatible with table motion, it is still possible, but the system needs to be re-docked at several points during the procedure.
- Start on the right side first: Robotic procedures generally work best by following a continuous path. I.e. Unnecessary changes from one quadrant to the next should be avoided as they interrupt the flow of the procedure and require repositioning of the small bowel that can result in iatrogenic injuries.
- Central vascular dissection for cancer: Transecting all vessels near the origin result in a small operation area which is generally easier with a robotic system. The stability and precision of robotic instruments also support such an approach.
- Use two right hands: The use of two right hands allows to use two graspers (right and left hand) at the same time. This is especially important in procedures where the small bowel needs to be repositioned several times.
- Repositioning robotic arms for left (and right) lower quadrant: the limitation of the suprapubic approach is to operate in the lower quadrants, as the instruments will start clashing against each other. Consider repositioning one arm into the Pfannenstiel incision to approach these areas if required!

Checklist

- Open cutdown use of a wound retractor for the Pfannenstiel incision
- Place robotic ports in a suprapubic fashion along the line between both anterior superior iliac spines
- Dock the robot with a target focus in the upper abdomen
- Use two right hands
- Use standard instruments (left hand bipolar grasper, right hand mono polar scissors/ Vesselsealer®, second right hand grasper)
- Start on the right subileal and/or at the ileocolic vessels

- Follow the SMV to take off all relevant vascular pedicels
- Complete the right side by hepatic flexure and lateral mobilisation
- Complete the supracolic compartment towards the left including the splenic flexure
- Resect the left transverse mesocolon from the pancreas
- Define the left prerenal fascia from medial and transection the IMV
- Transection the IMA and/or left ascending colic artery
- Mobilise the sigmoid from lateral
- Exteriorise and perform anastomosis

References

1. Mirnezami H, Mirnezami R, Venkatasubramaniam K, Chandrakumaran K, Cecil TD, Moran BJ. Robotic colorectal surgery: hype or new hope? A systematic review of robotics in colorectal surgery. Colorectal Dis. 2010;12:1084–93. https://doi.org/10.1111/j.1463-1318.2009.01999.x.
2. Araujo SEA, Seid VE, Klajner S. Robotic surgery for rectal cancer: Current immediate clinical and oncological outcomes. World J Gastroenterol. 2014;20:14359–70. https://doi.org/10.3748/wjg.v20.i39.14359.
3. Gallagher AG, McClure N, McGuigan J, Ritchie K, Sheehy NP. An ergonomic analysis of the fulcrum effect in the acquisition of endoscopic skills. Endoscopy. 1998;30:617–20. https://doi.org/10.1055/s-2007-1001366.
4. Association of Coloproctology of Great Britain and Ireland (ACPGBI). National Bowel Cancer Audit Annual Report 2020: An audit of the care received by people with bowel cancer in England and Wales. 2020.
5. Weber PA, Merola S, Wasielewski A, Ballantyne GH. Telerobotic-assisted laparoscopic right and sigmoid colectomies for benign disease. Dis Colon Rectum. 2002;45:1686–9. https://doi.org/10.1097/01.DCR.0000037657.78153.A8.
6. Petz W, Borin S, Fumagalli Romario U. Updates on robotic CME for right colon cancer: a qualitative systematic review. J Pers Med. 2021. https://doi.org/10.3390/jpm11060550.
7. Pietro BP, Salaj A, Giuliani G, Ferraro L, Formisano G. Feasibility of robotic right colectomy with complete mesocolic excision and intracorporeal anastomosis: short-term outcomes of 161 consecutive patients. Updates Surg. 2021;73:1065–72. https://doi.org/10.1007/s13304-021-01001-x.
8. Larach JT, Flynn J, Wright T, Rajkomar AKS, McCormick JJ, Kong J, Smart PJ, Heriot AG, Warrier SK. Robotic complete mesocolic excision versus conventional robotic right colectomy for right-sided colon cancer: a comparative study of perioperative outcomes. Surg Endosc. 2021. https://doi.org/10.1007/s00464-021-08498-8.
9. Hollandsworth HM, Stringfield S, Klepper K, Zhao B, Abbadessa B, Lopez NE, Parry L, Ramamoorthy S, Eisenstein S. Multiquadrant surgery in the robotic era: a technical description and outcomes for da Vinci Xi robotic subtotal colectomy and total proctocolectomy. Surg Endosc. 2020;34:5153–9. https://doi.org/10.1007/s00464-020-07633-1.
10. Ozben V, de Muijnck C, Karabork M, Ozoran E, Zenger S, Bilgin IA, Aytac E, Baca B, Balik E, Hamzaoglu I, Karahasanoglu T, Bugra D. The da Vinci Xi system for robotic total/subtotal colectomy versus conventional laparoscopy: short-term outcomes. Tech Coloproctol. 2019;23:861–8. https://doi.org/10.1007/s10151-019-02066-y.
11. McSorley ST, Steele CW, McMahon AJ. Meta-analysis of oral antibiotics, in combination with preoperative intravenous antibiotics and mechanical bowel preparation the day before surgery, compared with intravenous antibiotics and mechanical bowel preparation alone to reduce surgical-site infec. BJS Open. 2018;2:185–94. https://doi.org/10.1002/bjs5.68.

Chapter 17
Robotic Splenic Flexure Mobilization

Carmen Cagigas Fernandez, Marcos Gómez Ruiz, Lidia Cristobal Poch, and Natalia Suarez Pazos

Abstract Splenic flexure mobilization is a controversial issue during sigmoidectomy or anterior resection of the rectum. In the literature, it is not clear whether it is necessary to perform it routinely, nor is there a clear consensus regarding how to do it. Some surgeons would advocate performing this procedure only in selected cases, if there is no redundancy of the sigmoid colon or if the anastomosis will be in the upper rectum. Others would rather prefer to perform it systematically in order to standardize the procedure and gain experience. Similarly, its performance laparoscopically or robotically depends again on the preference of the surgeon, since to date it has not been shown in the literature whether one approach or another provides benefits for the patient or the surgeon. In this chapter we present our approach to this procedure as well as the step-by-step surgical technique for mobilizing the splenic flexure performed from medial to lateral with a robotic approach.

Keywords Robotic surgery · Splenic flexure · Left colon cancer · Diverticular disease

C. C. Fernandez (✉) · M. G. Ruiz · L. C. Poch · N. Suarez Pazos
General Surgery Department, Colorectal Surgery Unit, Marqués de Valdecilla University Hospital, 39008 Santander, Spain
e-mail: carmen.cagigas@scsalud.es

M. G. Ruiz
e-mail: marcos.gomez@scsalud.es

L. C. Poch
e-mail: Lidia.cristobal@scsalud.es

N. Suarez Pazos
e-mail: Natalia.suarez@scsalud.com

Valdecilla Biomedical Research Institute (IDIVAL), 39011 Santander, Spain

M. G. Ruiz
Medical School, University of Cantabria, 39011 Santander, Spain

Introduction/Indications

Splenic flexure mobilisation (SFM) is one of the fundamental surgical steps during colorectal procedures. SFM can be used in different cases, from oncological resection itself, Left colon cancer, transverse colon cancer, and reconstruction used in sigmoid or rectal cancer, involving more facts than the technique itself [1].

All colorectal procedures requiring SFM have been scored by surgeons with high difficulty ratings. Splenic flexure resection and transverse colectomy were two of the most challenging procedures in the laparoscopic approach [2]. However, laparoscopic SFM requires top-notch surgical skills since the surgical process is complex and demands an extensive dissection that preserves the retroperitoneal structures, including the pancreatic tail [3].

When deciding whether to mobilise the splenic flexure, one must assess the factors that influence this decision before embarking on a technically demanding and risky procedure [4].

SFM is one of the crucial steps in pelvic colorectal surgery with anastomosis. Tension-free anastomosis with good blood supply is facilitated by a complete mobilisation of letting colon and dividing IMV and IMA in origin, with a less chance of anastomotic stricture. We obtain potential advantages apart from those described previously, like less chance of anastomotic stricture [5].

Another potential benefit of SMF is the decreases in the rate of inadequate nodal staging. The failure to perform SFM may also be specifically associated with a shortening of the distal margin [6].

SFM is one of the most demanding surgical maneuvers in colorectal surgery, and the learning curve can be steep because of the complexity of the anatomical area and the possibility of intraoperative complications. With the introduction of robotics in the minimal invasive field, the surgeons have obtain some benefits along the evolution of it, like the stability of the surgical field, 3d vision or endowristed instruments.

Robotic systems introduced two decades ago were not designed for multi-quadrant abdominal dissection, as frequently required in the left-sided colon or rectal cancer surgery. Therefore, some surgeons developed the dual-docking method to take down the colonic splenic flexure robotically. The new platforms such as da Vinci Xi and X robotic systems have been specially designed for multi quadrant surgical access; narrower arms with greater reach, and lighter, slimmer endoscopes that can swap between ports [7].

Robotic surgery offers advantages over laparoscopic surgery, given the characteristics of robotic platforms.

- Filters physiologic tremor
- Stable camera control
- Endowristed instruments
- Haptic feedback
- Motion scaling
- 3D view

Compared to laparoscopic surgery: (two-dimensional visualisation).

- Amplification of physiological tremors
- Fulcrum effect (perception of stiffness)
- Restricted degrees of motion of the laparoscopic instruments
- Inversion of range and scaling of motion
- Friction at the incision point

During splenic flexure mobilization, robotic surgery might helps us better exposition mesocolon and vessels during the VMI dissection. It gives us a better vision during the pancreas and retroperitoneal dissection thanks to 3D and a stable surgical field and instruments in traction and countertraction during the mobilization/detachment of the colon from the spleen.

Procedural Cases

– Position of the patient

Patient is placed on the table in the modified Lloyd Davies position. For the specific mobilisation of the splenic flexure, the patient is positioned in a slight Tredelenburg and Tilt right to facilitate adequate visualisation of the medial aspect of the mesocolon.

– Theatre layout

The anesthesia team and anesthesiologist are positioned at the patient's bedside, the scrub nurse and assistant are positioned to the right of the patient. At the same time, the robot trolley enters from the left of the patient.

Care should be taken to avoid as far as possible the crossing of tubes and wires (pneumoperitoneum, monopolar/bipolar wires or sucker) on different sides of the patient as they may affect or be affected by the robot trolley or the arms (Fig. 17.1).

– Port position for X and Xi system

1. Port number 1(P1) is place 3–4 cm up from de Superior iliac spine and 3–4 cm medial. Port number 4 (P4) is placed 4 cm down from de xiphoid and 2 cm lateral. We draw a line and divide it in between 3 to place the rest of the trocars (Fig. 17.2).
2. Assistant trocar 12 mm high flow trocar is placed in RUQ.
3. Preferably use high flow insufflators, as they allow for more excellent stability of the pneumoperitoneum bell with slight variation, which facilitates lower pressure surgery.

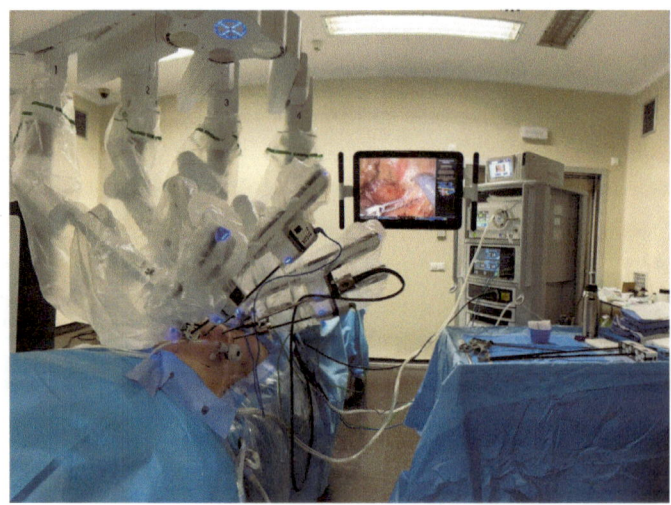

Fig. 17.1 Theater layout

Fig. 17.2 Port positioning

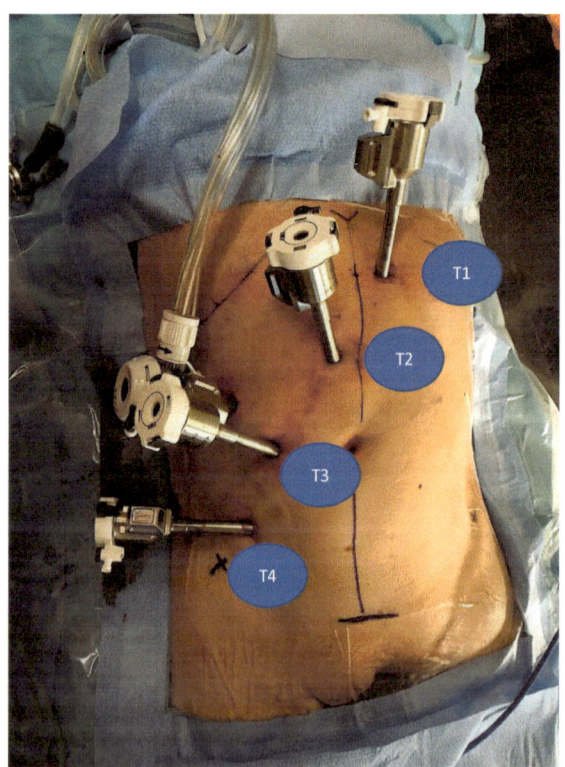

– Safety/adaptations versus lap or open

The patient must be protected from possible trauma caused by the robotic arms or possible injuries caused by forced positions. The arms are placed in an anatomical position with the aid of a glove to keep the hand in a neutral position, both arms are covered with protectors and padded shoulder pads, or a non-slip surface is applied.

– Equipment needed

A 30° camera is used to adapt to the mobilisation of the splenic flexure in different approaches.

Usually, in a standard patient, the camera is placed in arm 3, using two forceps in 1 and 2 (two left arms) and scissors or hook in arm 4 (one right). This allows us to maintain the necessary traction without collisions with the other two working arms [8].

– Graspers and alternatives

Usually, we will use an atraumatic tip up type grasper (Fig. 17.3).

Bipolar energy instrument, fenestrated grasper (Fig. 17.4) or vessel sealer (Fig. 17.5).

Monopolar energy instrument (scissors, Fig. 17.6 or hook, Fig. 17.7): The scissors have greater versatility than the hook, as we can use them with both functionalities.

For vessel ligation we use a robotic Hem-o-lock (Fig. 17.8). Usually medium-large, the use of it rather than the one use it by the assistant helps us to control it an a better orientation to clip the mayor vessels.

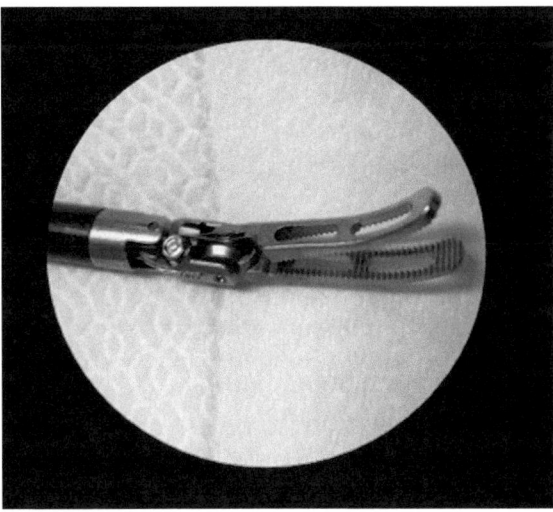

Fig. 17.3 Tip up type grasper

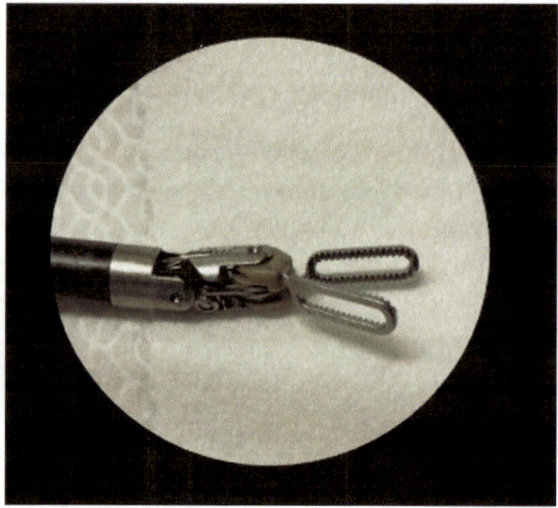

Fig. 17.4 Fenestrated grasper

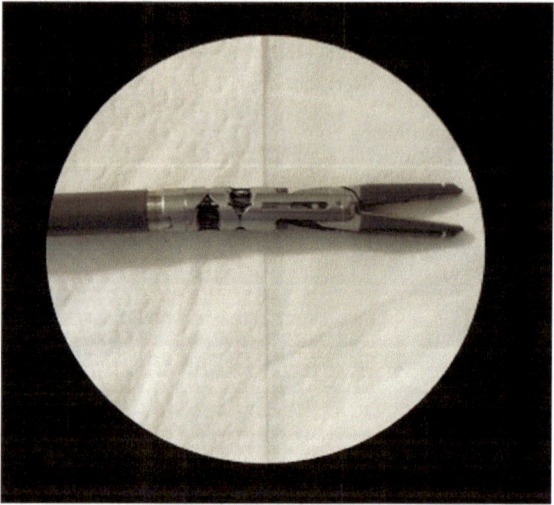

Fig. 17.5 Vessel sealer

Steps of Procedure

We routinely mobilised the colonic splenic flexure using the medial-to-lateral approach based on our experiences gained during the prime time of laparoscopic surgery and the Si robotic system. The procedure of complete mobilisation of colonic splenic flexure begins from the initial ligation of the inferior mesenteric vein (IMV).

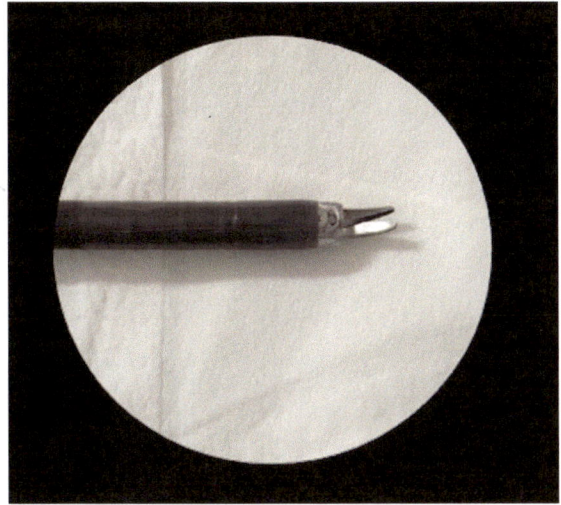

Fig. 17.6 Scissors

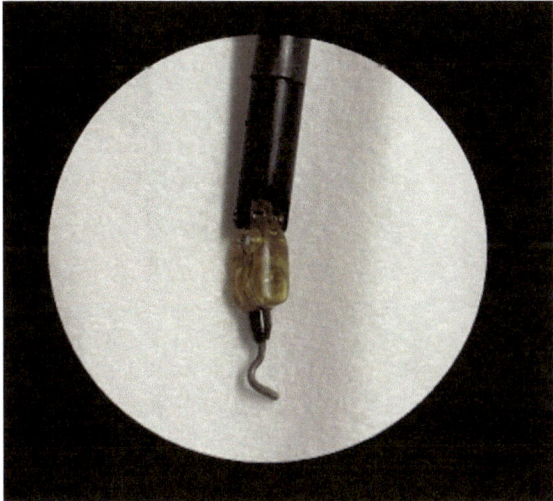

Fig. 17.7 Hook

Moreover, it ended in the complete separation descending colon. We divided SFM procedure into four steps.

1. IMV ligation
2. Medial to lateral dissection
3. Lateral dissection
4. Superior dissection.

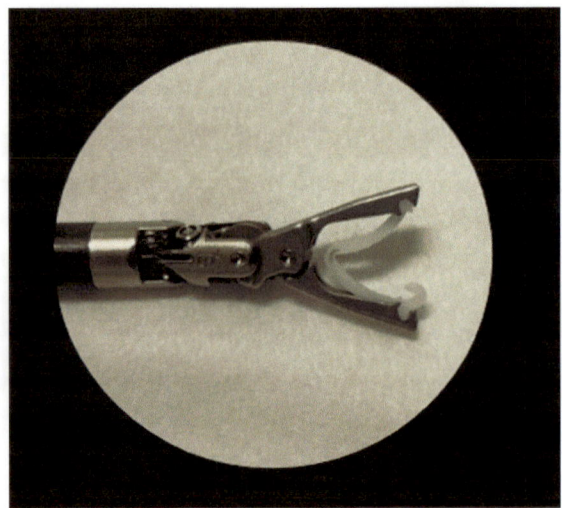

Fig. 17.8 Hem-o-lock

First of all, the small bowel is position towards the Right upper quadrant, which allows us to identify the origin of the IMV. DJ junction mobilisation is usually necessary for a correct visualisation and section of the vein at the level of the lower edge of the pancreas. We perform atraumatic traction from the left mesocolon with tip-up forceps (T1) up and lateral for adequate exposure. We made an incision at the medial aspect of the peritoneum of the left mesocolon to develop a surgical plane and proceed with the dissection cranially between the inferior mesenteric vein and the retroperitoneum (Fig. 17.9).

We do not go too far in the retroperitoneal dissection, as traction may cause injury to the non-dissected vessels. We dissect the tissue surrounding the inferior mesenteric vein at the inferior border of the pancreas. The vein is ligated between hem-o-locks, leaving at least one centimetre between them for a safe section, and all the tissues surrounding the vein are also sectioned (Fig. 17.10).

Once the vein has been sectioned, the traction of the atraumatic forceps is changed so that the Hem-o-lock is exposed; the traction must be anterior and lateral at the level of the left mesocolon with an atraumatic tip-up forceps. At the same time, the assistant's forceps perform traction at the transverse mesocolon level, cranially, allowing a safe dissection between the transverse mesocolon and the pancreas towards the lesser sac (Fig. 17.11).

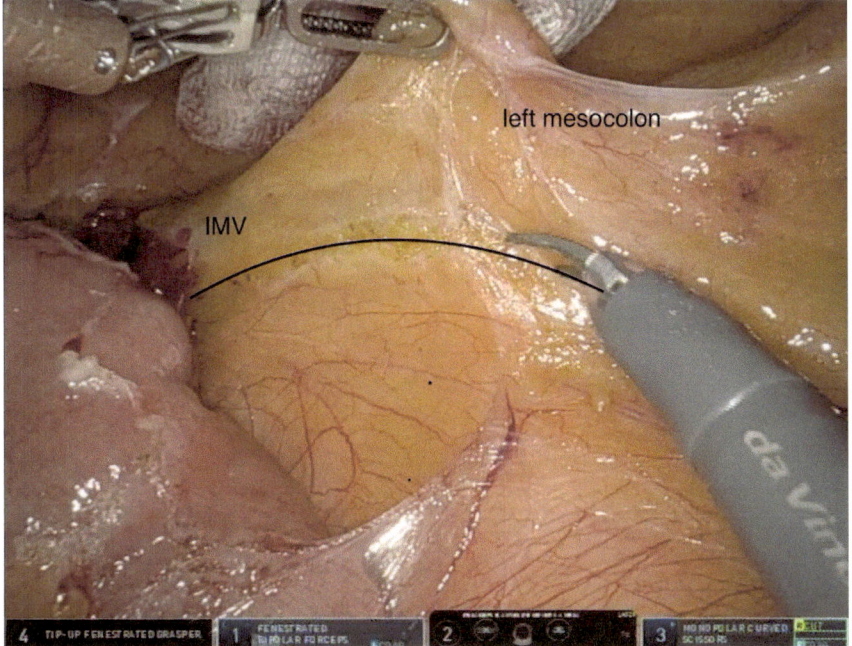

Fig. 17.9 IMV expousure

With monopolar and bipolar energy, the retroperitoneal dissection is progressed along the inferior border of the pancreas and laterally on the left Told's fascia. We continue in this plane until the posterior aspect of the descending colon is visualized, using constant traction with atraumatic forceps and with the help of gauze to reduce as much as possible the possible lesions that could be produced by the traction of the instruments, affecting the viability of the colon which has to reach the anastomosis (Fig. 17.12).

The upper edge of the pancreas is about 2 cm lateral and superior to the inferior mesenteric clip (origin of the IMV). A dissection plane is made on the ventral surface of the pancreas to access the lesser sac at this level. Once located, the assistant introduces the dissection forceps so that the transverse colon and the stomach are away from the dissection plane, and the dissection is carried out on the ventral surface of the pancreas towards the tail, typically not completed from the medial aspect due to possible lesions derived from splenic vessels (Fig. 17.13).

After completing these dissection planes, the left parietocolic attachment is released.

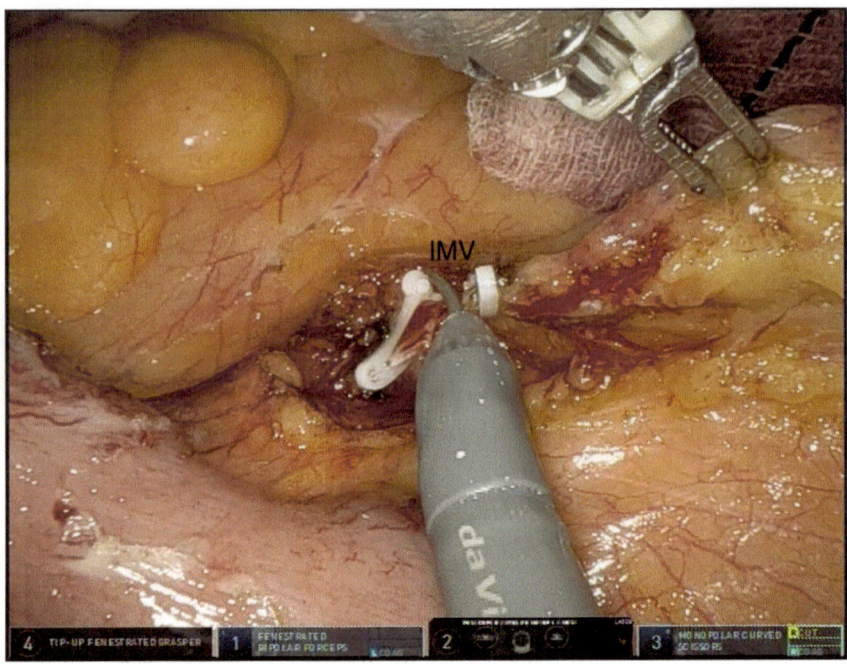

Fig. 17.10 IMV ligation and transection

With the atraumatic forceps(tip-up), medial traction and countertraction of the left parietal peritoneum are carried out, incising and dissecting this plane cranially until it converges medial–lateral dissection performed previously (Fig. 17.14). At the level of the splenic angle, where the greater omentum is anchored, dissection is performed below it, again using traction and countertraction, the greater omentum is dissected from the transverse colon, converging with the medial dissection plane that we had developed. With both dissection planes exposed, we finish the lysis of the pancreatocolic ligament at the level of the tail of the pancreas.

Finally, the rest of the omentum is separated from the transverse colon either from the medial or by continuing the dissection started from lateral to medial. Dissection starts from the middle transverse colon and advanced laterally. The aim is to separate the embryonic avascular plane between the greater omentum and the transverse colon (Fig. 17.15).

The lesser sac is entered from above (Fig. 17.16), and dissection is continued toward the splenic hilum, where the splenocolic ligament is encountered. The transverse mesocolon is not mobilised beyond the middle colic vessels.

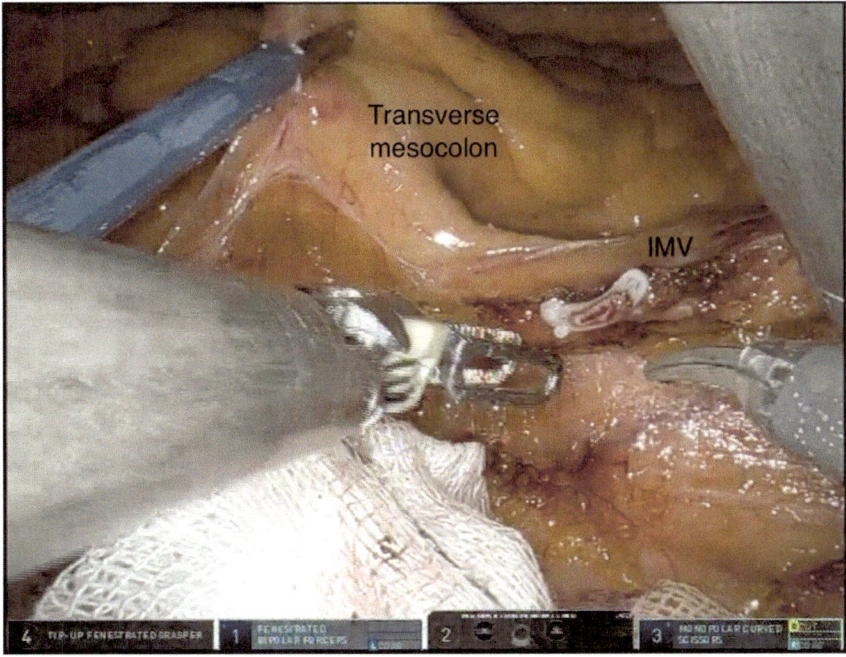

Fig. 17.11   Medial to lateral approach of splenic flexure

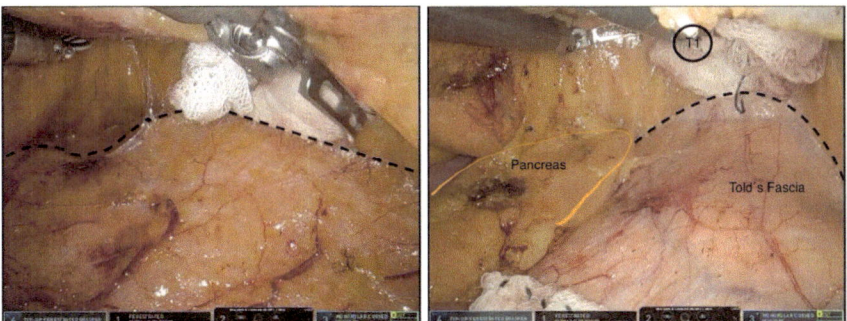

Fig. 17.12   Left Told's fascia disection

Top Tips

- Exposure with traction and countertraction is the Key
- Assistant's forceps perform traction at the transverse mesocolon level, cranially, allowing a safe dissection between the transverse mesocolon and the pancreas towards the lesser sac.
- Left a gauze at the lesser sac to find it out at the time of superior dissection and protect the pancreas from possible lesion (Fig. 17.16).

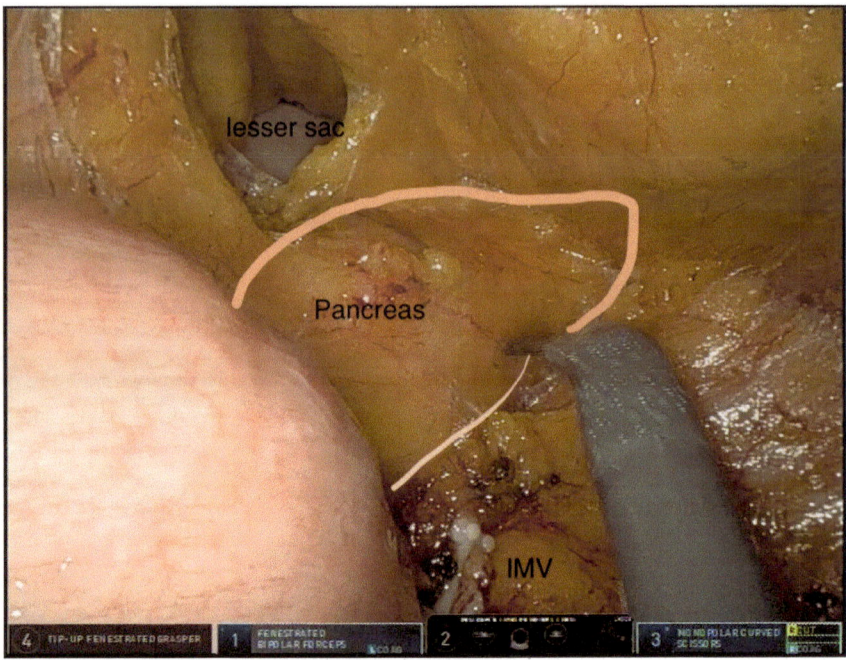

Fig. 17.13 Medial view of dissected pancreas and lesser sac

– Protect the specimen (left mesocolon) from robotic instruments traction with gauze in between the instrument and the tissue (Fig. 17.12).
– Systematize your procedure. Always try to perform it the same way.

Checklist

• Correct position and protection of the patient
• Table positioning (Tredelemburg and tilt right)
• 4 steps splenic flexure mobilisation
• IMV ligation
• Medial to lateral dissection
• Lateral dissection
• Superior dissection.

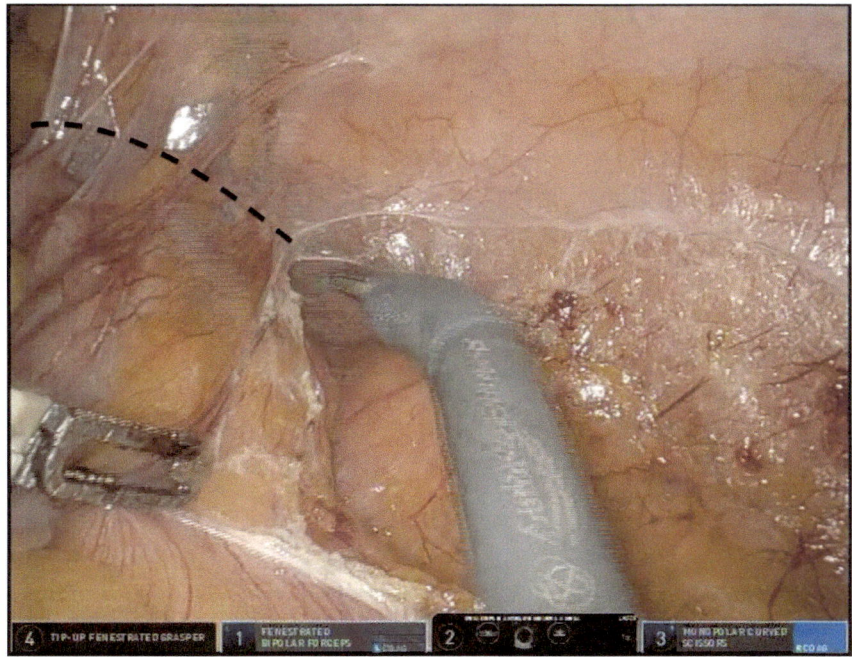

Fig. 17.14 Left parietocolic ligament transection

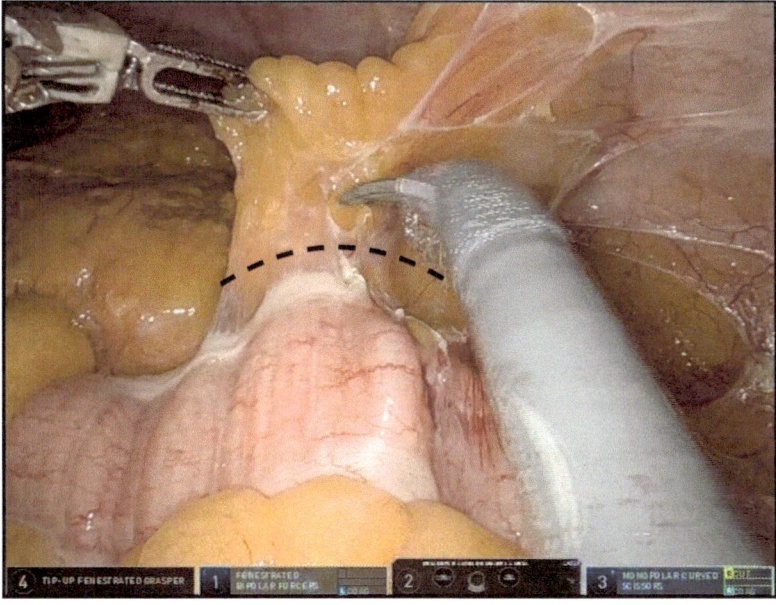

Fig. 17.15 Omental dissection from the splenic flexure

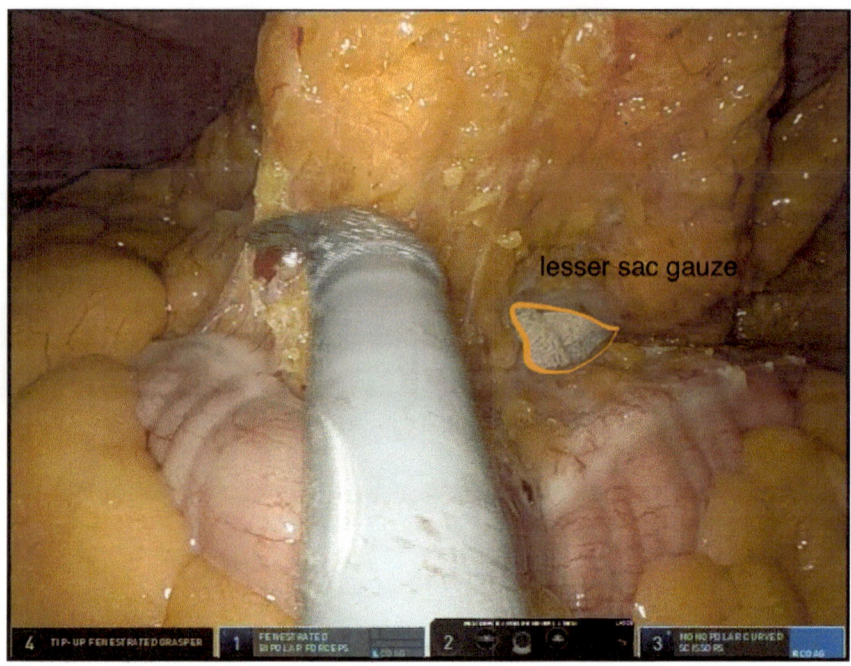

Fig. 17.16 Completion of omental transection from the transverse colon

References

1. Marsden MR, Conti JA, Zeidan S, Flashman KG, Khan JS, O'Leary DP, et al. The selective use of splenic flexure mobilization is safe in both laparoscopic and open anterior resections. Colorectal Dis. 2012;14(10):1255–61.
2. Jamali FR, Soweid AM, Dimassi H, Bailey C, Leroy J, Marescaux J. Evaluating the degree of difficulty of laparoscopic colorectal surgery. Arch Surg. 2008;143(8):762–7; discussion 8.
3. Kumamoto T, Shinohara H, Tomizawa K, Hanaoka Y, Toda S, Takemura N, et al. Inferior pancreatic approach for laparoscopic splenic flexure mobilization. Tech Coloproctol. 2018;22(1):71–2.
4. Chand M, Miskovic D, Parvaiz AC. Is splenic flexure mobilization necessary in laparoscopic anterior resection? Dis Colon Rectum. 2012;55(11):1195–7.
5. Hiranyakas A, Da Silva G, Denoya P, Shawki S, Wexner SD. Colorectal anastomotic stricture: is it associated with inadequate colonic mobilization? Tech Coloproctol. 2013;17(4):371–5.
6. Mouw TJ, King C, Ashcraft JH, Valentino JD, DiPasco PJ, Al-Kasspooles M. Routine splenic flexure mobilization may increase compliance with pathological quality metrics in patients undergoing low anterior resection. Colorectal Dis. 2019;21(1):23-9
7. Pai A, Marecik S, Park J, Prasad L. Robotic colorectal surgery for neoplasia. Surg Clin North Am. 2017;97(3):561–72.
8. Da Vinci X/Xi Instrument & Accessory Catalog. 2020.

Part IV
Miscellaneous

Chapter 18
Robotic Surgery for Perforated Diverticulitis

Ellen Van Eetvelde and Daniel Jacobs-Tulleneers-Tevissen

Abstract Diverticulitis complicated by diffuse purulent or fecal peritonitis should be treated surgically. This treatment usually consists of a sigmoid colon resection with or without primary anastomosis, depending on the general condition of the patient and the quality of the tissue. Technical difficulties arise when this type of surgery is approached laparoscopically, leading to a high percentage of patients undergoing upfront open surgery or being converted to laparotomy after initial laparoscopic exploration. In our experience, the robotic platform allows a minimally invasive approach in the emergency setting, with a conversion rate lower than laparoscopy, similar as documented for oncological resections. The current chapter presents the authors' personal step-by-step approach for surgical treatment of acute complicated diverticulitis using the robotic platform to perform emergency sigmoid colon resection with primary anastomosis or a Hartmann's resection. The detailed description of each operative step allows to adjust the chronology according to each specific case. Several tips and tricks to deal with difficulties during surgery, such as identification of the ureter, difficult mobilization of the splenic flexure, and presence of an inflammatory mass, are addressed.

Keywords Perforated diverticulitis · Emergency surgery · Hartmann's resection · Primary resection and anastomosis

Introduction

Treatment of acute diverticulitis depends on its severity reflected by the Hinchey classification. Surgical management is necessary in case of diverticulitis with purulent or fecal peritonitis (Hinchey III and IV). In these cases, a Hartmann's resection is often performed, especially in unstable or frail patients or when tissue quality is poor [1].

E. Van Eetvelde (✉) · D. Jacobs-Tulleneers-Tevissen (✉)
Department of Colorectal Surgery, UZ Brussel, Laarbeeklaan 101, 1090 Brussels, Belgium
e-mail: Ellen.VanEetvelde@uzbrussel.be

D. Jacobs-Tulleneers-Tevissen
e-mail: Ellen.VanEetvelde@uzbrussel.be

In order to avoid the important morbidity associated with a Hartmann's procedure as well as a permanent stoma rate as high as 60%, primary resection and anastomosis with or without protective ileostomy may be performed in hemodynamically stable immunocompetent patients [2, 3]. In highly selected cases with local peritonitis a simple laparoscopic peritoneal lavage can be considered as an emergency treatment to allow for an elective second-stage resection [4]. We therefore advocate to perform a laparoscopic exploration first to distinguish between a true Hinchey III and an occult Hinchey IV and choose the appropriate surgical treatment.

When diffuse purulent or fecal peritonitis or overt bowel perforation is observed, a resection is mandatory. However, performing a laparoscopic Hartmann's procedure or sigmoidectomy with primary anastomosis in emergency setting and under septic conditions is technically demanding even in experienced hands [5]. High conversion rates are noted associated with an increased postoperative morbidity such as wound infection, evisceration, or respiratory insufficiency. These findings explain the high rates of patients that are primarily treated by laparotomy [6].

There are several reasons why a robotic approach could offer a benefit over laparoscopy in these technically demanding procedures: articulating instruments and the aid of the third arm allowing for improved maneuverability in limited spaces, a visual stability of the operative field, and improved ergonomics [7, 8]. It is increasingly documented for oncological resections that these benefits may reduce conversion rate while keeping resection quality optimal [9–11]. Although we strongly believe in comparable benefits, such evidence is not yet available for benign colorectal disease such as emergency surgery for perforated diverticulitis or reversal of Hartmann's procedure.

Materials Needed

- 3D vision camera, 30° scope
- Cadiere Forceps or Tip-Up Grasper
- Monopolar Curved Scissors
- Fenestrated Bipolar Forceps or Vessel Sealer®
- Large or Medium Clip Applier
- Sureform® stapler 60 mm or 45 mm—blue or green reload depending on bowel thickness
- Needle Driver (stand-by)
- Suction/irrigation device
- Swabs
- Assistant port 12 mm
- Insufflation with AirSeal® (if available): it allows operating at a pressure of 8 cm H_2O with a stable pneumoperitoneum and a constant smoke evacuation
- Additional assistant port 5 mm (stand-by)
- Wound protector for specimen retrieval

Procedure Details

Theatre layout (Fig. 18.1)

The robotic patient cart is docked from the left side of the patient. A video screen is placed both at the feet of the patient and at the left side of the patient's head to facilitate pelvic exploration and possible splenic flexure mobilization. The first assist and scrub nurse are positioned at the patient's right side, as is the instrument table.

Patient preparation and positioning (Fig. 18.2a, b)

The patient is placed in a Lloyd-Davies position with the legs in stirrups and adequate padding at all pressure points. Depending on local practices, arms are placed adjacent to the body or in abduction on an arm board. A bladder catheter and a nasogastric tube are inserted. Monitoring is done according to preferences of the anesthesiologist. Eye shields are placed, and the face of the patient is protected from harm by the robotic arms using a cushion or a metal bar. Skin disinfection from nipple to the thighs, up to both posterior axillary lines and including the perineum. Sterile draping of the abdomen and installation of all cables. The patient is positioned in a Trendelenburg position (20°–25°) with right tilt (8°–10°).

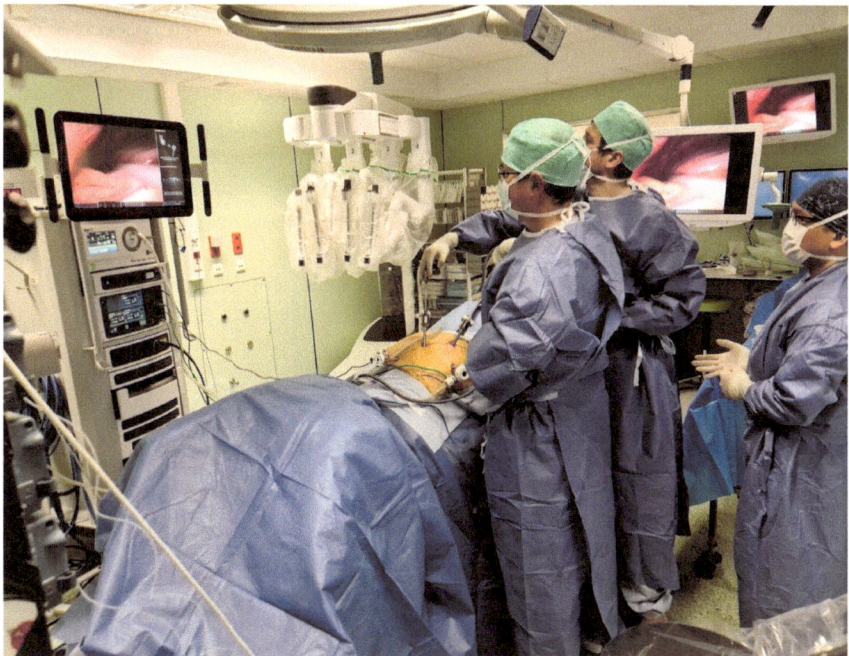

Fig. 18.1 Theatre layout. Robot is docked from the left side of the patient after laparoscopic exploration. Two monitors are positioned at the head and feet, respectively. Assistant and scrub nurse at the patient's right side

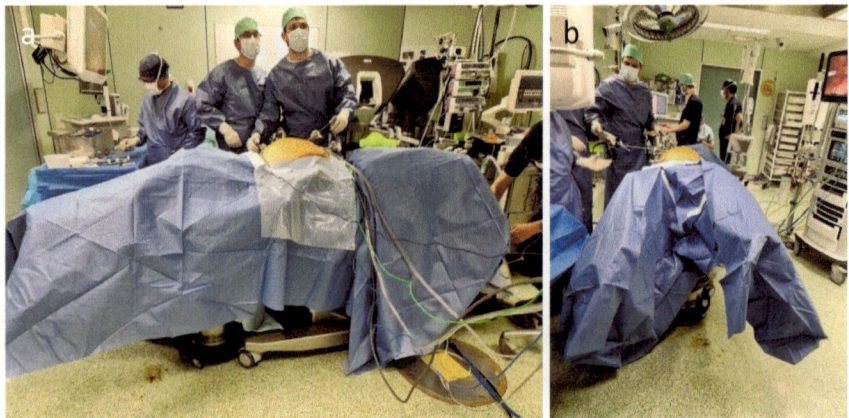

Fig. 18.2 a, b Patient positioning. The patient is installed in a Lloyd-Davies position and after draping placed in a Trendelenburg position (20–25°) (**a**) with right tilt (8–10°) (**b**)

Port placement (Fig. 18.3)

Three 8 mm robotic trocars and one 12 mm trocar for introduction of the stapler are used. The robotic trocars are placed in a diagonal line from the right anterior superior iliac spine to the subcostal margin on the left side with a space of 8–9 cm in between each port. The 12 mm trocar for stapling can be used as port 3 or 4, outlined in Fig. 18.3. This line may be moved towards the right side of the patient to keep enough distance (ideal at least 18–20 cm) between the port alignment and the target zone, being the sigmoid colon. It is important to place the ports at least 2 cm at distance from bony structures.

A 12 mm assistant port is placed in the right hypochondrium, triangulated between the robotic ports 2 and 3, at a distance of preferably 7 cm.

For the X-system the order of the port positions is, from left to right, 4–1–2–3 as the third arm needs to be positioned on the left side.

Laparoscopic phase

Creation of a pneumoperitoneum using the Verres needle technique at Palmer's point or via the open Hasson approach according to the surgeon's preference. Although not mandatory for insufflation, we advise the use of the AirSeal® insufflator to keep a stable pneumoperitoneum at low pressure, even when fluids are being aspirated. A pressure as low as 8 cm H_2O can be used while smoke is continuously evacuated.

Placement of port 3 (port 2 for X system) for camera introduction and initial exploration of the abdominal cavity to evaluate feasibility of a minimal invasive approach. If possible, placement of all additional trocars (Fig. 18.3).

Aspiration of fluid/pus for microbiological examination if needed. Peritoneal lavage of all quadrants using saline to reduce peritoneal contamination. Draping of the robotic system while positioning the patient in a Trendelenburg position (20°–25°) with right tilt (8°–10°) to facilitate bowel positioning and exposure of the

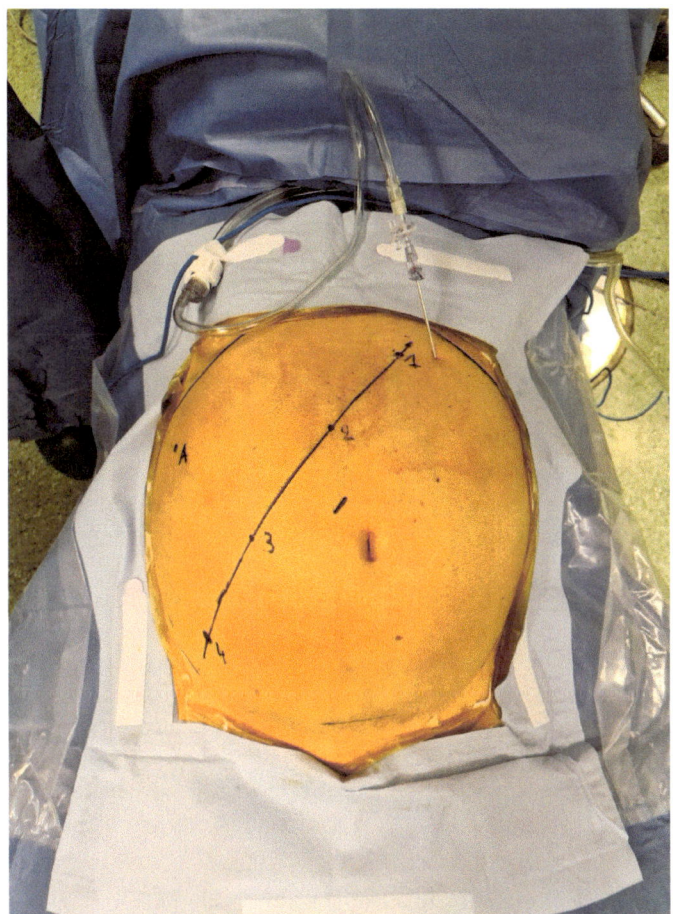

Fig. 18.3 Trocar placement. The trocars are placed in a diagonal line from the right anterior superior iliac spine to the subcostal margin on the left side (1–2–3–4). The 12 mm stapler trocar can be introduced at port 3 or 4. A 12 mm assistant port is placed triangulated between the robotic ports in the right hypochondrium (A). *Note: for the X-system the port numbers are 4–1-2–3 as the third arm needs to come from the left side*

operative field. Small bowel should be taken out of the pelvis and placed in the right hypochondrium.

Docking phase

X system: The robot cart is obliquely advanced over the patient's left leg aiming at port 2. Arm 2 is docked to port 2 with correct positioning in the so-called sweet spot. The remaining robotic arms are docked to the cannulas; the instruments are introduced under direct vision in the following order from left to right: Cadiere Forceps—Vessel sealer®—30° Camera—Scissors. The tension on the abdominal wall is released.

Xi system: The robotic cart is approached from the left side with the robotic cart prepared for '*lower abdominal surgery, patient left*'. The laser cross is oriented on the camera port (port 3), arm 3 is then docked to the camera port and the camera is introduced. Release the tension on the cannula. Target on the sigmoid colon with alignment of arm 3 according to targeting. The boom will orientate to the target zone. The other cannulas are then docked with proper adjustment of the spacing between the arms. Tension on the abdominal wall is released. Instruments are introduced under direct vision in the following order from left to right: Cadiere Forceps—Vessel sealer®—30° Camera—Scissors.

Console phase

Exploration of the abdomen: First, the degree of pelvic sepsis is evaluated, and safety and feasibility of primary colorectal anastomosis is determined. If a primary anastomosis is considered inappropriate, a Hartmann's resection should be performed. This decision will guide further surgical approach. When a primary anastomosis is attempted, the colonic length proximal to the diverticular perforation determines to what extent a splenic flexure mobilization is needed to create a tension-free anastomosis.

The different steps of sigmoidectomy for acute diverticulitis are described. Their chronology should be adapted on a case-by-case basis depending on difficulties encountered during the procedure; if splenic flexure mobilization is necessary, our preference is to perform this first. In case of severe inflammation in the pelvis with the need for conversion to laparotomy, the incision can be reduced in size if mobilization of the splenic flexure was already performed.

In case a Hartmann's resection is performed, splenic flexure mobilization is unnecessary and should be limited to avoid compromising a future Hartmann's reversal.

Splenic flexure mobilization: Complete splenic flexure mobilization is not always necessary. The degree of splenic flexure mobilization depends on the bowel length needed to create a tension free anastomosis or ostomy. In case of complete splenic flexure mobilization, this is done by a medial to lateral approach (MTL). The ligament of Treitz is exposed by lifting the inferior mesenteric vein (IMV) with the Cadiere Forceps. The assistant aids exposure by keeping the small bowel loops out of the surgical field with the use of a swab (Fig. 18.4a, b). The peritoneum is incised at the posterior part of the IMV, and the correct dissection plane is identified: this is the avascular plane between the left mesocolic fascia and the retroperitoneal fascia. Sharp dissection is then continued in cephalad direction towards the inferior border of the pancreas, and to the lateral side of the abdomen at the level of the descending colon (Fig. 18.5). During this step, the Cadiere Forceps lifts the dissected mesocolon towards the abdominal wall to provide exposure, while traction with the use of the Vessel Sealer® and countertraction by the assistant pressing the retroperitoneal surface further aids identification of the correct dissection plane. The splenic flexure is fully mobilized by incising the mesocolon along the caudal border of the pancreas, thus entering the lesser sac from below. At this stage, we prefer ligation of the

IMV using clips to avoid accidental rupture due to traction, while also providing extra bowel length to ensure a tension free anastomosis. It should be noted that it is not always feasible to enter the lesser sac at this point due to inadequate exposure, especially in obese patients. If this is the case, a swab can be left at the level of the pancreas for future identification when entering the lesser sac from anterior as described below.

The splenic flexure mobilization is continued by opening the lesser sac from the anterior side by transecting the gastrocolic ligament. This is facilitated using the Cadiere Forceps to lift the omentum with counter traction given on the transverse colon by the first assist, holding an epiploic appendix (Fig. 18.6). Sharp dissection with scissors or energy-sealing with a Vessel Sealer® can be used. The splenocolic ligament is divided, taking care to avoid iatrogenic lesions to the lower pole of the spleen. If the mesocolon was mobilized from the pancreas from below, mobilization of the splenic flexure is complete at this stage. If not, the swab left at the level of the pancreas will guide correct separation of the mesocolon from the inferior border of the pancreas.

Mobilization of the sigmoid and descending colon: This is achieved with lateral to medial dissection (LTM). The line of Toldt is incised at the level of the descending colon. Incision is continued cephalad towards the splenic flexure with transection of the phrenocolic ligament and caudal towards the sigmoid colon, which is most often the site of diverticular perforation. Mobilization is continued in a LTM way by further developing the dissection plane between the mesocolon and Gerota's fascia. The left gonadal vessels and ureter should be visualized, and care should be taken not to harm them, especially if the perforation is at the level of the left iliac fossa (Fig. 18.7a, b).

Exposure of the recto-sigmoidal junction and transection of the mesocolon: This is frequently the most challenging part of the intervention: a pelvic abscess is often present and an adhesive and inflammatory sigmoid might be folded over the rectum,

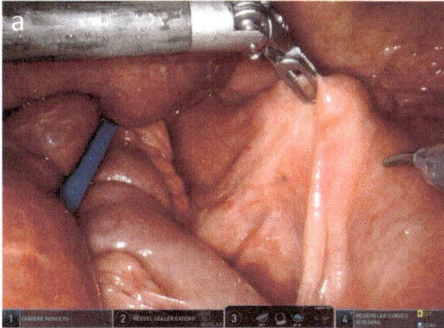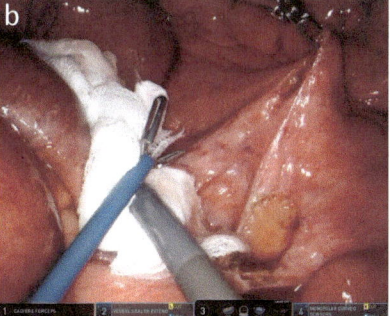

Fig. 18.4 a, b Exposure of Treitz ligament and the IMV (**a**); the use of a gauze may help exposure (**b**)

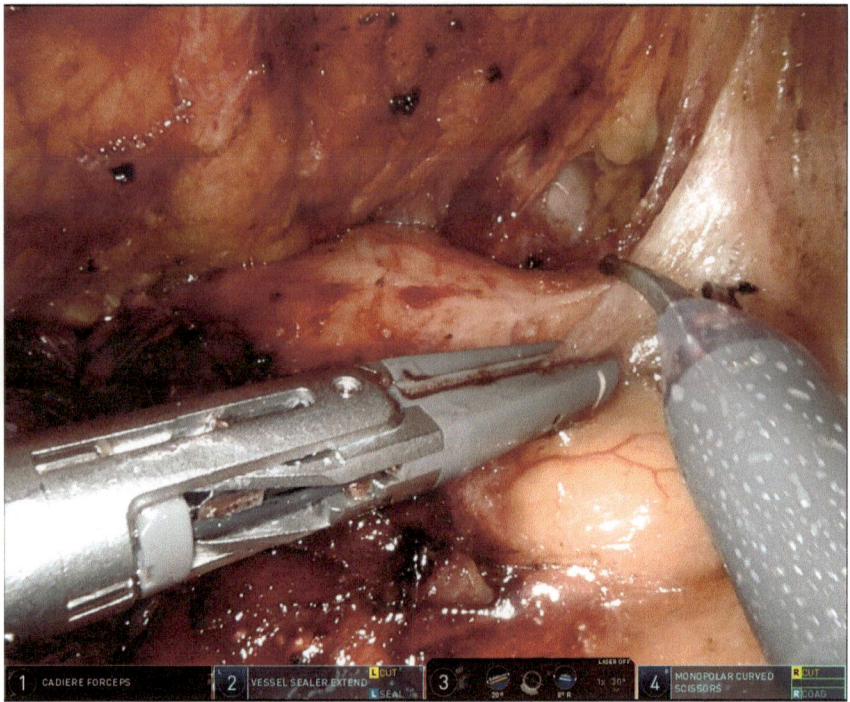

| 1 | CADIERE FORCEPS | 2 | VESSEL SEALER EXTEND | 3 | | 4 | MONOPOLAR CURVED SCISSORS |

Fig. 18.5 Dissection towards the descending colon by separating the retroperitoneal fascia (Gerota's fascia) and the mesocolic fascia using sharp dissection with the scissors

rendering exposure of the recto-sigmoidal junction difficult. Dissection with identification of rectum and sigmoid colon should be done stepwise and a good exposure with the aid of the Cadiere Forceps and the first assist is mandatory.

After the recto-sigmoidal junction is liberated, vascular division is performed. We perform in general a close colon dissection. This is done by lifting the recto-sigmoidal junction towards the anterior abdominal wall using the Cadiere Forceps and exposing the inferior mesenteric artery (IMA). The peritoneum is incised at the level of the proximal rectum and a tunnel is created exposing its posterior surface. A transection line on the mesocolon towards the descending colon proximal of the diseased sigmoid colon is marked using scissors (Fig. 18.8a, b). Care should be taken to select a non-inflamed bowel segment suited for anastomosis. A close colonic mesentery division with preservation of the superior rectal artery is then performed using the Vessel Sealer® and clips, starting at the proximal rectum towards the marked proximal colon. During this step, the Cadiere Forceps holds up one end of the bowel, while the first assist exposes the opposite side. It should be noted that although close colon dissection might be sufficient in case of a benign pathology such as diverticulitis, this might be complicated due to inflammatory thickening of the mesentery. In case

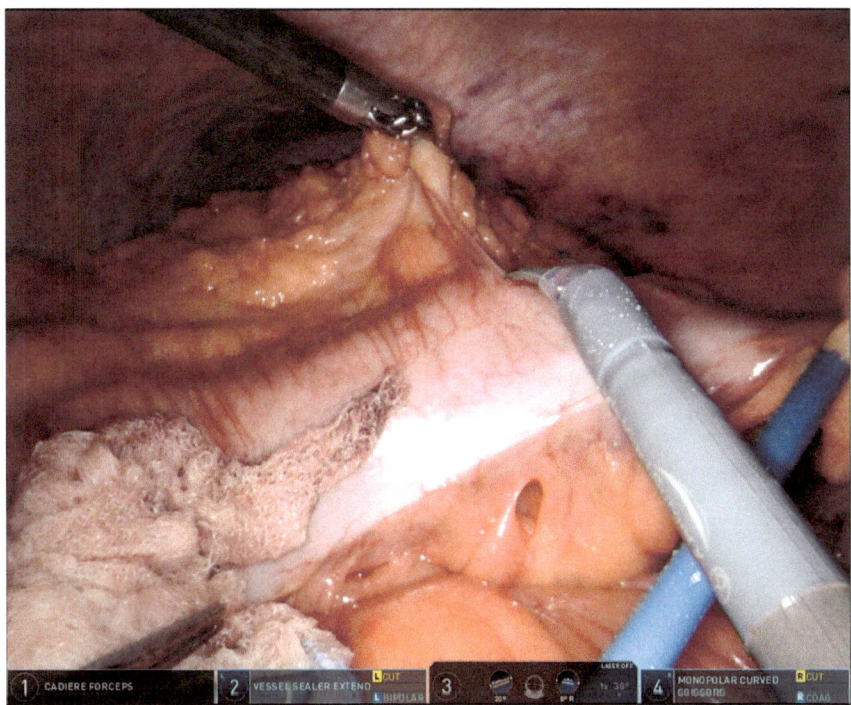

Fig. 18.6 Opening of the lesser sac. The assistant takes an epiploic appendix while the Cadiere Forceps holds the omentum to facilitate separation of the gastrocolic ligament

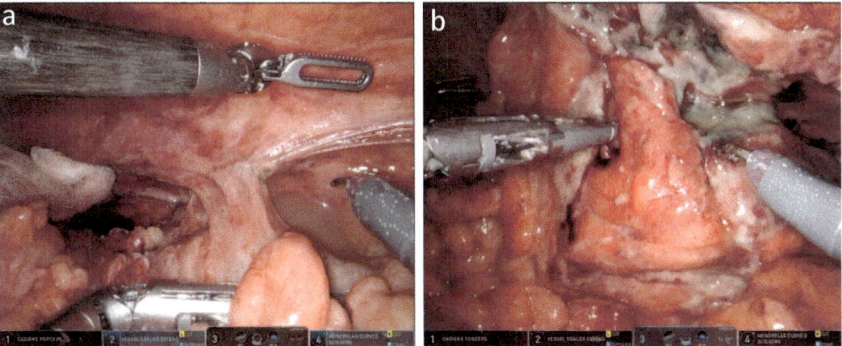

Fig. 18.7 **a**, **b** Incision of Toldt's line and LTM mobilization of the sigmoid colon (**a**). If the perforation is at the level of the iliac vessels, care should be taken not to harm the left gonadal vessels or ureter (**b**)

of uncertainty about underlying malignancy, an oncological correct dissection is advised with ligation of the IMA at its origin.

After completion of the mesenteric division, the Firefly® technology is used with intravenous injection of 5 mg of indocyanine green (ICG) to check adequate bowel perfusion of both proximal colon and distal rectum (Fig. 18.9a, b). Rectal transection is performed using the Sureform® 60 mm stapler. If the bowel is inflamed with a thickened bowel wall, a green reload is preferred over a blue one.

The specimen is now ready for extraction.

Primary anastomosis

If a primary anastomosis is performed, extraction of the specimen can be done depending on the bowel length either through a Pfannenstiel incision (typically in cases where splenic flexure mobilization was done), or through a transabdominal incision in the left iliac fossa. We advocate the use of a wound protector to avoid wound infection.

The bowel is prepared for anastomosis with introduction of the stapler anvil. The choice between and end-to-end or latero-terminal anastomosis depends on bowel quality. The bowel is then placed in the abdomen and after re-insufflation the circular transanal anastomosis is made. An air leak test is performed.

Finally, all quadrants are inspected and rinsed with saline until clear fluid is observed. The use of drainage is at the surgeon's discretion, as is the creation of a temporary loop ileostomy. Bowel and omentum are repositioned. All trocars are removed under direct vision and the abdomen is desufflated. Closure of the wounds and aseptic draping.

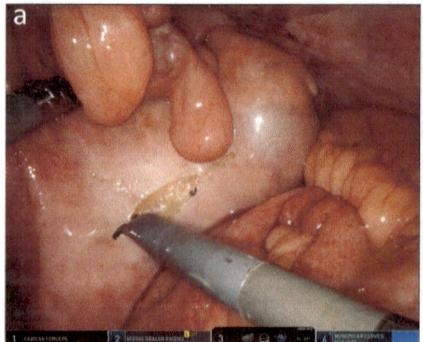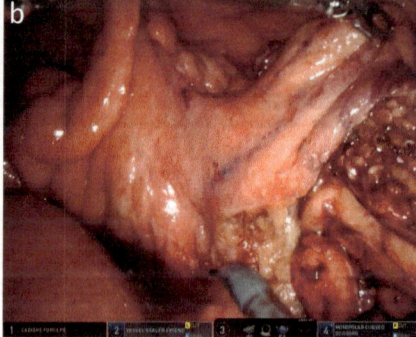

Fig. 18.8 a, b Lifting the recto-sigmoidal junction and incising the peritoneum to expose the posterior rectal surface (**a**). Stepwise close colon dissection towards a non-inflamed bowel segment suited for anastomosis (**b**)

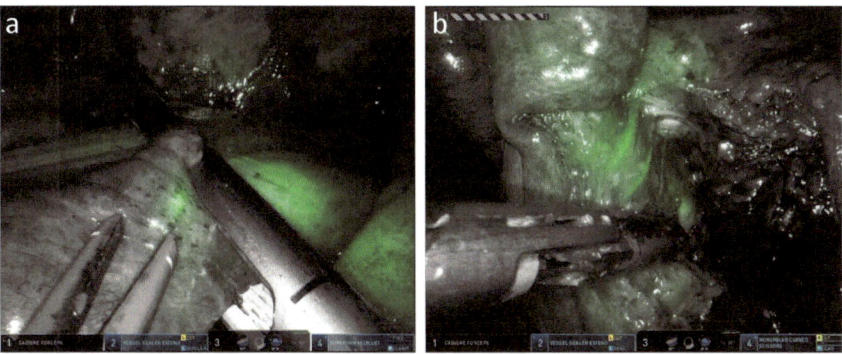

Fig. 18.9 a, b Intraoperative use of indocyanine green (ICG) to check adequate bowel perfusion of both rectal (**a**) and colonic transection site (**b**)

Hartmann's resection

If primary anastomosis is considered inappropriate, an ostomy is created at the left side of the abdomen. Specimen extraction can be done through the stoma site or through a Pfannenstiel incision, as needed.

The rectal stump might be marked with non-absorbable sutures for future identification during Hartmann's reversal.

Difficulty—Tips and Tricks

While using a standardized approach is advised for robotic surgery, this is not always applicable in emergency surgery such as for perforated diverticulitis. One should always be ready to think outside of the box and have alternative plans and bailouts ready in case it is not possible to follow a standard procedure. We will now discuss some difficult situations and provide tips and tricks to deal with each situation.

Small bowel blocks operative field

Not seldom there might be dilation of bowel loops due to peritonitis which makes access to the operative field difficult. Insertion of a gauze or swab, together with an additional 5 mm trocar for the first assist, may help to ensure adequate exposure of the surgical field.

Identifying the left ureter

The presence of severe inflammation with involvement of the ureter in the inflammatory process, may make dissection at the level of left iliac artery tricky. In robotic surgery the placement of a temporary ureter stent is not sufficient to visualize the ureter due to the lack of tactile feedback and injection of ICG directly in the ureter may help its identification during the procedure.

Difficult splenic flexure mobilization

In case of difficulty during splenic flexure mobilization, switch the sequence of mobilization. Start at the Treitz ligament with dissection posterior of the IMV. Alternatively, start with opening the lesser sac after partial dissection at the lateral side. Use table motion to reverse Trendelenburg to facilitate splenic flexure mobilization. If not available, do not hesitate to undock the robot, place the patient in reversed-Trendelenburg position, and redock the system. Although this may take a few minutes, this time is easily regained because of better exposure for splenic flexure mobilization.

Inflammatory mass in pelvis and left fossa, lateral mobilization difficult

If perforation is at the site of the left iliac fossa, starting LTM dissection might be too difficult. Alternatively, mobilization of the sigmoid colon can be performed MTL with the creation of a tunnel under the IMA for identification of the correct dissection plane and the left ureter and gonadal vessels, similar for oncological resections. The level of vascular transection can be determined afterwards. Transection of the colon proximal to the perforation might further aid the exposure of the lateral side by pulling the transected bowel medially.

Pelvic sepsis, inadequate exposure of the recto-sigmoidal junction

Surgery for perforated diverticulitis is often complicated by the presence of an inflammatory mass in the pelvis due to adhesions of the sigmoid loop to the recto-sigmoid junction. In this case, it might be better to lift the entire inflamed mass by pushing it towards the anterior abdominal wall using the Cadiere Forceps. Second, develop the posterior TME-plane at the proximal rectum from MTL. Dissection is then continued towards the IMA followed by transection of the proximal mesorectum and then by transection of the rectum itself. Next, a classic MTL approach for mobilization of the sigmoid colon can be performed towards a non-inflamed bowel segment for proximal transection. Splenic flexure mobilization, if needed, is best performed before starting the pelvic dissection.

Use of the Vessel Sealer®

Exposure of the operative field is often the main issue in robotic surgery. As described before, the placement of an additional trocar for the first assist helps, as does the insertion of gauzes to hold back bowel loops. However, exposure is further aided using the Vessel Sealer®, due to its size and maneuverability, in combination with the fact that it grasps bowel gently. At first sight, it might seem a bulky instrument that lacks precise grasping, but in case of inflammatory conditions, a larger sealing device is superior to a Fenestrated Bipolar Forceps in our experience.

Acknowledgements The authors would like to thank Marian Vanhoeij and Jasper Stijns for critical review of the manuscript.

References

1. Horesh N, Rudnicki Y, Dreznik Y, Zbar AP, Gutman M, Zmora O, Rosin D. Reversal of Hartmann's procedure: still a complicated operation. Tech Coloproctol. 2018;22:81–87.
2. Hall J, Hardiman K, Lee S, Lightner A, Stocchi L, Paquette IM, Steele SR, Feingold DL, Surgeons P on behalf of the CPGC of the AS of C and R. The American society of colon and rectal surgeons clinical practice guidelines for the treatment of left-sided colonic diverticulitis. Dis Colon Rectum. 2020;63:728–47.
3. Schultz JK, Azhar N, Binda GA, et al. European Society of Coloproctology: guidelines for the management of diverticular disease of the colon. Colorectal Dis. 2020;22:5–28.
4. Swank HA, Vermeulen J, Lange JF, et al. The ladies trial: laparoscopic peritoneal lavage or resection for purulent peritonitisA and Hartmann's procedure or resection with primary anastomosis for purulent or faecal peritonitisB in perforated diverticulitis (NTR2037). Bmc Surg. 2010;10:29.
5. Lambrichts DPV, Vennix S, Musters GD, et al. Hartmann's procedure versus sigmoidectomy with primary anastomosis for perforated diverticulitis with purulent or faecal peritonitis (LADIES): a multicentre, parallel-group, randomised, open-label, superiority trial. Lancet Gastroenterol Hepatology. 2019;4:599–610.
6. Lee YF, Brown RF, Battaglia M, Cleary RK. Laparoscopic versus open emergent sigmoid resection for perforated diverticulitis. J Gastrointest Surg. 2020;24:1173–82.
7. Lanfranco AR, Castellanos AE, Desai JP, Meyers WC. Robotic surgery. Ann Surg. 2004;239:14–21.
8. Koerner C, Rosen SA. How robotics is changing and will change the field of colorectal surgery. World J Gastrointest Surg. 2019;11:381–7.
9. Bhama AR, Wafa AM, Ferraro J, Collins SD, Mullard AJ, Vandewarker JF, Krapohl G, Byrn JC, Cleary RK. Comparison of risk factors for unplanned conversion from laparoscopic and robotic to open colorectal surgery using the Michigan surgical quality collaborative (MSQC) database. J Gastrointest Surg. 2016;20:1223–30.
10. Khan JS, Ahmad A, Odermatt M, Jayne DG, Ahmad NZ, Kandala N, West NP (2021) Robotic complete mesocolic excision with central vascular ligation for right colonic tumours—a propensity score-matching study comparing with standard laparoscopy. Bjs Open 5:zrab016
11. Bianchi PP, Ceriani C, Locatelli A, Spinoglio G, Zampino MG, Sonzogni A, Crosta C, Andreoni B. Robotic versus laparoscopic total mesorectal excision for rectal cancer: a comparative analysis of oncological safety and short-term outcomes. Surg Endosc. 2010;24:2888–94.

Chapter 19
Robotic Urological Surgery for Colorectal Surgeons

Arjun K. Nambiar, Paul Gravestock, and Rakesh Heer

Abstract Urological applications of robotic laparoscopic surgery have been pioneered since its widespread inception at the start of the twenty-first century, with its use and applications continuing to expand. One such development is the increasing role of minimally invasive multivisceral pelvic exenteration. These complex combined urology/colorectal cases often require some form of urinary diversion and we use this chapter to primarily discuss the formation of an ileal conduit. We discuss our own set up for robotic urological surgery including preoperative considerations, patient and port positioning and common equipment used. Further to this we discuss the steps involved in ileal conduit formation including identification and detachment of the ureters, transposition of the left ureter, cystectomy/cystoprostatectomy and isolation of a small bowel segment. We discuss the main two ureteric anastomosis techniques; Wallace and Bricker's, and the subsequent formation of a urostomy. Finally we discuss aspects of post operative care and give our top tips on a successful procedure.

Keywords Robotic surgical procedures · Urinary diversion · Pelvic exenteration

Introduction

Robotic minimally invasive surgery using a master–slave robotic system has been around since the late 1980's [1], but it was the year 2000 when the da Vinci system became the first robotic surgical system approved for laparoscopic surgery by the

A. K. Nambiar (✉) · P. Gravestock · R. Heer
Department of Urology, Freeman Hospital, Newcastle-upon-Tyne, England
e-mail: arjun.nambiar@nhs.net

P. Gravestock
e-mail: paul.gravestock@nhs.net

R. Heer
e-mail: rakesh.heer@nhs.net

A. K. Nambiar
Department of Urology, Newcastle University, Newcastle, UK

© The Author(s), under exclusive license to Springer Nature Switzerland AG 2022   221
P. Coyne and J. Khan (eds.), *Robotic Colorectal Surgery*,
https://doi.org/10.1007/978-3-031-15198-9_19

FDA. Since then, urology has embraced the use of robotic systems more widely than most surgical specialties, with robotic-assisted laparoscopic prostatectomy (RALP) being one of the most frequently performed robotic procedures worldwide. Robotic-assisted radical cystectomy (RARC) is also becoming the standard of care for surgical management of muscle-invasive bladder cancer.

RARC and open cystectomy have been found to have comparable oncological outcomes. A 2018 randomised phase 3 trial [2] and a 2019 systematic review [3] of robotic assisted radical cystectomy vs open cystectomy found no difference in rate of disease progression (up to 2 years), major complications or quality of life. RARC was associated with lower peri-operative transfusion rates and marginally shorter hospital stay, but longer mean operative time [2]. The downsides of RARC have traditionally been the large initial investment and maintenance expenditure, and the steep learning curve.

Minimally-invasive multi-visceral pelvic exenteration is less widely performed but increasing and shows similar trends. A systematic review in 2018 which included 170 patients showed similar oncological outcomes with a significantly increased operative time (83 min), lower median blood loss (1750 ml) and shorter length of stay (6 days shorter) for the minimally-invasive approach. A trend towards reduced morbidity in the robotic group was observed but was not significant. This study confirmed feasibility of minimally invasive pelvic exenteration in selected cases with favourable anatomy and tumour characteristics [4].

It should be noted that the data on robotic surgery for pelvic exenteration is probably not yet mature. A number of centres are still on the learning curve and it is likely that outcomes will continue to improve as surgical teams become more familiar and proficient with the technique. Given that existing data already suggests non-inferiority compared to open surgery, the authors think it is highly probable that future studies will show superior outcomes with the robotic approach.

There are, of course, some caveats. A proportion of these patients will have had multiple previous laparotomies and require extensive adhesiolysis to gain abdominal access, precluding minimally invasive surgery. Surgeon experience is also a critical factor—robotic pelvic exenterations are generally not training cases and wide experience in other forms of robotic pelvic surgery is desirable before taking on these complex procedures.

Combined urology/colorectal cases usually involve some form of urological reconstruction, the most common being an ileal conduit urinary diversion, or a ureteric reimplantation. For purposes of this chapter, we will focus on the ileal conduit diversion, it being the more complex form of reconstruction.

Pre-operative Checks

As with any minimally-invasive surgery, equipment checks should be carried out prior to starting the procedure. Staff should be familiar and trained in emergency response scenarios to convert quickly to an open procedure if required. Use of the WHO surgical safety checklist [5] is recommended.

Patient Positioning

Patients are positioned supine on a robotic operating table in steep Trendelen-burg position (30° head-down tilt) to aid working in the pelvis, using gravity to aid bowel retraction cranially. Potential complications associated with this position include raised intra-cranial pressure and cerebral oedema/hypoperfusion/ischaemia, rare retinal detachment, increased middle ear pressure, compartment syndrome (especially in those with established peripheral vascular disease), pressure sores and nerve injuries (e.g., brachial nerve traction in poorly positioned cases) [6]. Neurological complications are rare and tend to occur when patients have been maintained in continuous steep head-down position for over 6–7 h, hence it is our practice to level-off every 3–4 h for at least 20 min.

At the point of isolating a section of small bowel to create the conduit, the degree of head-down is reduced as this helps manipulation of the bowel segment in the desired operative field.

Theatre Layout

Layouts will vary depending on resources available and size of operating rooms in each individual centre. However, certain basic principles should be kept in mind.

– Hard-wired connections between robotic consoles are still used on many units, and can form a significant trip hazard.
– Although surgeon consoles can theoretically be placed quite remote from the patient cart, and even in separate rooms, in our experience it is safer and more convenient to have the surgeon consoles in the same operating room to aid communication between team members.
– The vision stack and robotic arms do have a relatively large footprint, and along with the other standard trays and equipment required will necessitate an operating room of adequate size to accommodate safely.

Additional Points

VTE prophylaxis should be considered which may include intraoperative Sequential Compression Devices (SCDS) or thromo-embolic deterrent stockings and the prescription of post-operative low molecular weight heparin (LMWH) if safe to do so.

Port Positioning

Port placements for robotic systems vary slightly depending on the system being used. The Intuitive Surgical systems are the most widely used, and the Da Vinci Si™ system is currently in use at our centre. The Da Vinci Xi™ system is the current version and allows for camera placement in any of the standard robotic ports, allowing for a more symmetrical positioning.

Standard port placement for pelvic surgery using the Si system involves a centrally placed supra-umbilical 12 mm camera port, a RIF 12 mm assistant Airseal (CONMED, US) port, three 8 mm robotic ports (one on the right and two on the left) and one 5 mm assistant port. For RARC and pelvic exenterations these ports are placed slightly higher than for RALP, to allow for bowel manipulation. Generally, the camera port is placed about 5 cm above the umbilicus, with the rest of the ports fanning out from this port in an arc (except the 5 mm port). (Fig. 19.1).

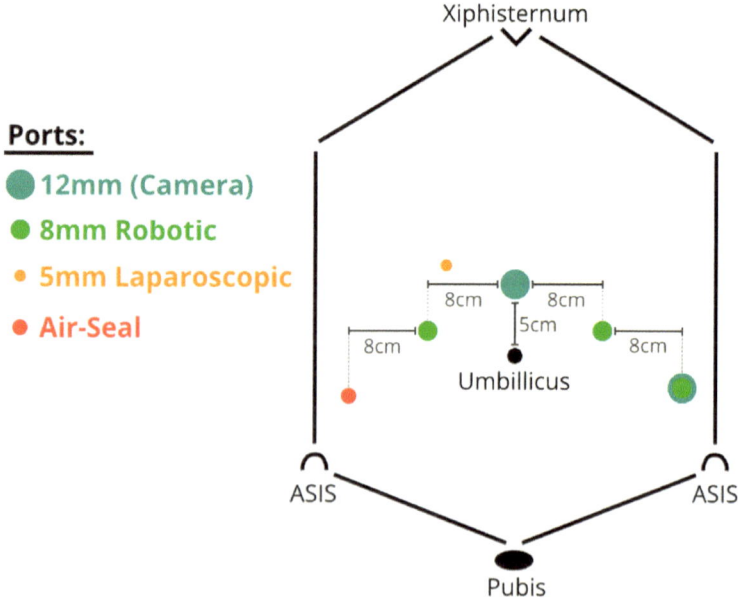

Fig. 19.1 Port placement (schematic)

Some centres may use a 12 mm LIF port with a long robotic port placed through it. This allows the assistant to remove the robotic port and use the 12 mm port to pass the bowel stapler manually at the relevant time. In centres that use the robotic stapler this is not necessary.

Safety/Adaptations Versus Lap or Open Surgery

Robotic surgery allows improved visualisation of structures over open surgery, and even over laparoscopic surgery due to the 3D vision enabled by the binocular lenses. However, there is no haptic feedback through the instruments, and this needs to be taken into account particularly when handling delicate structures such as bowel and ureters. Vision is also entirely dependent on the single camera, which therefore needs to be kept clean and mist-free at all times.

Pressure required to maintain pneumoperitoneum has been a topic of debate recently, with some articles suggesting lower pressures are associated with better outcomes (less post-op pain and hospital stay) [7]. In general, we recommend keeping pressures at 12 mmHg or below, with pressure increase to 15 used temporarily when urgent haemostasis is required.

Equipment Needed

We have already discussed the robotic console components, so in terms of disposable equipment the general requirements for these cases, from a urological perspective, are:

- Monopolar curved scissors × 1
- Bipolar forceps × 1
- Prograsp forceps × 1
- Cadiere forceps × 2
- Vessel sealer × 1
- Needle holder × 2
- Bowel stapler such as endo-GIA or TLC with reloads

Specific varieties/brands of these instruments may vary based on surgeon-preference or institutional factors. For example, some centres will choose to use laparoscopic bowel staplers controlled by the assistant, whereas others may use the robotic stapler.

Steps of Procedure

A common indication for robotic pelvic exenteration is a colorectal cancer invading the bladder/ureter. The initial dissection is therefore guided by the primary pathology, and is detailed in the relevant chapter of this book. Here we will discuss the steps of the cystectomy and ileal conduit urinary diversion.

Once the colonic tumor has been identified and the colon disconnected proximally, the main steps of the procedure are as follows:

- **Identification of the ureters**: the ureters can consistently be identified where they cross anteriorly over the bifurcation of the common iliac vessels at the pelvic brim. An incision in the retroperitoneum at this point will aid identification of the tubular structure which 'vermiculates' or peristalses, usually spontaneously, sometimes requiring a gentle nudge. Once identified, the ureter can be dissected free by releasing the fascial attachments on either side, from a few centimetres above the crossing of the iliacs, down as far as possible close to the bladder. The important thing to note here is not to de-vascularise the ureter, by maintaining peri-ureteric adventia tissue that contains blood supply. The blood supply to the distal ureter comes from the branches of the internal iliac lateral to the ureter. As the ureter is ultimately transected distally, it is important to preserve peri-ureteric vessels transmitting antegrade perfusion from the renal blood supply.
- **Clip and detach the ureters**: 2 weck clips are placed on the ureter as close to bladder as possible, with a further weck clip (marked with a vicryl tie) placed more proximally. The ureter is then divided between this more proximal clip and the distal ones. Note that in cases of ureteric involvement in tumor, the ureter may need to be divided more proximally, and in these cases the principle is to retain as much ureteric length as possible without sacrificing oncological control.
- **Transposition of the left ureter**: to enable both ureters to be anastomosed to a bowel segment, the left ureter needs to be transposed to the right side. This is done through a small window in the sigmoid mesocolon. This window is created at a point so as to minimize tension on the left ureter as it is pulled through. Generally, this will be at the level or just above the aortic bifurcation, initially developed by incising just above the sacral promontory and proceeding along the common iliac vessels. The main pitfall to avoid here is injury to the iliac veins and the median sacral vessels. Always check for any tension or kinks in the ureter once it has been pulled through, and release/adjust as necessary.
- **Clip isolated ureters to abdominal wall in RIF**: the vicryl ties on the weck clips placed on the ureteric ends can be used as anchors to clip the ureters to the RIF side wall peritoneum, so they remain out of the way and less prone to injury during subsequent bowel manipulation.
- **Cystectomy/cystoprostatectomy**: an incision is made in the peritoneum posterior to the bladder to allow entry to the recto-vesical space. The lateral bladder pedicles are then mobilized and taken with the vessel sealer, using weck clips sparingly as required. The bladder pedicle continues as the prostatic pedicle, which is also taken down. The endopelvic fascia is punctured to allow mobilization of the prostate

and the posterior plane between prostate and rectum dissected. This leaves the attachments anteriorly, along with the urethra. The anterior bladder attachments are then dropped and the dorsal venous complex (between the prostate and posterior pubis) either ligated or cut with diathermy. Finally, the urethra is isolated and cut (after removing the catheter) and a large 3-way catheter placed through the urethral stump as a pelvic drain.

In females the procedure is largely the same, except that posterior dissection usually proceeds in the plane behind the uterus until the posterior fornix of the vagina is opened, following which a portion of the anterior vaginal wall is excised along with the specimen, that is ultimately extracted through the vagina. The vaginal vault is then closed with continuous sutures.

- **Isolation of small bowel segment**: to create a conduit a length of small bowel needs to be isolated and disconnected on a mesenteric pedicle. To reduce the risk of malabsorption of bile acids, B12 and folate, the segment is taken at least 20–30 cm from the ileo-caecal valve. The length of the conduit will vary depending on patient habitus and thickness of the abdominal wall, but a general guide of 15 cm is usually a good starting point, and adjustments made from there on an individual patient basis. Intra-corporeal surgery makes identification of mesenteric vessels difficult, but it is possible with either the use of a firefly scope (passed through the assistant port to trans-illuminate the vasculature, as would be done in open surgery) or by IV administration of indocyanine green (ICG) at a dose of 1–5 ml of 2.5 mg/ml solution in saline [8]. In our experience, it is safe to blindly mobilise tangentially to the bowel segment, parallel to the mesenteric vascular arcades, to avoid devascularization. The bowel segment is isolated using 45 or 60 mm stapler (our preference is 60 mm), and the bowel re-anastomosed using a trouser-leg technique, with the bowel anastomosis over the conduit segment to prevent strain on the conduit (the classical "water under the bridge" description). The distal end of the conduit is then marked with a loose 3–0 vicryl stitch to aid identification of the distal (stoma) end.

  Pitfalls: a conduit that is too long results in urinary stasis, recurrent infections and possibly renal impairment in the long term. Too much tension on the mesentery can also cause conduit ischaemia and resultant complications. Large mesenteric defects can result in internal herniation, so these should be closed if necessary.

- **Ureteric anastomoses**: there are two classical techniques to anastomose the ureters to the small bowel segment, and the choice of technique varies between countries and between centres [9]. The first is the Wallace technique [10], in which both ureters are brought together and spatulated, then the medial aspects of each ureteric spatulation are stitched together (using 4–0 PDS or vicryl) to create a ureteric 'plate'. This plate is then stitched to the proximal conduit segment in an end-to-side fashion (Fig. 19.2). The alternative is the Bricker technique [12], in which each ureter is anastomosed separately to the bowel through separate enterotomies on the proximal part of the conduit (Fig. 19.2). Whichever technique is adopted, the ureters are typically stented prior to completion of the anastomotic suturing with urinary diversion stents (by convention the blue stent to the left ureter and the red stent to the right). These stents are inserted through the 12 mm

RIF assistant port and advanced over a wire to the renal pelvis by feel (resistance felt once the tip is in the renal pelvis). Some surgeons advocate securing the stents to the ureter with a 4–0 vicryl rapide stitch to prevent them falling out too early, but this is not universally adopted as the stent pigtail in the renal pelvis is enough to secure the stent in position. The ends of the stent are then pulled through the conduit before completing the ureteric anastomosis.

Pitfalls: too many sutures on the ureter, or applying sutures too tight, causing ischaemic stricturing of the anastomosis [11].

- **Specimen extraction**: at this point the procedure reverts to completion of the excision of the primary specimen and removal, either through the vagina (in women) or through a separate pfannensteil incision.

Bricker Anastamosis

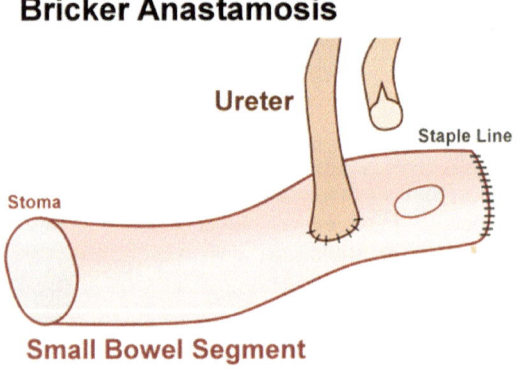

Wallace Anastamosis

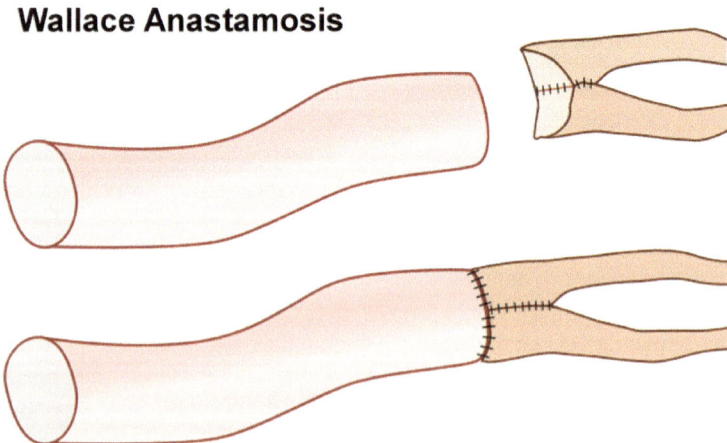

Fig. 19.2 Bricker and Wallace uretero-ileal anastomosis

- **Creation of urostomy**: the premarked urostomy site is prepared as for any stoma – the skin and fat excised elliptically and a cruciate incision made in the rectus sheath. Four vicryl sutures are applied to the corners of the sheath to help anchor the conduit. After a muscle-splitting incision and incising the peritoneum the distal conduit segment is brought through and anchored. A spout is created and the conduit fixed to the skin with 3–0 undied vicryl.

Pitfalls: a hole in the abdominal wall that is too tight can result in poor drainage and even ischemia of the conduit, whereas if too loose will result in a parastomal hernia. Getting this right is challenging! Avoid stitches through the mesentery of the conduit as this can also result in distal ischaemia and sloughing of the conduit.

Post-op Care

The important considerations in the immediate post-op period are to promote bowel motility, monitor urine output and prevent wound and chest infections. Early mobilization is key to all of these, as well as early institution of light diet as tolerated. Enhanced recovery protocols have helped improve recovery times in general and can be beneficial [13].

From a urological perspective, monitoring urine output is of course essential, as well as documenting drain outputs. If drain outputs are high the possibility of a urine leak should be considered, and a sample of drain fluid sent for assessment of electrolyte content. A creatinine level in the fluid exponentially greater than serum creatinine indicates the presence of urine in the fluid. Cross-sectional imaging may be necessary to establish the degree of leakage, but in general most small leaks will heal spontaneously with a prolonged period of stenting. In most cases, where no leak is suspected, the diversion stents can be removed at post-op day 7–10.

In the longer term, patient will require monitoring for electrolyte disturbances and should have at least annual U/E, B12 and folate level assessment.

5 Top Tips

- Leave adequate periureteric tissue to reduce the risk of ureteric ischaemia and strictures
- Ileal conduits are generally the preferred option for diversion in cases of locally advanced pelvic malignancy
- Pick a healthy segment of bowel for the conduit—watch out for radiation change!
- As in all anastomoses—tension free, well vascularised healthy tissue, over a stent and with a drain alongside are keys to success.
- Use the multidisciplinary team—a technically excellent operation can be let down by poor pre-operative counselling and post-operative care

References

1. Lane T. A short history of robotic surgery. Ann R Coll Surg Engl. 2018;100(6_suppl):5–7. https://doi.org/10.1308/rcsann.supp1.5.
2. Parekh DJ, Reis IM, Castle EP, et al. Robot-assisted radical cystectomy versus open radical cystectomy in patients with bladder cancer (RAZOR): an open-label, randomised, phase 3, non-inferiority trial. Lancet. 2018;391(10139):2525–36. https://doi.org/10.1016/S0140-673 6(18)30996-6 PMID: 29976469.
3. Sathianathen NJ, Kalapara A, Frydenberg M, et al. Robotic assisted radical cystectomy vs open radical cystectomy: systematic review and meta-analysis. J Urol. 2019;201(4):715–20. https://doi.org/10.1016/j.juro.2018.10.006 PMID: 30321551.
4. Collaborative PelvEx. Minimally invasive surgery techniques in pelvic exenteration: a systematic and meta-analysis review. Surg Endosc. 2018;32(12):4707–15. https://doi.org/10.1007/s00 464-018-6299-5 Epub 2018 Jul 17 PMID: 30019221.
5. Haynes AB, Weiser TG, Berry WR, Lipsitz SR, Breizat AH, Dellinger EP, Herbosa T, Joseph S, Kibatala PL, Lapitan MC, Merry AF, Moorthy K, Reznick RK, Taylor B, Gawande AA, Safe Surgery Saves Lives Study Group. A surgical safety checklist to reduce morbidity and mortality in a global population. N Engl J Med. 2009;360(5):491–9. https://doi.org/10.1056/NEJMsa0810119. Epub 2009 Jan 14. PMID: 19144931.
6. Balbay MD, Koc E, Canda AE. Robot-assisted radical cystectomy: patient selection and special considerations. Robot Surg. 2017;4:101–6. Published 2017 Oct 19. https://doi.org/10.2147/RSRR.S119858.
7. Foley CE, Ryan E, Huang JQ. Less is more: clinical impact of decreasing pneumoperitoneum pressures during robotic surgery. J Robot Surg. 2021;15(2):299–307. https://doi.org/10.1007/s11701-020-01104-4 Epub 2020 Jun 22 PMID: 32572753.
8. Pathak RA, Hemal AK. Intraoperative ICG-fluorescence imaging for robotic-assisted urologic surgery: current status and review of literature. Int Urol Nephrol. 2019;51:765–71. https://doi.org/10.1007/s11255-019-02126-0.
9. Hautmann RE, Abol-Enein H, Lee CT, Mansson W, Mills RD, Penson DF, Skinner EC, Studer UE, Thueroff JW, Volkmer BG. Urinary diversion: how experts divert. Urology. 2015;85(1):233–8. https://doi.org/10.1016/j.urology.2014.06.075 Epub 2014 Nov 8 PMID: 25440985.
10. Wallace DM. Uretero-ileostomy. Br J Urol. 1970;42(5):529–34. https://doi.org/10.1111/j.1464-410x.1970.tb04498.x PMID: 5475799.
11. Lobo N, Dupré S, Sahai A, et al. Getting out of a tight spot: an overview of ureteroenteric anastomotic strictures. Nat Rev Urol. 2016;13:447–55. https://doi.org/10.1038/nrurol.2016.104.
12. Bricker EM. Bladder substitution after pelvic evisceration. Surg Clin North Am. 1950;30(5):1511–21. https://doi.org/10.1016/s0039-6109(16)33147-4. PMID: 14782163.
13. Azhar RA, Bochner B, Catto J, Goh AC, Kelly J, Patel HD, Pruthi RS, Thalmann GN, Desai M. Enhanced recovery after urological surgery: a contemporary systematic review of outcomes, key elements, and research needs. Eur Urol. 2016;70(1):176–87. https://doi.org/10.1016/j.eururo.2016.02.051. Epub 2016 Mar 9. PMID: 26970912; PMCID: PMC5514421.

Chapter 20
Robotic Approach
for Ileal-Pouch-Anal-Anastomosis

Solafah Abdalla and David W. Larson

Abstract The robotic approach for ileal pouch anal anastomosis (IPAA) has increasingly gained popularity over laparoscopy due to its technical superiority in the pelvic region. The robotic platform provides articulated instruments and three-dimensional vision, allowing improved identification of anatomic structures and nuanced dissection. However, the learning curve is still steep and requires solid experience in minimally invasive colorectal surgery. This chapter aims to guide surgeons step by step along with robotic proctectomy completion and IPAA procedure and give them tips and tricks to make it safe and easy. The main steps consist of J-pouch construction, followed by proctectomy and IPAA in one robotic docking.

Keywords Robotic · Ileal pouch anal anastomosis · Restorative ·
Proctocolectomy · Minimally invasive surgery

Abbreviations

EEA	End-to-end anastomosis
IPAA	Ileal pouch anal anastomosis
MIS	Minimally invasive surgery
TME	Total mesorectal excision

Introduction

Ileal pouch anal anastomosis (IPAA) is indicated in ulcerative colitis and familial adenomatous polyposis. Laparoscopic IPAA progressively became the standard approach due to its associated improved short-term and long-term outcomes [1].

S. Abdalla · D. W. Larson (✉)
Division of Colon and Rectal Surgery, Mayo Clinic, Rochester, MN, United States
e-mail: larson.david2@mayo.edu

© The Author(s), under exclusive license to Springer Nature Switzerland AG 2022
P. Coyne and J. Khan (eds.), *Robotic Colorectal Surgery*,
https://doi.org/10.1007/978-3-031-15198-9_20

However, laparoscopy is limited by unenhanced camera technology and restricted instruments' maneuverability in narrow regions such as the pelvis. Therefore, the current opportunity is to transition to an approach that facilitates dissection in the anatomical demands of the pelvis.

The robotic-assisted platform, such as the da Vinci® robot (Intuitive Surgical Inc, Sunnyvale, CA), was introduced to overcome these limitations and has been increasingly used in colorectal surgery [2]. The articulated robotic instruments and the surgeon-controlled three-dimensional camera allow improved ergonomics, dexterity, exposure, and visualization. The robotic platform is particularly adapted to IPAA as this surgery occurs in the narrow pelvic space with challenging operating angles. The vascular and nervous structures are more easily identified, with improved optics, and protected with a more nuanced dissection. These mechanical improvements are expected to translate into optimal postoperative and functional results in these predominantly young patients in a relatively good general health status.

Our previous laparoscopic experience in IPAA performed in 600 patients [3] highlighted minimally invasive surgery's (MIS) potential improvement in this indication. Compared to open surgery, laparoscopy provided significantly improved short-term recovery outcomes [4] and was associated with better functional results [5], sexual function, body image, and quality of life [6]. Therefore, the decision to transition from laparoscopy to robotics for IPAA procedures was integrated into a logical pathway to optimize the MIS benefits in this indication. Between 2015 and 2021, we have performed a hundred robotic IPAA using a standardized technique [7]. Our experience in robotic IPAA procedures is encouraging, as shown in our previously published cohort study [8] including 74 robotic and 58 laparoscopic IPAA. Although requiring a longer operative time, we demonstrated that the robotic approach was as safe as the laparoscopic approach and was associated with decreased intraoperative blood loss, decreased pelvic sepsis, and improved length of hospital stay. These results are consistent with the few existing small studies on robotic IPAA [9].

We believe that the robotic approach demonstrates its full potential when integrated into enhanced recovery pathways. This multimodal strategy is based on pre- intra- and postoperative parameters aiming to optimize postoperative pain control and nausea, limit fluid input, and speed up returning to regular daily activity [10, 11]. This strategy is of utmost interest in young and healthy patients undergoing IPAA.

The learning curve for safe robotic rectal surgery [12], IPAA included, is steep, and the optimal postoperative outcomes are obtained when it is performed in high-volume centers (>10 pouches per year) [13, 14], underlining the importance of the technical aspects. This chapter aims to provide practical tips and tricks following a standardized step-by-step description of performing a robotic IPAA safely. Although the technique can be transposed to prophylactic total proctocolectomy for familial adenomatous polyposis, we will focus in this chapter on IPAA in the context of proctectomy completion after subtotal colectomy for acute severe ulcerative colitis, with end ileostomy and rectal stump, requiring stapled IPAA without mucosectomy.

Procedural Case

Cautionary Note: Safety and Adaptations to Laparoscopic and Open Surgery

The learning curve for robotic rectal surgery is steep. Surgeons should have solid experience in laparoscopic rectal surgery before attempting their first robotic rectal resection. It is advised to perform the first robotic IPAA in a "favorable" context, with a proctor or an experienced colleague in robotic rectal surgery. In challenging cases or intraoperative complications, conversion to laparoscopy or open approach should not be delayed and are not considered a failure. For this purpose, laparoscopic and open instruments should be ready to use for any robotic intervention. A high-functioning team can, if trained, perform emergency undocking when required. All the general safety measures for robotic surgery apply to robotic IPAA. Notably, all robotic instruments must remain under visual control, especially when replaced, to prevent any organ or vascular injury. This is even more critical given the absence of haptic feedback.

Theater Layout

The Operating Room layout for robotic IPAA is similar to any other robotic rectal surgery. The anesthetic team and machines are placed at the head of the patient. The robot is placed on the left side of the patient and docked over his left hip. The monitor and adjunct energy device cart are placed at the level of the patient's left shoulder. Two monitors are placed on both sides of the patient. The assistant and the scrubbing nurse remain on the patient's right side while the primary surgeon is at the console (Fig. 20.1).

Patient's Position and Trocar Placement

The patient is placed in a modified lithotomy position with both arms along the body to access the perineum. Before doing any robotic work, the first step consists of ileostomy takedown and pouch construction. These steps are performed while the table is horizontal. After ileostomy takedown and pouch construction, trocars can be placed. A 15-mm assist balloon trocar is placed into the previous ileostomy site, and insufflation is achieved through this trocar. Other trocars are placed under direct visual control. The four robotic trocars are aligned in a transverse fashion (Fig. 20.2). Classically the 8-mm camera robotic port is placed just above the umbilicus (Arm 3). The other two 8-mm robotic ports are placed on the same transverse line on the left at the level of the mid-clavicular line (Arm 2) and the left anterosuperior iliac

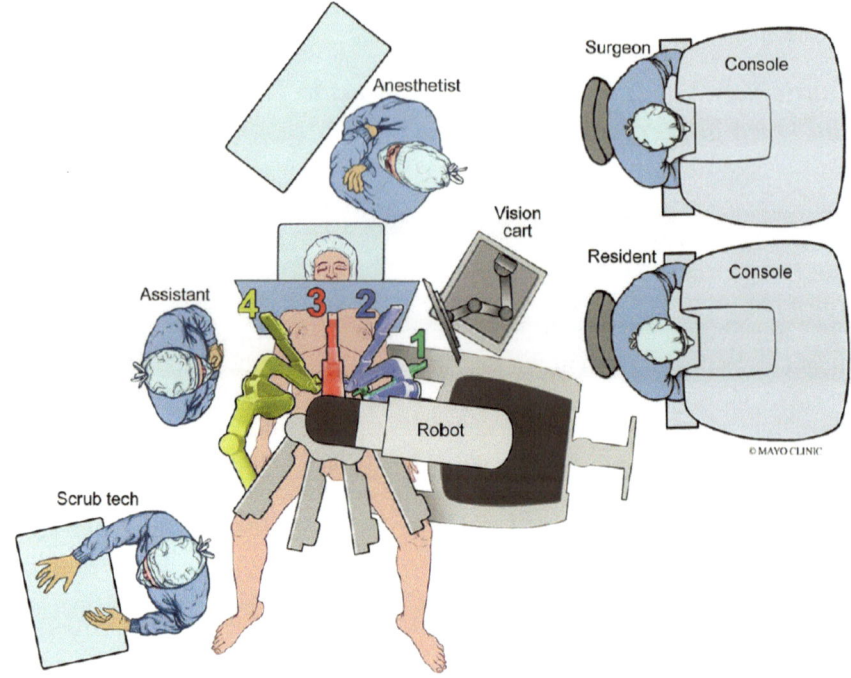

Fig. 20.1 Theater layout for robotic IPAA

spine (Arm 1). The 12-mm robotic port (Arm 4) is placed on the right side at the level of the mid-clavicular line. A 5-mm assist port is placed on the right upper quadrant. Another 5-mm suprapubic assist port can also be added if the pelvic exposure is problematic. The patient is then placed in steep Trendelenburg to allow the small bowel to fall cephalad and expose the pelvis. In the case of a long rectosigmoid stump, a slight tilt right side down can be added to allow an easy dissection of the left side of the stump.

Tips and Tricks

Position for trocars placement is determined after insufflation. For the Xi robot, a 6–8 cm distance between each robotic trocar is maintained to avoid arms collision, and the camera port is placed 15–20 cm from the target anatomy. In patients with a long torso, trocars placed too cephalad will make the pelvic floor challenging to reach, the sacral promontory acting as a fulcrum. If the trocars are placed too laterally (particularly in men with a narrow straight pelvis), the low pelvic dissection will be difficult secondary to collisions with the lateral pelvic sidewall. In obese patients, the usual landmarks for port placement can be misleading as the umbilicus is pulled downwards. The most consistent landmark is to keep a 15 cm distance between the camera port and the rectal stump. The other ports are placed under direct visual control.

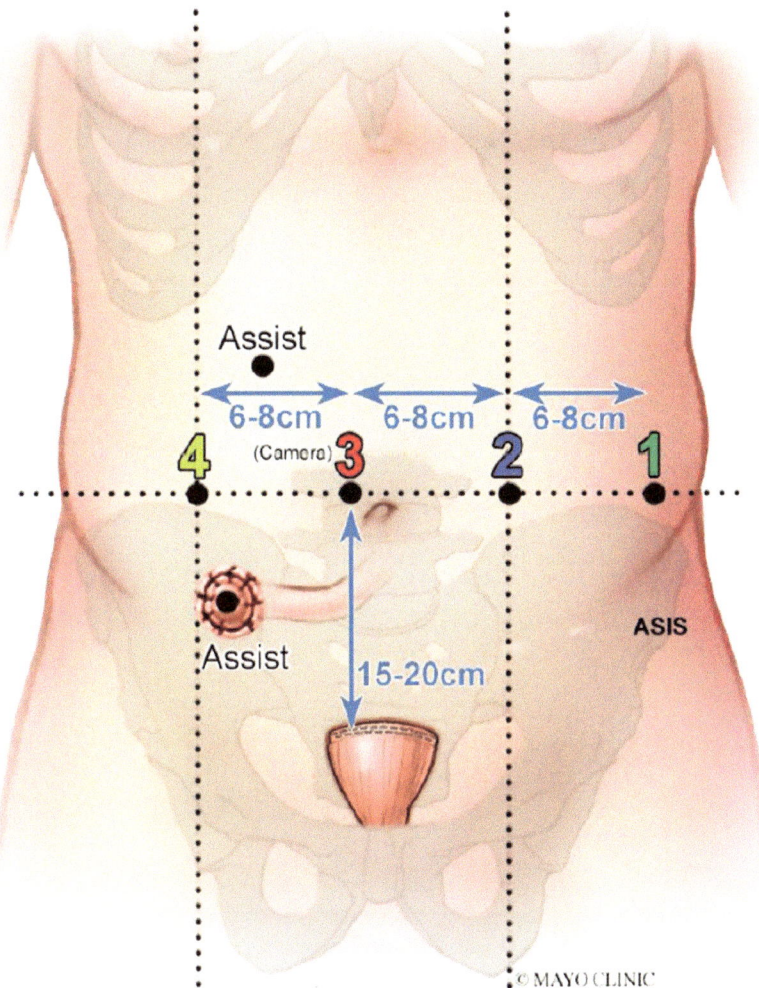

Fig. 20.2 Port placement for one docking robotic IPAA. The four robotic trocars are aligned in a transverse fashion (horizontal dotted line). Classically the 8-mm camera robotic port is placed just above the umbilicus (Arm 3). Ports for Arm 2 (8-mm) and 4 (12-mm) are placed at the level of the midclavicular lines (vertical dotted lines) and port for Arm 1 (8-mm) at the level of the ASIS. A 5-mm assist port is placed on the right upper quadrant. A 15-mm assist balloon trocar is placed into the previous ileostomy site. ASIS Anterior superior iliac spine

Robot Docking

Only one docking is necessary for this procedure. The robot is docked over the patient's left hip (Fig. 20.3), aligning the targeting icon over the Arm 3 (camera port). The most distal aspect of the camera arm and port should be in line with the patient's spine. The Small Graptor™ is placed in Arm 1, the fenestrated bipolar forceps in Arm 2, the camera in Arm 3, and the monopolar-curved scissors in Arm 4.

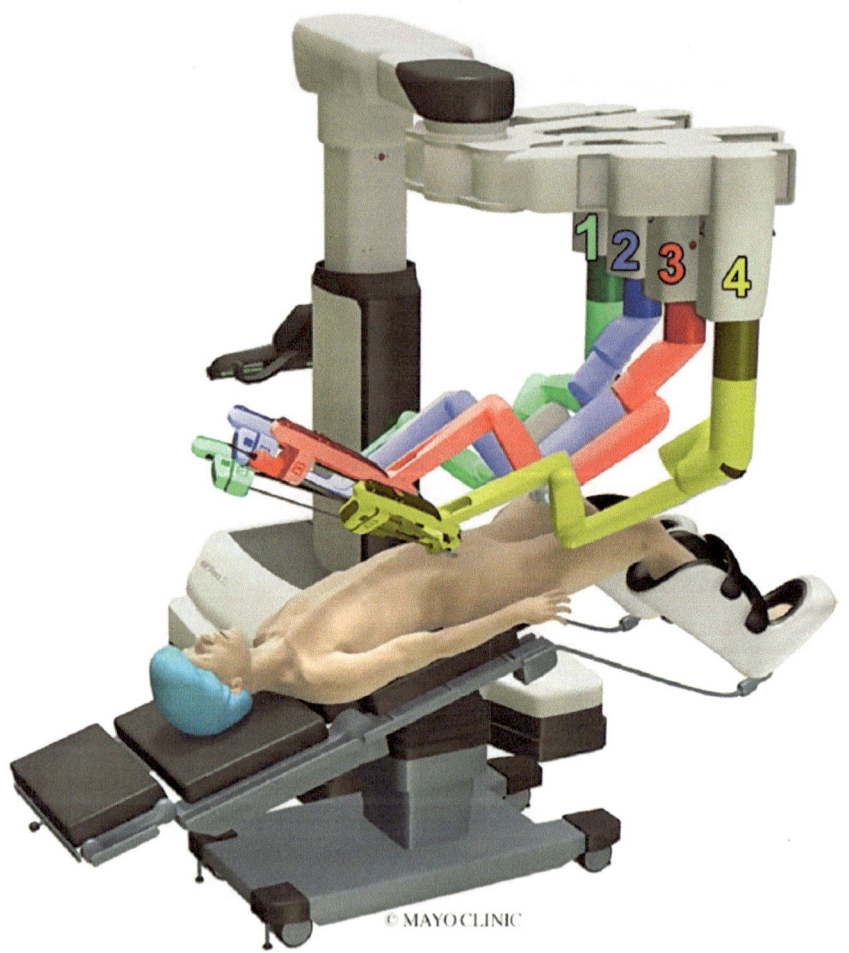

Fig. 20.3 Robot docking for IPAA procedure. After the trocars' placement, the robot is docked over the patient's left hip, aligning the targeting icon over the Arm 3 (camera port)

Equipment

We describe the technique with the model Xi of the da Vinci Robot platform. The instruments used here are valid for the previous S and Si models.

Instruments for Pouch Construction

- **One 80-mm extracorporeal linear stapler (GIA™ 80, Covidien, Boulder, CO) and three 80-mm blue loads:** one load is used for ileal division, two loads for pouch construction. Instead of 80-mm loads, 100-mm loads can be used.
- **One 28 or 29-mm end-to-end anastomosis (EEA™ Circular stapler, Covidien, Boulder, CO) stapler:** for stapled IPAA, the diameter depends on the anal dilatation capacity.

Robotic Instruments

Camera

- **One 8-mm 30° robotic camera:** the ease of switching from up to down with the Xi model increases the opportunity to provide optimal visual exposure.

Trocars

- **Three 8-mm and one 12-mm robotic trocars:** the four robotic arms are used in this procedure.
- **One 15-mm balloon laparoscopic trocar:** placed at the site of the previous ileostomy. This adds a potential alternative and useful trocar.
- **Two 5-mm laparoscopic trocars:** used as assist trocars if needed.

Energy

- **Monopolar scissors:** used for both blunt and sharp dissection.
- **Fenestrated bipolar and vessel sealer (da Vinci® EndoWrist® One™ Vessel Sealer, Intuitive Surgical Inc., Sunnyvale, CA):** in a thick inflammatory mesentery, we like to use multiple overlapping burn techniques, with bipolar energy to skeletonize the vessels and vessel sealer for optimal control of the bleeding.

Graspers

- **One Small Graptor™ (da Vinci® EndoWrist® Small Graptor™, Intuitive Surgical Inc., Sunnyvale, CA):** this is critical to provide the kind of atraumatic bite force to limit injury to an inflamed rectum but also to provide the instrument surface area to move structure out of the surgeon's way providing needed exposure.

Staplers

- **One EndoWrist® 60-mm stapler and one or two EndoWrist® 60-mm green loads (da Vinci®, Intuitive Surgical Inc., Sunnyvale, CA):** most healthy patients can have their rectum divided successfully with a single load.

Laparoscopic Instruments

- **Monopolar scissors and fenestrated bipolar:** for mesentery mobilization.
- **Two atraumatic bowel graspers:** any atraumatic grasper can be used (fenestrated, Babcock's, etc.).
- **One 10-mm suction/irrigator:** essential, is also helpful for exposure.
- **AirSeal® System (ConMed, Utica, NY):** very helpful for the confined pelvic region to maintain a stable pneumoperitoneum and continuous smoke evacuation along with the procedure.

Operative Steps

J-Pouch Construction

The J-pouch construction is performed first. Performing the J-pouch allows an early assessment of the mesentery length and potential need for further lengthening maneuvers. It is crucial not to take the rectum out before assessing the pouch's reach to the anus without tension. Also, once the pouch is fashioned, only one docking will be necessary to finish the procedure. Here, we describe the technique to fashion a J-pouch, which is the current standard reconstruction after total proctocolectomy.

The first step consists of dissecting free the terminal end ileostomy from the fascia. The terminal ileum is divided with a linear stapler and extracted from the abdominal wall defect. Then, the mesentery length is assessed: the small bowel is folded at 15 cm from its end and pulled over the pubis. The mesentery and pouch length are considered appropriate when the apex of the pouch reaches ≥ 1 cm past the lower side of the pubic symphysis (Fig. 20.4).

If the pouch's mesentery is too short, several methods can increase the pouch's mesentery length. Usually, performing superficial relaxing incisions on both sides of the mesentery and high ligation of the ileocolic pedicle is sufficient to ensure the IPAA reaches the pelvis (Fig. 20.5A–C).

Otherwise, the division of the distal branches of the superior mesenteric pedicle (Fig. 20.6) and full mobilization of small bowel mesentery (Fig. 20.7) may be added to obtain adequate mesentery length.

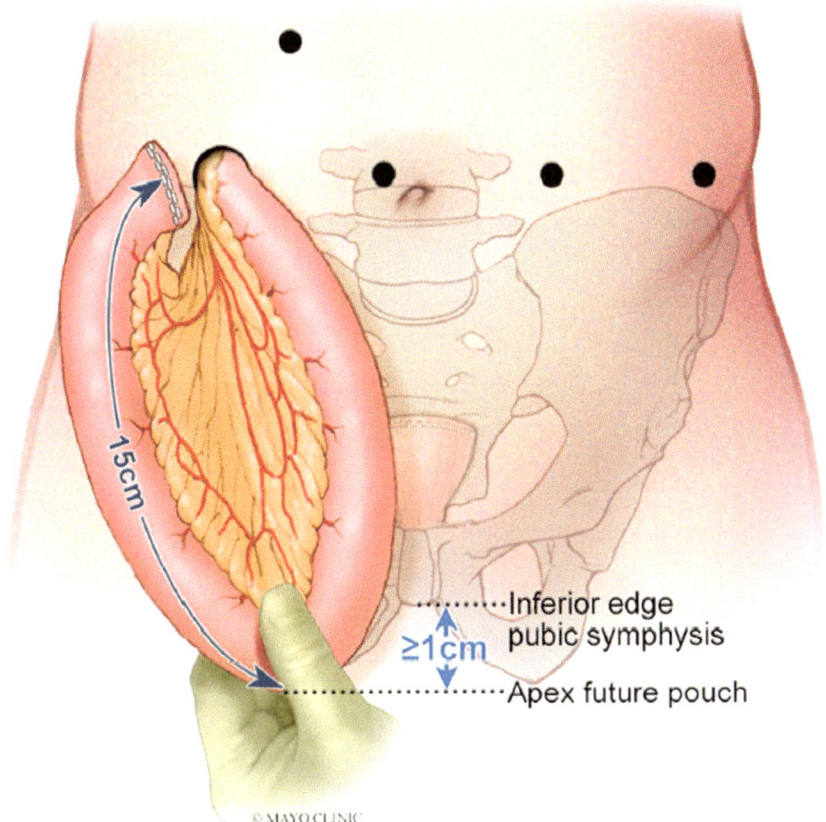

Fig. 20.4 Assessment of adequate mesentery length for J-pouch construction

To fashion the pouch, the ileum is folded 15–20 cm from the stapled end (this will be the apex of the pouch), the stapled end being oriented on the patient's right side, and the mesentery placed posteriorly. The ileal stapled line is oversewn utilizing multiple interrupted 3–0 silks. Three interrupted 3–0 silk sutures are placed on the antimesenteric side of the bowel to align both limbs of the pouch. The stitch most proximal to the pouch apex is cut long enough to be held by a grasper (Fig. 20.8A).

It will be helpful for the anastomotic construction step. The pouch's apex is opened on the anti-mesenteric side with a horizontal incision using electrocautery. The pouch is constructed using 2 firings of the 80-mm blue load extracorporeal linear stapler (Fig. 20.8B). The internal staple line hemostasis is controlled. The anvil (EEA 28 or 29 mm) is then secured to the pouch's apex opening using a 2–0 Prolene® (Ethicon, Inc, Somerville, NJ) in a pursestring fashion (Fig. 20.8C). The pouch is then returned to the abdomen cavity, and a 15-mm balloon trocar is placed into the ileostomy site. Pneumoperitoneum is established, the other ports are placed.

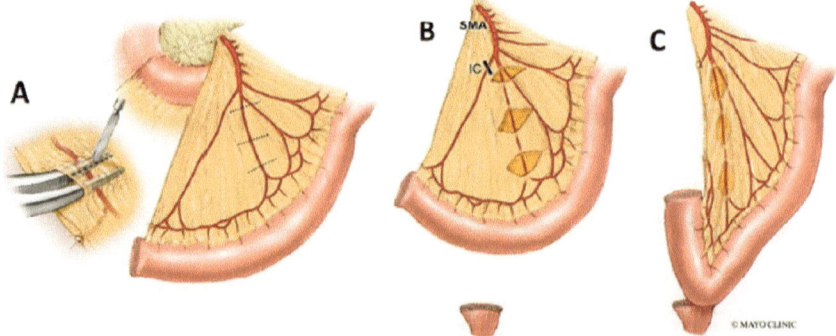

Fig. 20.5 Mesentery lengthening maneuvers: relaxing incisions and high ligation of the ileocolic pedicle. **A**. Superficial stepwise relaxing incisions are performed on both sides of the mesentery. **B**. The origin of the ileocolic artery (IC) is identified to perform a high ligation of the ileocolic pedicle. **C**. Most frequently, adequate mesentery length is obtained after these two maneuvers. IC Ileocolic artery, SMA Superior mesenteric artery

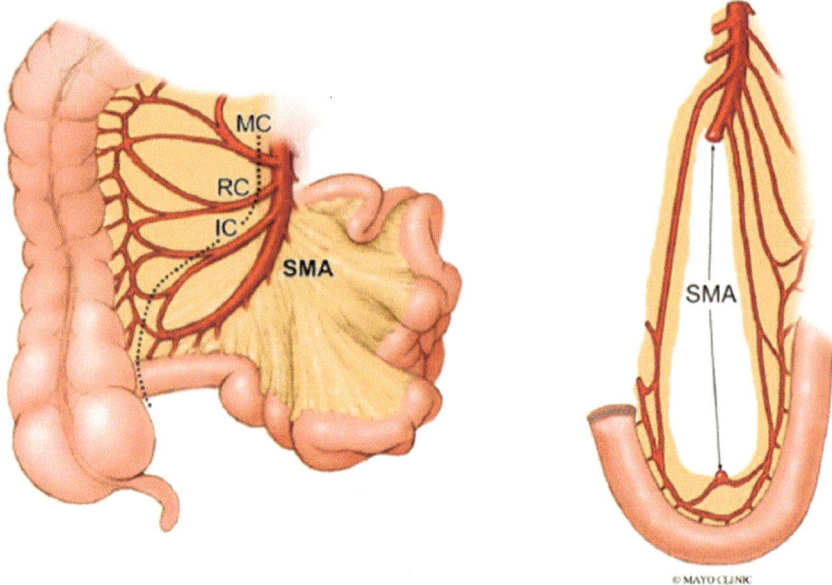

Fig. 20.6 Mesentery lengthening maneuvers: ligation of the superior mesenteric artery's distal branches. If the ileocolic pedicle was preserved during the previous subtotal colectomy, distal branches of the superior mesenteric artery could be performed to lengthen the mesentery. IC Ileocolic artery, MC Middle colic artery, RC Right colic artery, SMA Superior mesenteric artery

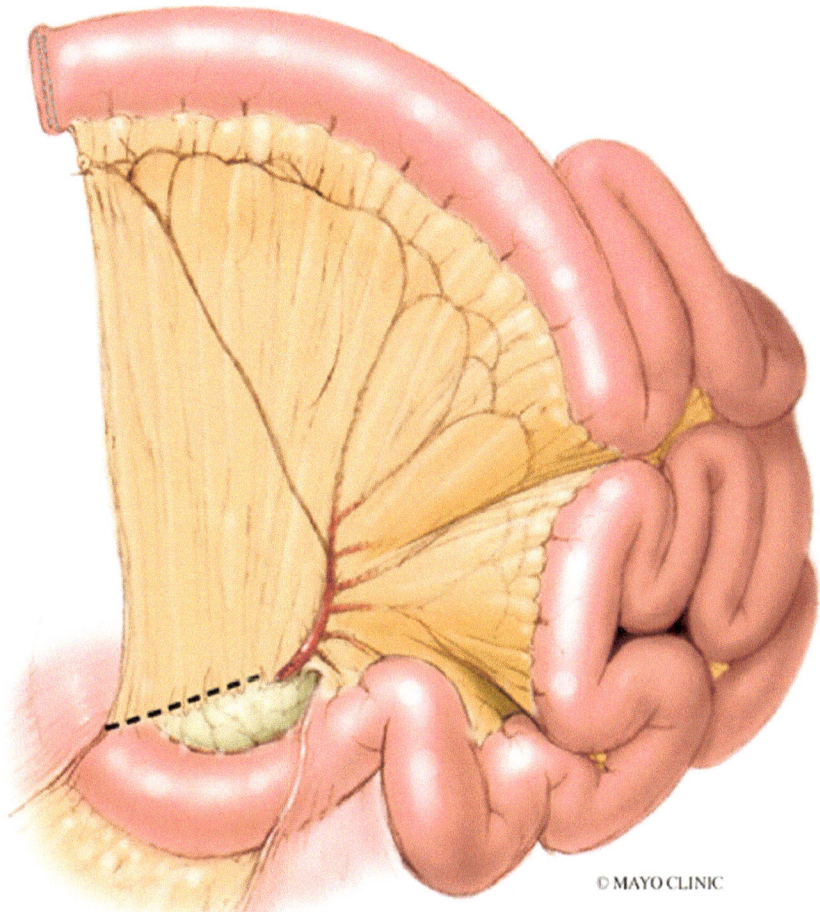

Fig. 20.7 Complete mobilization of the small bowel mesentery. The mesenteric root (dotted line) is taken down at the second and third portions of the duodenum level

Proctectomy Completion

The robot is docked over the patient's left hip. The patient is placed into a steep Trendelenburg position so that the small bowel falls cephalad and exposes the pelvis. The scissors are placed in Arm 4, the camera in Arm 3, the fenestrated bipolar in Arm 2, and a Small Graptor™ in Arm 1.

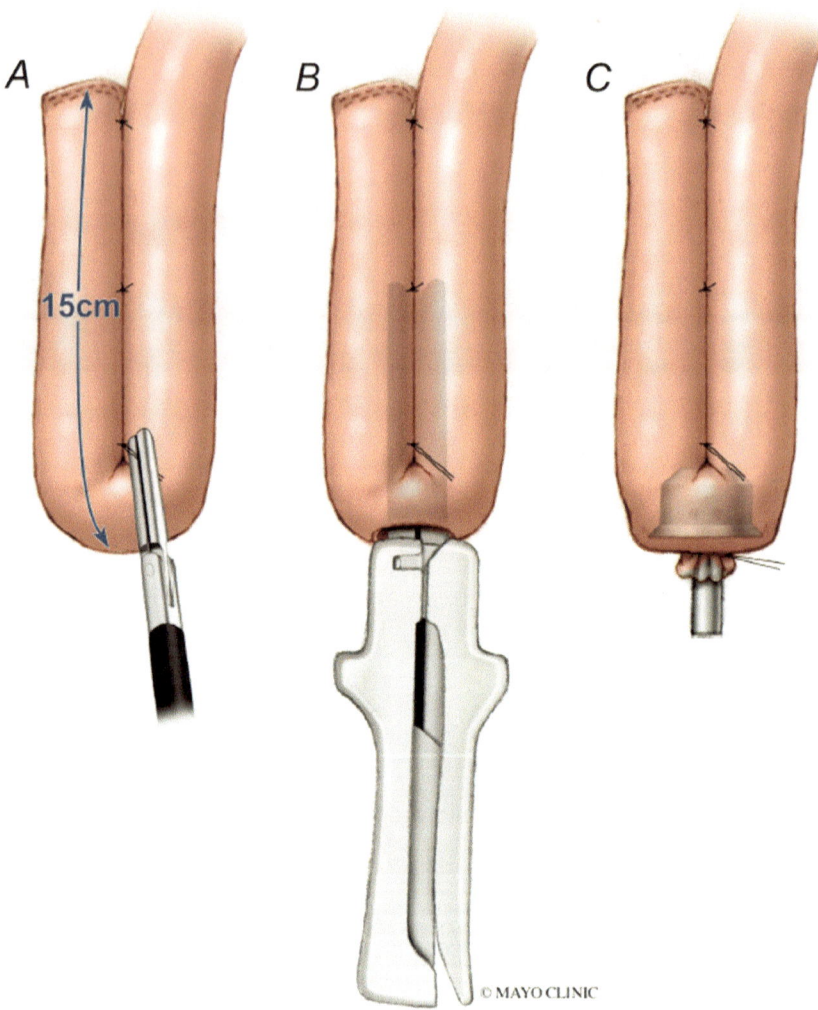

Fig. 20.8 Construction of the ileal J-pouch. **A**. The ileum is folded 15 cm from the stapled end, and both limbs are secured together with stitches. The stitch most proximal to the pouch apex should be cut long enough to be held by a grasper. **B**. The pouch is constructed using 2 firings of the 80-mm blue load extracorporeal linear stapler. **C**. The anvil is secured to the pouch's apex opening in a pursestring fashion

Tips and Tricks

Pelvic exposition: in female patients, the uterus can block adequate exposure of the low part of the rectal stump. Using a straight needle, a transfixing stitch through the abdominal wall and the uterus or around both tubes can help to pull forward the uterus and liberate the pelvic vision (Fig. 20.9).

The tip of the rectal stump is identified and freed from eventual adhesions. At this point, it is also important to divide the adhesions between the small bowel and the retroperitoneum to ensure adequate subsequent pouch placement in the pelvis.

Before rectal stump dissection, several landmarks need to be identified. For this purpose, it is helpful to picture the pelvis as a field with "humps" and "valleys" (Fig. 20.10).

"Humps" contain critical structures such as the superior rectal artery, the iliac vessels, the ureters. For example, suitable planes are found in the "valleys", between the mesentery and the mesocolon.

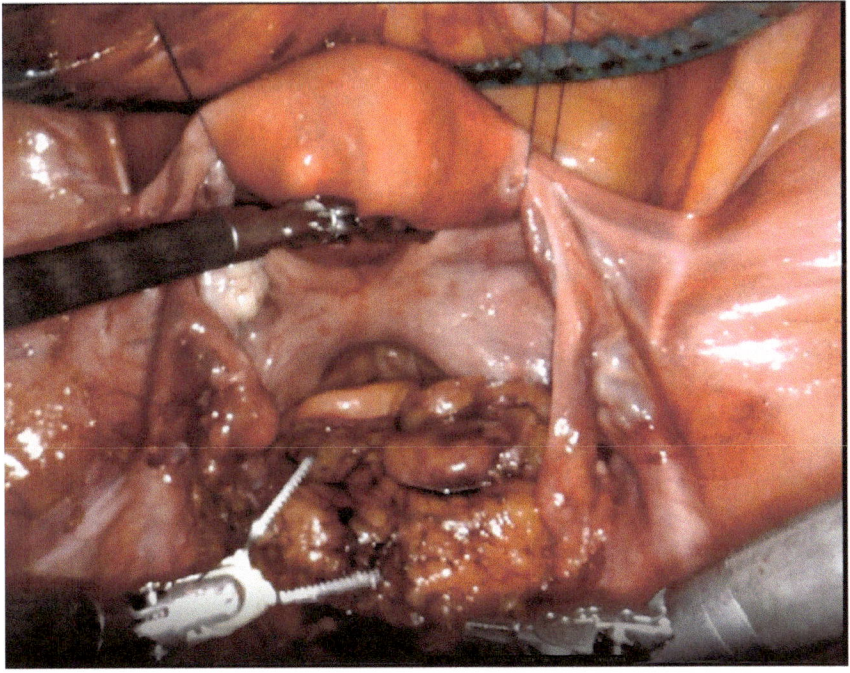

Fig. 20.9 Uterus suspension. Transfixing stitches through the abdominal wall and around the fallopian tubes are helpful to pull forward the uterus

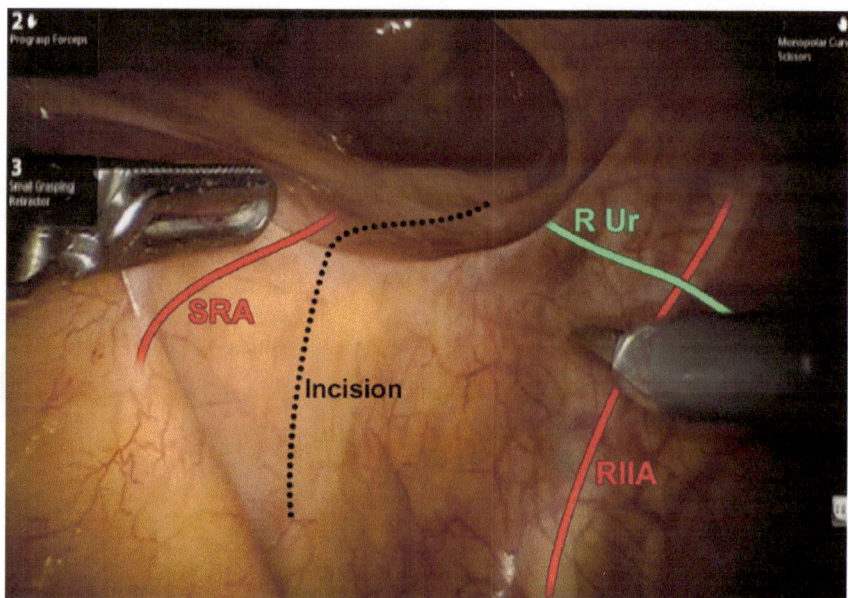

Fig. 20.10 Landmarks for rectal stump liberation. The incision plan (dotted black line) is situated at the junction between the mesentery and the mesocolon. The landmark arteries are figured in red lines, and the right ureter is figured in a green line. RIIA Right internal iliac artery, RUr Right ureter, SRA Superior rectal artery

Our typical dissection of the rectal stump is first performed on the right side and then on the left side, posterior to anterior (Fig. 20.11). We usually perform the proctectomy completion with total mesorectal excision as it is safe and easy without any risk of bleeding.

The tip of the rectal stump is grasped with the Small Graptor™ in Arm 1, and the rectum is retracted out of the pelvis, initially to the left side. Critical landmarks are identified: the sacral promontory, the right ureter, the suitable iliac vessels. Using the scissors (Arm 4), a superficial incision is made on the right side of the rectal stump, at the junction of the mesorectum and the mesentery, just under the level of the sacral promontory. This small incision allows the air to enter the presacral plane and ease the dissection. At this point, the bipolar in Arm 2 is placed posterior to the rectum and elevated anteriorly. This right posterolateral dissection is carried as far to the left pelvic sidewall as possible to decrease the dissection necessary from the left side. Be sure here to identify the left ureter to avoid any injury. The superior hypogastric nerves are identified and preserved by gently sweeping them posteriorly toward the sacrum. The bipolar vessel sealer then replaces the scissors to take the lateral stalks and the mesentery with the remaining superior artery. The rectal stump is then pulled to the right side, and the exact steps are followed on the left side of the rectal stump. The instrumentation in Arms 1 et 4 may be exchanged to complete the dissection along the left side of the rectum. The left ureter is identified so that

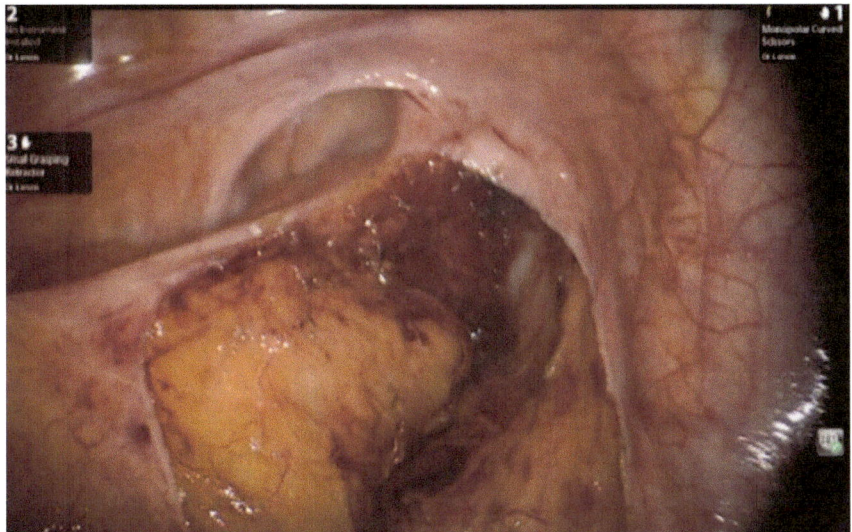

Fig. 20.11 Presacral dissection along the posterior right side of the rectal stump

the rectal dissection doesn't go beyond laterally. If the dissection is too lateral, the nervous structures are at risk for injury, leading to erectile dysfunction.

Tips and Tricks

"Dissection is geometry: open your angles!": working inside obtuse angles ensures safe and easy dissection, especially in rectal surgery. For most efficient exposure, the traction vectors of your instruments should be orientated in a way that you work into an open angle (Fig. 20.12).

The anterior dissection is undertaken last. Arm 1 is used to pull the rectal stump down and out of the pelvis to provide proper tension on the anterior structures. The assistant helps the dissection by placing a suction device or a grasper anterior at the seminal vesicle or posterior vagina level and lifting anteriorly. As the anterior dissection proceeds distally down to the pelvic floor just posterior to the Denonvilliers's fascia, the Small Graptor™ or the fenestrated bipolar in Arm 2 is left in an open position and used to provide strong anterior countertraction. In contrast, Arm 1 places gentle traction on the rectum in a posterior direction (Fig. 20.13). This is particularly useful in a deep narrow male pelvis.

Once the pelvic floor is reached, the rectum is digitized transanally to ensure that the anastomosis will be performed just above the anorectal junction. The rectum is pulled posteriorly and divided with the robotic 60-mm stapler (Fig. 20.14A and B).

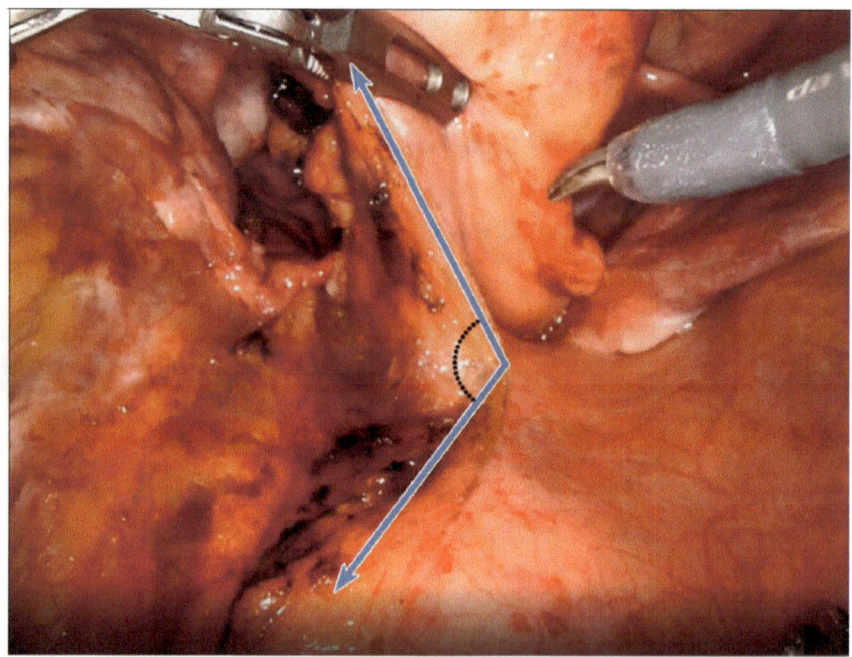

Fig. 20.12 The obtuse angle between dissected structures. Working inside obtuse angles (dotted line) between the structures makes the dissection safe and more straightforward. Traction vectors are figured with blue arrows

Anastomosis Construction

The transected rectum is moved out of the pelvis up to the left side. The anvil and the pouch are brought toward the pelvis.

> **Tips and Tricks**
> "The Tom Thumb move": if the pouch is challenging to find among the small bowel loops, just reach the mesentery root and follow it, it will directly lead you to the pouch.

The anvil is held with the right-hand grasper, while the left-hand grasper has the most proximal stitch to the pouch apex to keep it in the right direction and prevent any twist during the anastomosis. Once the EEA stapler is inserted transanally, the pin is deployed in the central staple line and connected to the anvil under robotic visualization (Fig. 20.15).

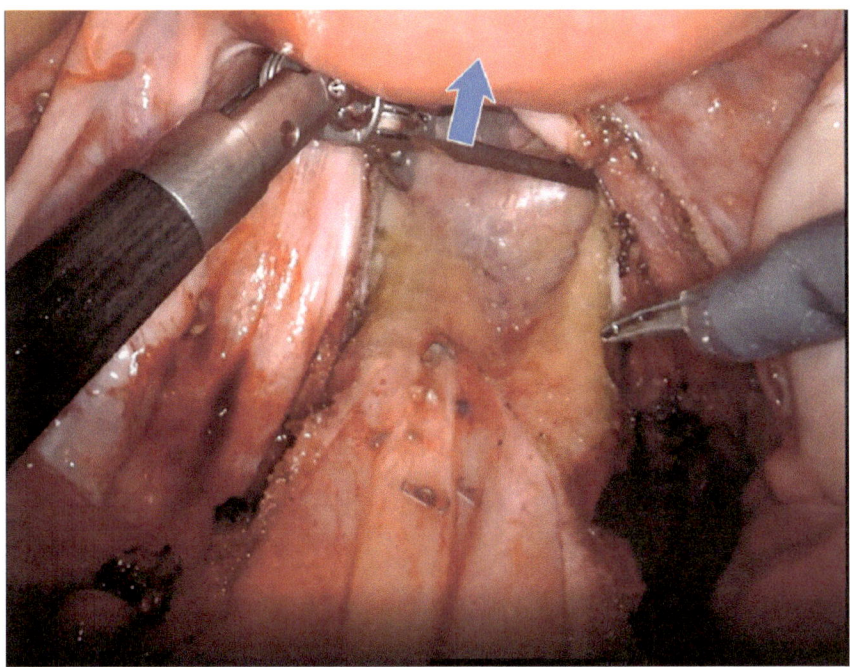

Fig. 20.13 Exposition for anterior dissection. The grasper is left in an open position and provides strong anterior countertraction (blue arrow)

Anastomosis Testing

The patient is placed into a reverse Trendelenburg position, the pelvis is irrigated, and a grasper pushes on the pouch inlet to clamp it. The pouch is insufflated through proctoscopic visualization to control the absence of an anastomotic leak.

What do I do if a leak is identified?

A small anastomotic defect can be managed by adding interrupted 2–0 stitches through the transanal approach. Broader defects require refashioning the anastomosis or even the whole pouch.

Specimen Extraction and Diverting Loop Ileostomy Construction

The rectum is removed through the ileostomy site. The diverting loop ileostomy is placed in the previous ileostomy site. The absence of a twisted loop and the correct

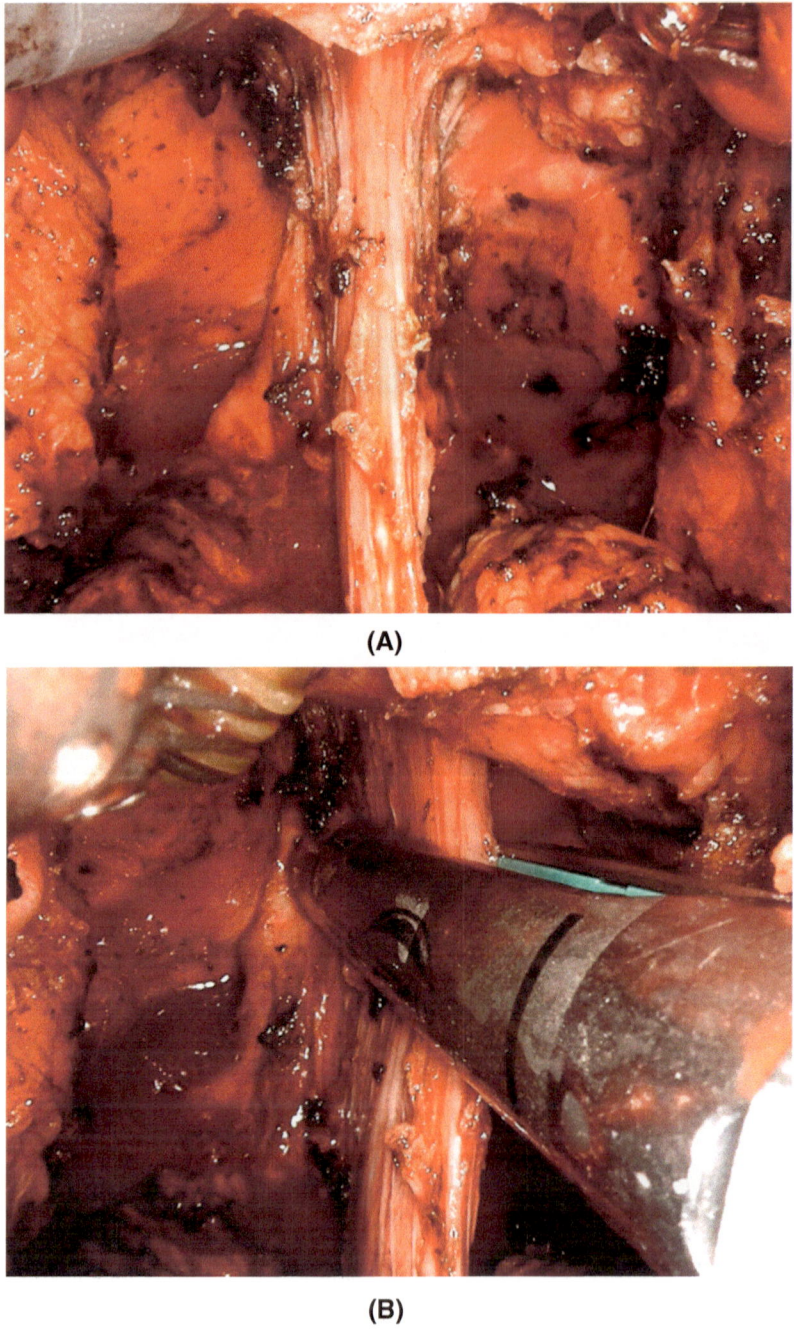

(A)

(B)

Fig. 20.14 Rectal exposition and stapling. The rectum is exposed **A** and stapled just above the anorectal junction **B**

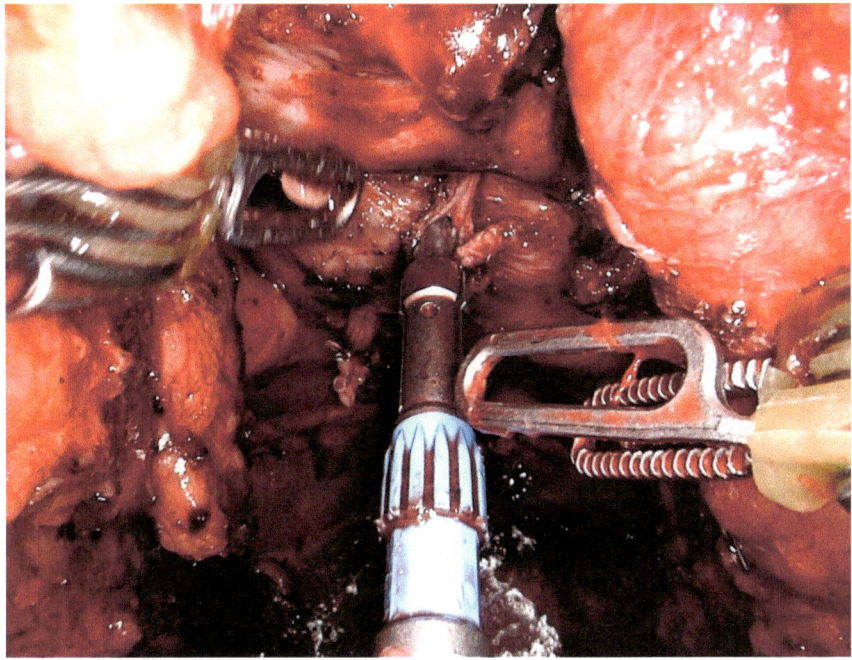

Fig. 20.15 Preparation for anastomosis. The pin of the EEA stapler is deployed in the central staple line of the rectum. Source: Mayo Clinic Rochester

orientation of the ileal loop is controlled (afferent outlet situated on the upper part of the ileostomy). The enterotomy is fashioned within a minimal distance of 30 cm from the pouch inlet to prevent any tension between the stoma site and the pouch.

Five top tips:

1. **Pouch construction:** the stitch most proximal to the pouch apex should be cut long enough to be held by a grasper. It will be easier to maintain the pouch in the right direction during the pouch-anal anastomosis.
2. **Trocar placement:** after insufflation, optimal port placement is obtained when robotic trocars are placed at 6–8 cm from each other, with the camera port placed 15–20 cm from the rectal stump.
3. **Pelvis exposition:** transfixing stitches through the abdominal wall and around both fallopian tubes can help to pull forward the uterus and liberate the pelvic vision.
4. **Finding the right dissection plan with "humps" and "valleys":** it is helpful to picture the rectal stump and the pelvis as a field with "humps" and "valleys." "Humps" contain critical structures such as the superior

rectal artery, the iliac vessels, the ureters. The correct planes are found in the "valleys", for example, between the mesentery and the mesocolon.

5. **Safe and easy dissection plans:** working inside obtuse angles between structures makes the dissection safe and easy.

Aide-memoire—final preoperative checklist:

1. First step is J-pouch construction. Do not take the rectum out before assessing the pouch's reach to the anus without tension.
2. Only one docking is necessary for proctectomy completion.
3. Place the trocars after insufflation, with an ideal distance of 6–8 cm between each port and 15–20 cm between the camera port and the rectal stump.
4. For safety, always have your robotic instruments under direct visual control, especially when they are replaced.
5. Proctectomy completion is performed in the TME plan. Be sure to identify and preserve ureters and nerves along with the dissection.
6. During J-pouch anal anastomosis, be careful of the pouch's orientation: the stapled ileal end is oriented on the right, and the mesentery is posterior.

References

1. Ahmed Ali U, Keus F, Heikens JT, Bemelman WA, Berdah SV, Gooszen HG, et al. Open versus laparoscopic (assisted) ileo pouch anal anastomosis for ulcerative colitis and familial adenomatous polyposis. Cochrane Database Syst Rev. 2009:CD006267. https://doi.org/10.1002/146 51858.CD006267.pub2.
2. Kim MJ, Park SC, Park JW, Chang HJ, Kim DY, Nam BH, et al. Robot-assisted versus laparoscopic surgery for rectal cancer: a phase II open label prospective randomized controlled trial. Ann Surg. 2018;267:243–51. https://doi.org/10.1097/SLA.0000000000002321.
3. Baek SJ, Dozois EJ, Mathis KL, Lightner AL, Boostrom SY, Cima RR, et al. Safety, feasibility, and short-term outcomes in 588 patients undergoing minimally invasive ileal pouch-anal anastomosis: a single-institution experience. Tech Coloproctol. 2016;20:369–74. https://doi.org/10.1007/s10151-016-1465-z.
4. Larson DW, Cima RR, Dozois EJ, Davies M, Piotrowicz K, Barnes SA, et al. Safety, feasibility, and short-term outcomes of laparoscopic ileal-pouch-anal anastomosis: a single institutional case-matched experience. Ann Surg. 2006;243:667–70. https://doi.org/10.1097/01.sla.000021 6762.83407.d2.
5. Baek SJ, Lightner AL, Boostrom SY, Mathis KL, Cima RR, Pemberton JH, et al. Functional outcomes following laparoscopic ileal pouch-anal anastomosis in patients with chronic ulcerative colitis: long-term follow-up of a case-matched study. J Gastrointest Surg. 2017;21:1304–8. https://doi.org/10.1007/s11605-017-3411-4.

6. Larson DW, Davies MM, Dozois EJ, Cima RR, Piotrowicz K, Anderson K, et al. Sexual function, body image, and quality of life after laparoscopic and open ileal pouch-anal anastomosis. Dis Colon Rectum. 2008;51:392–6. https://doi.org/10.1007/s10350-007-9180-5.
7. Lightner AL, Kelley SR, Larson DW. Robotic platform for an IPAA. Dis Colon Rectum. 2018;61:869–74. https://doi.org/10.1097/DCR.0000000000001125.
8. Lightner AL, Grass F, McKenna NP, Tilman M, Alsughayer A, Kelley SR, et al. Short-term postoperative outcomes following robotic versus laparoscopic ileal pouch-anal anastomosis are equivalent. Tech Coloproctol. 2019;23(3):259–66. https://doi.org/10.1007/s10151-019-019 53-8.
9. Flynn J, Larach JT, Kong JCH, Warrier SK, Heriot A. Robotic versus laparoscopic ileal pouch-anal anastomosis (IPAA): a systematic review and meta-analysis. Int J Colorectal Dis. 2021. https://doi.org/10.1007/s00384-021-03868-z.
10. Khreiss W, Huebner M, Cima RR, Dozois ER, Chua HK, Pemberton JH, et al. Improving conventional recovery with enhanced recovery in minimally invasive surgery for rectal cancer. Dis Colon Rectum. 2014;57:557–63. https://doi.org/10.1097/DCR.0000000000000101.
11. Larson DW, Lovely JK, Cima RR, Dozois EJ, Chua H, Wolff BG, et al. Outcomes after implementation of a multimodal standard care pathway for laparoscopic colorectal surgery. Br J Surg. 2014;101:1023–30. https://doi.org/10.1002/bjs.9534.
12. Lee JM, Yang SY, Han YD, Cho MS, Hur H, Min BS, et al. Can better surgical outcomes be obtained in the learning process of robotic rectal cancer surgery? A propensity score-matched comparison between learning phases. Surg Endosc. 2021;35:770–8. https://doi.org/10.1007/s00464-020-07445-3.
13. Oresland T, Bemelman WA, Sampietro GM, Spinelli A, Windsor A, Ferrante M, et al. European evidence based consensus on surgery for ulcerative colitis. J Crohns Colitis. 2015;9:4–25. https://doi.org/10.1016/j.crohns.2014.08.012.
14. Parc Y, Reboul-Marty J, Lefevre JH, Shields C, Chafai N, Tiret E. Restorative proctocolectomy and ileal pouch-anal anastomosis. Ann Surg. 2015;262:849–53. https://doi.org/10.1097/SLA.0000000000001406.

Chapter 21
Robotic Parastomal and Perineal Hernia Repair

Enda Hannan and Colin Peirce

Abstract Both parastomal hernia repair and perineal hernia repair represent two of the most dreaded procedures that colorectal surgeons may encounter. Not only do they represent unfortunate post-operative complications that can be highly debilitating and distressing for patients, but they also present therapeutic challenges, with high recurrence rates reported in many of the described approaches to repair. However, both of these pathologies may benefit from robotic surgery. With regards to parastomal hernia repair, it has been demonstrated that concurrent fascial closure with mesh placement is superior to mesh placement alone. The robotic platform is ergonomically advantageous with regards to intracorporeal suturing when compared with laparoscopy, and thus may allow for this step to be more consistently performed. Laparoscopic approaches to perineal hernia repair are also highly challenging, with difficulties encountered in mesh placement and suturing with rigid instruments in the narrow bony pelvis. The ergonomic advantages and dexterity offered by robotic surgery may allow the surgeon to overcome such difficulties. In this chapter, the authors describe robotic approaches to both parastomal and perineal hernia repair.

Keywords Robotic · Parastomal hernia repair · Sugarbaker · Perineal hernia repair

Abbreviations

PSH   Parastomal hernia
PH   Perineal hernia
APR   Abdominoperineal resection
eAPR   Extralevator abdominoperineal resection

E. Hannan (✉) · C. Peirce
Department of Colorectal Surgery, University Hospital Limerick, St. Nessan's Road, Dooradoyle, Limerick, Ireland
e-mail: endahannan@rcsi.ie

C. Peirce
School of Medicine, University of Limerick, Limerick, Ireland

© The Author(s), under exclusive license to Springer Nature Switzerland AG 2022
P. Coyne and J. Khan (eds.), *Robotic Colorectal Surgery*,
https://doi.org/10.1007/978-3-031-15198-9_21

253

Part 1: Robotic Parastomal Hernia Repair

Introduction

Parastomal herniation is a common complication. Approximately 1 in 500 people live with a stoma, and up to 75% will develop a parastomal hernia [1, 2]. Risk factors include obesity, smoking, older age, malnutrition, emergency surgery and immunocompromisation [1, 3]. It can cause chronic pain, bowel strangulation and obstruction [1], troublesome leakage from the stoma site, peristomal skin irritation and interfere with daily activities [1, 3]. Thirty to 50% of patients will require repair which can be challenging, with a recurrence rate of up to 70% reported in those managed by fascial closure alone [1]. For this reason, the placement of mesh is recommended in parastomal hernia repair [1, 2].

The two most common approaches to parastomal hernia repair are the Sugarbaker and keyhole techniques [2]. It has been demonstrated by meta-analysis that the Sugarbaker technique is more effective, with a lower recurrence rate [4]. Outcomes have also been shown to be more favourable in laparoscopic repair compared to open approaches [1]. However, the use of laparoscopy may prove challenging, where attempting to close the fascial defect using conventional rigid laparoscopic instruments can create difficulty that may compromise the quality of repair [1]. For this reason, most laparoscopic hernias are repaired without fascial closure [1]. However, it has been demonstrated that concurrent fascial closure with mesh placement reduces recurrence rates in laparoscopic ventral hernia repair [5]. Thus, being able to consistently perform fascial closure in parastomal hernia repair may improve outcomes [1, 2]. The robotic platform is ergonomically advantageous for fascial closure compared with laparoscopic approaches, with a 40% higher rate of fascial closure reported in ventral hernia repair compared with laparoscopic approaches [5, 6]. Here, the authors describe their technique of robotic Sugarbaker repair with fascial closure.

Procedural Cases

Indications for Repair

The most common indications for surgery are issues relating to quality of life such as chronic discomfort, issues with stoma bag appliance or prior bowel obstruction as a result of the hernia. Asymptomatic patients should be managed non-operatively due to the risk of recurrence and other potential postoperative complications.

Preoperative Workup

A thorough evaluation including history, physical examination, baseline laboratory investigations and cross-sectional imaging is essential prior to surgery. A recent computed tomography (CT) study of the abdomen and pelvis is useful for diagnosis, assessment of anatomy, preoperative planning and measurement of the fascial defect. In all patients, consider if stoma reversal is possible prior to proceeding with hernia repair. All prior operative notes need to be thoroughly reviewed to anticipate the intra-abdominal anatomy. For those with a history of malignancy or symptoms that could relate to colonic pathology, ensure that recent endoscopic evaluation has been performed. The patient's comorbidities should be optimised by a multidisciplinary approach prior to repair. Patients with a smoking history must cease smoking for at least 4 weeks prior to surgery. Obese patients should be strongly encouraged to lose weight prior to surgery as this will reduce risk of recurrence and potentially reduce intra-abdominal adiposity. For diabetic patients, a glycated haemoglobin (HbA1c) level below 7% should be achieved. The patient should be thoroughly counselled on the risks and benefits of surgery, especially the risk of potential recurrence.

Operating Theatre Setup

The patient is placed in the supine position with both arms tucked and the umbilicus overlying the table break, so that the table may be flexed to allow greater exposure of the abdomen and thus increase the working room for the robotic arms. Appropriate prophylactic intravenous antibiotics should be given prior to commencing surgery. The stoma is covered with gauze and an occlusive dressing to avoid contamination during the case.

Port Placement

Three 8 mm robotic ports and one 12 mm AirSeal® assistant port are used for this technique. All 8 mm ports are placed on the side contralateral to the stoma in a line along the lateral abdominal wall through the transversus abdominal muscle, with a 6–8 cm distance between each robotic port tailored to each patient. The 12 mm AirSeal® port is placed in the right upper quadrant and will be used for the introduction of mesh and sutures under vision. Entry to the abdomen can be achieved either by placement of an 8 mm port by direct cutdown at the same level as the stoma on the contralateral side, or by use of an optical entry port or Veress needle if preferred. Under vision via the da Vinci® camera, two further 8 mm ports and the 12 mm AirSeal® port are placed and numbered as shown in the diagram (Image 21.1). The robot is docked from the side of the stoma.

Image 21.1 Port placement
for robotic PSH repair

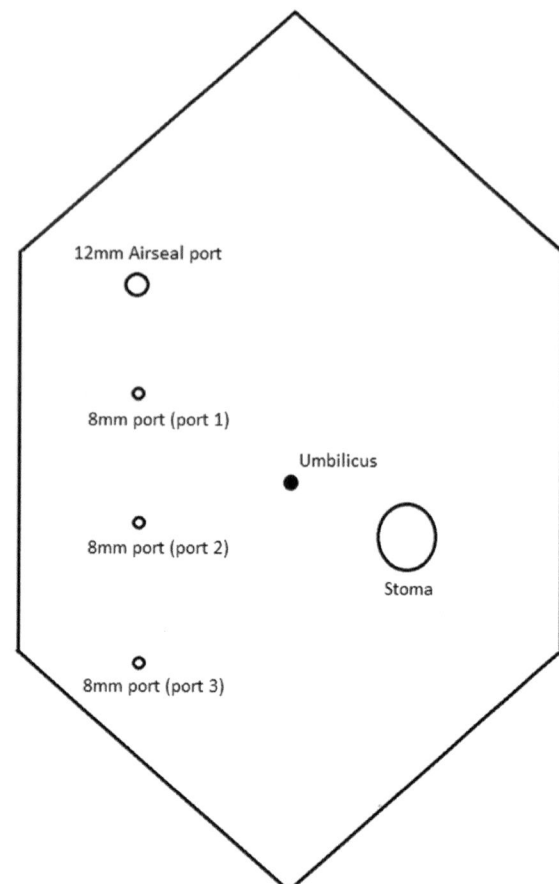

Equipment Needed

Our technique is described utilising the da Vinci® Xi Surgical System by Intuitive Surgical®

Camera

- mm 30° da Vinci® Xi robotic camera with Firefly™ Fluorescence Imaging (port 2)
  - Fluorescence guidance can aid in identifying the stoma conduit and associated mesenteric blood supply

Ports/trocars

- Three Intuitive Surgical® 8 mm robotic trocars
- 12 mm AirSeal® port

- For assistance and insertion of sutures and mesh
- Provides stable pneumoperitoneum and constant smoke evacuation

Robotic instruments for dissection

- Fenestrated bipolar forceps (port 1)
- Monopolar scissors (port 3)

Robotic instruments for suturing

- Fenestrated biopolar forceps (port 1)
- Mega Suture Cut™ needle driver (port 3)

Laparoscopic instruments

- Atraumatic grasper
- Suction/irrigation available
- Laparoscopic tacker
- Laparoscopic suture passer

Sutures and mesh

- 1.0 V-Loc™ barbed suture
- 2.0 non-absorbable suture for mesh placement, such as nylon or polypropelene
- Mesh selection based on operating conditions

  - If the operative field may be contaminated, a biologic mesh is used. Otherwise, a synthetic mesh is used.

Other

- Measuring tape/ruler

  - Introduced via the 12 mm assist port to measure the size of the fascial defect intraoperatively

- Urinary catheter

  - Can be inserted into the lumen of the stoma which will help identify a full thickness bowel injury by the catheter becoming visible

Procedural Steps

The procedure commences with the fenestrated bipolar forceps in the left hand (port 1) and the monopolar scissors in the right hand (port 3). Following an inspection of the abdomen for abnormal findings, the stoma orifice and parastomal hernia are inspected. Adhesiolysis is performed if required, using the monopolar scissors to divide the adhesions and the bipolar forceps for haemostasis. Following this, the contents of the hernia are gently reduced into the abdominal cavity, which will also allow delineation of the fascial edges. Any adhesions between intra-abdominal contents to the fascial edges or hernia sac should be gently dissected to allow complete reduction, taking care not to injure the bowel going toward the stoma. Ideally, the bowel should not be handled with the forceps if possible and instead the back of the instrument used to push the bowel away on tension allowing dissection of the relevant plane with the scissors. Firefly™ Fluorescence Imaging can be used to help identify the stoma conduit during this stage.

Following hernia reduction, the defect that is to be covered by the mesh is measured by means of a ruler inserted into the abdomen via the assistant port. The greatest diameter of the defect measured is used to size the mesh. It is essential that a 5 cm overlap is achieved in all directions based on these measurements. The most likely location for recurrence of a parastomal hernia is at the lateral aspect, and thus any additional overlap that can be obtained laterally will be beneficial.

At this point, the monopolar scissors is replaced by the Mega Suture Cut™ needle driver. A 1–0 V-Loc™ barbed permanent suture is inserted by the assistant through the 12 mm port and passed to the robotic needle driver. The fascial defect at the stoma is then narrowed using this stitch in a running manner, with care taken not to narrow the defect to the point where stoma outflow is compromised. The initial bites are taken close to the bowel and then stitching proceeds away from the bowel to the far extent of the fascial defect. In the case of end stomas, the mesentery of the bowel should be 'pexied' to the lateral abdominal wall with a permanent suture, either interrupted or running, to prevent this loop of bowel from elongating into the defect and resulting in re-herniation.

Prior to insertion into the abdomen, the mesh should be appropriately trimmed to size to ensure adequate cover and is marked for orientation purposes. Anchoring nonabsorbable sutures are placed at the superior, inferior, medial and middle aspects of the mesh with the tails left long. Using these pre-placed sutures, the mesh is then secured to the abdominal wall by use of the suture passer by the assistant, with the suture at the middle aspect of the mesh secured first at the medial fascia edge by the stoma. This allows the mesh to be suspended from the abdominal wall and centred to ensure adequate overlap. Following this, the remaining preplaced sutures should also be secured in a similar manner via the suture passer at the medial, inferior and superior aspects. (It must be noted that the authors think this aids in precision mesh placement, albeit some surgeons do not use any pre-placed sutures in the mesh).

A long Sugarbaker tunnel is then created by placement of 2 nonabsorbable sutures at the lateral edges of the mesh superior and inferior to the bowel within the Sugarbaker tunnel. These sutures should be placed in a proximal-to-distal manner, first placing the needle approximately 0.5–1 cm from the edge of the mesh and then through the abdominal wall at a position that is close enough to the conduit so that there is no potential space for herniation between the stoma and mesh, but also not so close that it may impede flow of stoma contents. These rows of sutures are extended along the length of the Sugarbaker tunnel back to the level of the stoma orifice so that the mesh is then secured circumferentially around the bowel conduit. This can be done by further interrupted robotic suturing or, given the large size of the mesh, the surgeon can transition to laparoscopy and use a tacking device which may be a time-saving manoeuvre. The entire mesh should then be secured around the perimeter in a manner so that the interrupted sutures or tackers are close together so that there is no potential for small bowel or omental herniation between the mesh and abdominal wall. Following this, the mesh should be inspected to ensure that it is taut with the abdominal wall, but not so tight that it is obstructing the stoma.

The fascia at the 12 mm trocar site is closed with a 1.0 polydioxanone suture. The remaining 8 mm ports are then removed and the abdomen is desufflated. Prior to camera removal, the 8 mm port sites should be checked as they might require primary closure, especially in patients with hernias who have weaker fascia potentially. The skin is closed using a 4.0 absorbable monofilament suture and sterile dressings are applied. A transversus abdominus plane block should be considered to help reduce opioid use and shorten length of stay.

The authors do not recommend the keyhole technique, which has a higher recurrence rate, nor do the authors have experience with combining the Sugarbaker technique with transversus abdominis release, which is sometimes utilised in recurrent cases or cases with very large defects.

Top 5 Tips

1. An experienced assistant that is familiar with the setup required in robotic surgery is essential. This will allow the assistant to deal with basic troubleshooting issues such as arms clashing and the requirement to change robotic instruments mid-procedure, such as when the robotic needle driver is required. The assistant should also have at least basic laparoscopic skills, as these will be required to insert sutures and the mesh via the assistant port.
2. One of the most important steps is the preparation and sizing of the mesh. It may be valuable for the primary operator to step away from the robotic console and scrub for this stage to ensure that the mesh is appropriately marked with sutures placed correctly to ensure appropriate coverage.
3. The main benefit that a robotic platform offers to enhance the Sugarbaker technique is that it allows the surgeon to consistently suture the fascial defect. Once this has been achieved, it is possible to complete the remainder of the procedure laparoscopically by securing the mesh via laparoscopic tacking, which may save time, should the surgeon prefer (but we would advocate a complete robotic approach, negating the need and expense of a laparoscopic tacker).
4. At the end of the case, digitally examine the stoma to ensure that it has not been rendered too tight by the Sugarbaker tunnel or by fascial closure.
5. Placing a urinary catheter in the stoma is a useful adjunct as a full thickness injury of the bowel will become evident by the catheter becoming visible in the operative field.

Checklist

- Full preoperative workup
- Thorough patient counselling and consent
- Consider if a non-operative approach is a viable option
- Consider if the stoma can be reversed
- Check that all required equipment is available in theatre
- Ensure the availability of an assistant with appropriate experience
- Review cross-sectional imaging pre-procedure
- Establish pneumoperitoneum via the 8 mm robotic trocar using direct cutdown at the same level as the stoma on the contralateral side
- Place the other two 8 mm robotic trocars as shown in the diagram with at least a 6 cm distance between trocars
- Place the 12 mm AirSeal® port in the upper abdomen under vision
- Commence adhesiolysis and reduction of the hernia contents
- Close the fascial defect using a running 1.0 V-Loc™ barbed suture
- Measure the maximum diameter of the hernia defect
- Appropriately mark and size the mesh to ensure 5 cm coverage from all aspects
- Secure the mesh using the suture passer with preplaced sutures
- Ensure that the mesh is secured circumferentially around the conduit to fashion the Sugarbaker tunnel and then around the entire perimeter
- Ensure that the mesh is taut with the abdominal wall but not occluding the lumen
- Close the fascia at the 12 mm port and close the skin.

Part 2: Robotic Perineal Hernia Repair

Introduction

Perineal hernia (PH) is defined as a pelvic floor defect through which intra-abdominal viscera protrude [7]. PH is a rare complication following conventional abdominoperineal resection (APR), with an incidence of less than 1% [8]. However, an incidence as high as 26% has been reported following extralevator APR (ELAPE), which creates a much wider perineal defect [8]. Since the introduction of ELAPE, a sharp increase in the number of reported cases of PH in the literature has been noted [9]. The advent of neoadjuvant chemoradiotherapy for rectal cancer may have also contributed to this increased incidence in PH, which is recognised to impair wound healing [9]. Asymptomatic PH should be managed non-operatively. However, a PH may cause symptoms such as perineal pain, difficulty walking and/or sitting, and may be complicated by skin erosion, urinary dysfunction and bowel obstruction [10].

Surgical repair of PH is challenging, with high rates of recurrence and significant risk of morbidity [11]. Currently, there is no gold standard technique for PH repair, although numerous techniques have been described in the literature, including open abdominal, perineal, laparoscopic or hybrid approaches [11]. Open abdominal and perineal techniques provide adequate exposure for mesh and suture placement, but come with significant postoperative pain, slower recovery and risk of further wound complications [7–10]. Laparoscopic surgery reduces length of stay and wound complications, but mesh placement and suturing with rigid instruments in the narrow bony pelvis can by highly challenging [7–10]. The improved ergonomics and dexterity offered by robotic surgery allow for ease of suturing and mesh placement in the pelvis while maintaining the advantages of a minimally invasive approach on recovery and morbidity [7–9]. Here, the authors describe their technique of robotic PH repair.

Steps of the Procedure

Indications for Repair

Repair should be offered in symptomatic patients with significant impact on quality of life or those with complications such as bowel obstruction.

Preoperative Workup

Full history, examination, baseline laboratory investigations and cross-sectional imaging should be completed prior to surgery. Up to date CT and magnetic resonance imaging if indicated are important for surveillance as well as for delineating hernia anatomy, including the size of the defect and hernia contents. As described in the PSH repair section, all comorbid conditions should be optimised using a multidisciplinary approach.

Operating Theatre Setup

The patient should be placed in the lithotomy position with both arms tucked. A urinary catheter should be inserted, the stoma covered by gauze and an occlusive dressing and appropriate prophylactic intravenous antibiotics administered.

Port Placement

The initial 8 mm robotic trocar (port 2) which will act as the endoscope port is placed in the subumbilical position by Hasson technique, after which pneumoperitoneum is established. A further 8 mm port (port 1) is placed left lateral 8 cm away from this port, while two further 8 mm ports (ports 3 and 4) are placed right lateral from the initial port 8 cm away from each other. Particular care and attention should be taken

Image 21.2 Port placement
for robotic PH repair

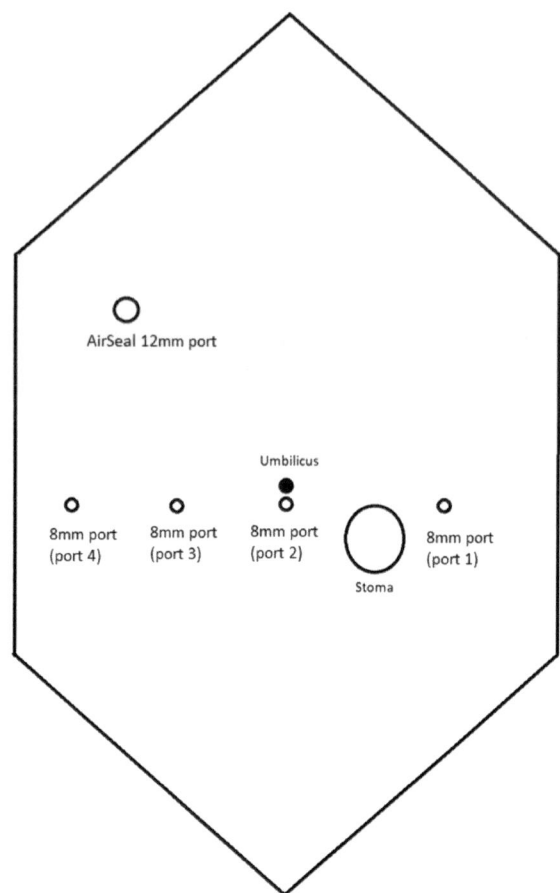

on insertion of port 1 which will be in close proximity to the colostomy following
APR, with the position adjusted to be lateral to the stoma and taking care to avoid
injury to potential parastomal hernia contents. Port position can vary from 6 to 10 cm
between trocars, with this range used to ensure appropriate placement of port 1 in
relation to the colostomy. A 12 mm assistant port is placed in the right upper quadrant
between the longitudinal axis of ports 3 and 4 (Image 21.2). The robot is docked from
the patient's left with the centre of the perineal defect used as the target anatomy.

Equipment Needed

Our technique is described utilising the da Vinci® Xi Surgical System by Intuitive
Surgical®

Camera

- 8 mm 30° da Vinci® Xi robotic camera (port 2)

Ports/trocars

- Three 8 mm robotic trocars
- 12 mm AirSeal® port

   - For assistance and insertion of sutures and mesh
   - Provides stable pneumoperitoneum and constant smoke evacuation

Robotic instruments for dissection

- Fenestrated bipolar forceps (port 1)
- Monopolar scissors (port 3)
- Tip-up fenestrated grasper (port 4)

Robotic instruments for suturing

- Fenestrated biopolar forceps (port 1)
- Mega Suture Cut™ needle driver (port 3)

Laparoscopic instruments

- Atraumatic grasper
- Suction/irrigation

Sutures and mesh

- 1.0 V-Loc™ barbed sutures
- 2.0 Ethibond Excel® sutures
- 1.0 Silk suture on a straight needle
- Non-absorbable synthetic mesh

Other

- Measuring tape/ruler

Procedural Steps

The procedure commences with a diagnostic laparoscopy to assess for potential disease recurrence. The patient is then placed in steep Trendelenberg position and tilted to the right to mobilise the small bowel out of the perineal hernia defect and to facilitate adhesiolysis. Adhesiolysis is performed with the fenestrated bipolar grasper in port 1 and the monopolar scissors in port 3, with the laparoscopic assistant port and tip-up grasper in port 4 used to provide gentle retraction and care taken to avoid enterotomy. Once this is completed, the small bowel should be allowed to fall into the upper abdomen. A similar approach should be taken to displace any adherent omentum into the upper abdomen to clear the operative field.

Once the pelvis has been cleared of adhesions, the perineal defect should be examined. In female patients where the uterus is still present, the uterus should be temporarily suspended to the anterior abdominal wall by a 2.0 Silk stitch on a straight needle introduced by the assistant in the suprapubic region to improve visualisation of the defect. A ruler is introduced via the 12 mm assistant port to measure the maximum diameter of the perineal defect which will aid with sizing of the mesh. Both ureters should also be identified in the pelvis. If there is concern about risk of ureteric injury or difficulty in identifying the ureters, transilluminating ureteric stents may be placed. The neck of the hernial sac of the PH should also be noted as well as the presence or absence of adequate levator plates that may facilitate levatorplasty, which will not be possible following ELAPE.

Due to the risk of iatrogenic injury to pelvic structures and the potential for creating a defect in the perineal skin, we do not recommend attempting to excise the hernial sac. Rather, the hernial sac is closed at its neck by a running 1.0 V-Loc™ barbed suture from anterior to posterior. Sutures are introduced via the 12 mm assistant port, and the instrument in port 3 replaced with the Mega Suture Cut™ needle driver. Following this, if there is sufficient levator muscle tissue left to close the muscular defect, this should be performed using a running 1.0 V-Loc™ barbed suture, starting anteriorly and finishing posteriorly. If levatorplasty is not possible, then the surgeon should move on to mesh placement.

The mesh should be sized according to the maximum diameter measured by the ruler and trimmed accordingly, maintaining a circular shape and aiming for an overlap of 3 cm in all directions. The mesh is then introduced via the 12 mm assistant port and placed in an appropriate position in the pelvis covering the defect; directly onto the levatorplasty if this step was possible or covering the defect if not. The mesh is then sutured in position by interrupted 2.0 Ethibond Excel® sutures. The mesh is secured anteriorly to the symphysis pubis and pelvic brim, posteriorly to the sacrum and coccyx, and laterally to the origins of the divided levators, or to their lateral insertion point if still present. Single interrupted sutures should be placed at the anterior, posterior and most lateral points of fixation initially to ensure the mesh is appropriately positioned and anchored before placing further interrupted sutures between these points so that there is no potential space for small bowel or omentum to herniate under the mesh into the pelvis. The sutures should be placed through the mesh first at its edge and then into the corresponding point of fixation, with approximately 1 cm spaces between sutures.

Once the mesh has been secured, the pelvis should be thoroughly inspected to ensure haemostasis, and appropriate suction and irrigation performed via the assistant port. A one-quarter inch Redivac™ drain should be placed in the pelvis to avoid haematoma formation. If possible, the omentum should be placed in the pelvis to act as a barrier to avoid small bowel adhesions to the mesh. The 12 mm trocar site is closed with a 1.0 polydioxanone suture. The remaining 8 mm ports are then removed and the abdomen is desufflated. The skin is closed using a 4.0 absorbable monofilament suture and sterile dressings are applied.

Top 5 Tips

1. Robotic PH repair is challenging as it is re-operative pelvic surgery. As with PSH repair, an experienced assistant familiar with assisting in robotic colorectal surgery that also has adequate laparoscopic skills is essential.
2. Port placement may vary according to preference, and one may find it more appropriate to adapt their typical port setup employed for a robotic APR or robotic low anterior resection. However, care must be taken to position the ports so that the instruments do not pose the risk of damaging the colostomy in the left iliac fossa. The port placement we describe allows the internal aspect of the trocar to emerge just inferolateral to the colostomy to protect it from injury.
3. While the operation would be technically feasible with just three robotic arms, we recommend using four. The fourth arm is particularly useful in initial adhesiolysis of the pelvis, where the extra retraction may be highly useful to identify safe planes of dissection where small bowel is adherent to the pelvis.
4. If possible, the omentum should be placed in the pelvis (i.e. an omentoplasty) upon completion of mesh repair to avoid small bowel adhesions to the mesh. It may be useful to perform an omentopexy by suturing the omentum loosely to the pelvic brim if it can reach the pelvis without tension.
5. We recommend the use of interrupted sutures to secure the mesh in the pelvis as opposed to running sutures as this will allow for better positioning and potential adjusting of the mesh placement.

Checklist

- Full preoperative workup
- Thorough patient counselling and consent
- Consider if a non-operative approach is a viable option
- Check that all required equipment is available in theatre
- Ensure the availability of an assistant with appropriate experience
- Review cross-sectional imaging pre-procedure
- Position the patient in lithotomy position with a urinary catheter in-situ
- Establish pneumoperitoneum via an 8 mm robotic trocar placed sub-umbilically via the Hasson technique
- Place 3 further 8 mm ports and the 12 mm assistant port as shown in Image 21.2.
- Use the perineal defect as the target anatomy and position the patient in steep Trendelenberg
- Clear the small bowel from the pelvis and perform adhesiolysis
- Measure the perineal defect with a ruler
- Close the peritoneal defect by a running 1.0 V-Loc™ barbed suture
- Perform a levatorplasty if possible by a running 1.0 V-Loc™ barbed suture
- Size and secure the mesh by means of interrupted 2.0 Ethibond Excel™ sutures
- Ensure haemostasis and place a drain in the pelvis

- Place the omentum in the pelvis if possible
- Close the fascia at the 12 mm port and close the skin.

References

1. Ayuso SA, Shao JM, Deerenberg EB, Elhage SA, George MB, Heniford BT, Augenstein VA. Robotic Sugarbaker parastomal hernia repair: technique and outcomes. Hernia. 2020. (Epub ahead of print).
2. Addo A., Lu R, Belyansky I, LeBlanc KA. Robotic-assisted parastomal hernia repair: sugarbaker repair (With and Without Component Release). In: LeBlanc K, editor. Robotic Assisted Hernia Repair. Cham; Springer; 2019.
3. Shah N, Craft R, Harold K. Parastomal hernia repair. Surg Clin North Am. 2013;93(5):1185–98.
4. Hansson BME, Slater NJ, van der Velden AS, et al. Surgical techniques for parastomal hernia repair. Ann Surg. 2012;255:685–95.
5. Nguyen DH, Nguyen MT, Askenasy EP, et al. Primary fascial closure with laparoscopic ventral hernia repair: systematic review. World J Surg. 2014;38:3097–104.
6. Prabhu AS, Dickens EO, Copper CM, Mann JW, Yunis JP, Phillips S, Huang LC, Poulose BK, Rosen MJ. Laparoscopic vs robotic intraperitoneal mesh repair for incisional hernia: an americas hernia society quality collaborative analysis. J Am Coll Surg. 2017;225(2):285–93.
7. Maurissen J, Schoneveld M, Van Eetvelde E, Allaeys M. Robotic-assisted repair of perineal hernia after extralevator abdominoperineal resection. Tech Coloproctol. 2019;23(5):479–82.
8. Rajabaleyan P, Dorfelt A, Poornoroozy P, Vadgaard AP. Robot-assisted laparoscopic repair of perineal hernia after abdominoperineal resection: a case report and review of the literature. Int J Surg Case Rep. 2019;55:54–7.
9. Balla A, Batista Rodríguez G, Buonomo N, Martinez C, Hernández P, Bollo J, Targarona EM. Perineal hernia repair after abdominoperineal excision or extralevator abdominoperineal excision: a systematic review of the literature. Tech Coloproctol. 2017;21(5):329–36. https://doi.org/10.1007/s10151-017-1634-8.
10. Li D, Zhang S, Zhang Z, Li Y. A new method of robot-assisted laparoscopic repair of perineal hernia after abdominoperineal resection: a case report. Int J Colorectal Dis. 2020;35(4):775–8. https://doi.org/10.1007/s00384-020-03506-0 Epub 2020 Feb 4 PMID: 32020267.
11. Goedhart-de Haan AMS, Langenhoff BS, Petersen D, Verheijen PM. Laparoscopic repair of perineal hernia after abdominoperineal excision. Hernia. 2016;20:741–6.